Surgical Ethics

SURGICAL ETHICS

Edited by

LAURENCE B. McCULLOUGH

JAMES W. JONES

BARUCH A. BRODY

Baylor College of Medicine
Houston, Texas

New York   Oxford
OXFORD UNIVERSITY PRESS
1998

Oxford University Press

Oxford   New York
Athens   Auckland   Bangkok   Bogota   Bombay
Buenos Aires   Calcutta   Cape Town   Dar es Salaam
Delhi   Florence   Hong Kong   Istanbul   Karachi
Kuala Lumpur   Madras   Madrid   Melbourne
Mexico City   Nairobi   Paris   Singapore
Taipei   Tokyo   Toronto   Warsaw

and associated companies in
Berlin   Ibadan

Copyright © 1998 by Oxford University Press

Published by Oxford University Press, Inc.
198 Madison Avenue, New York, New York 10016

Oxford is a registered trademark of Oxford University Press

Library of Congress Cataloging-in-Publication Data
Surgical ethics /
edited by Laurence B. McCullough, James W. Jones, Baruch A. Brody ;
with a foreword by Paul A. Ebert.
p.   cm.
Includes bibliographical references and index.
ISBN 0-19-510347-5
1.   Surgeons—Professional ethics.
I. Jones, James W. (James Wilson), 1941– .
II. Brody, Baruch A.
[DNLM: 1. Ethics, Medical.   2. Surgery.
WO 21 S961 1998]   RD27.7.S87   1998
174'.2—dc21
DNLM/DLC   for Library of Congress   97-29008

9 8 7 6 5 4 3 2

Printed in the United States of America
on acid-free paper

For Joan, Linda, and Dena

Foreword

The surgical profession, which traces its history to the earliest advanced civilizations on earth, has always had a profound concern for the ethical practice of medicine as essential to the quality of care it provides. From the notorious Babylonian Code of Hammurabi through the Hippocratic writings, to Paracelcus in the sixteenth century and the technologically sophisticated surgery of the twentieth, surgeons have understood their responsibility to proceed with care, minimize the pain and risk of their operations, and accept a rigorous program of intellectual training to insure their legitimacy. The American College of Surgeons believes that the ethical practice of surgery promotes an environment in which all patients are treated with dignity, tolerance, and respect for their wishes. Surgeons accepting Fellowship in the College are asked to place the welfare and the rights of their patients above their own, and to treat each patient as they would wish to be treated, were they to become patients themselves. Value each individual, and do unto others as you would have them do unto you. Not new or unusual concepts, but the stronger for having endured and prevailed across centuries of shifting opinion about how people can best negotiate their relationships. We honor the most refined of these relationships with the term "ethical," by which we mean that they have achieved an ideal measure of fairness, compassion, and integrity, with self-interest subordinated to a greater good. The book you are about to read is the first extensive examination of applied ethics in surgery.

The contributors to this volume about surgical ethics have addressed many of the contending imperatives we confront in daily practice. The basic concept of informed consent, for example, now a matter of law as well as a cornerstone of medical ethics throughout the United States, tests the patient's right to adequate disclosure of risks and benefits, and authority to accept or reject medical procedures based upon that information, against the physician's necessarily superior fund of specialized knowledge, experience, and traditional beneficence of the medical profession. The ethical resolution of the problem lies in the incorporation of all those elements within the process of informed consent. Advance directives are usually intended to give the patient proper control of his disposition as the end of life approaches, but may not adequately anticipate events as they actually unfold; the exercise of the surgeon'a judgment in such cases, and particularly a medical decision to limit compliance with the advance directive, may appear to create a conflict between the patient's decision-making authority and the physician's duty to treat. The scarcity of such resources as transplantable organs means that some patients will be chosen as recipients and others will not, but the lives of all are in the balance; the determining factors in the decision to make an organ available to one patient and not another are subject to broad interpretation. Clinical research is essential to the improvement of surgical therapy, but may not benefit, and can even harm, individual patients who participate in clinical trials. Difficult ethical dilemmas arise from these competing interests. The exigencies of emergency treatment, advancing technology, the role of trainees, and many other elements of surgical care all require sensitivity to their ethical implications. This book disscusses the theoretical structure and practical application of principles necessary to evaluate ethical problems bearing upon our work.

Although the American Medical Association and the American College of Surgeons have published position papers on the basic ethical standards expected of their members, prior to this book, there has been no treatment of the specific conditions under which surgeons are called upon to make ethical determinations, and no clear guide to a process with which to make ethical judgments in surgery. The editors have asked teams of surgeons and ethicists to describe here their detailed considerations of ethical problems and resolutions as references and intellectual stimulants for the surgical profession. I am pleased that they have been able to do so comprehensively, authoritatively, and interestingly. There is little question in my mind that all surgeons will benefit from reading *Surgical Ethics,* and that it will help all of us as we face the emerging problems of surgical practice in the twenty-first century.

Paul A. Ebert

Preface

Patients know intuitively and physicians by experience that surgery harms before it heals. Without specifically pronouncing themselves ethicists in so doing, surgeons have always attempted to limit the harm that they do to their patients and extend the healing power of their craft. Through many ages this was a unilateral action, with the surgeon accepting the role of the paternalistic wise man, whose decisions concerning acceptable risk, patient choice, and right and wrong were always assumed to be correct, regardless of outcome.

In the latter part of this century, radical changes in how we all perceive one another's personal rights and authority, astonishing advances in medical technology, and vibrant debate about what constitutes right and wrong have complicated choices that surgeons and their patients once considered self-evident. While surgeons are still largely and accurately perceived as honest, highly trained, and highly intelligent healers who regularly place the needs of their patients before their own and accept responsibility for their actions, the entry of these changes into the arena of surgical thought and practice has made surgical care more complex, particularly as it is affected by non-medical considerations in which surgeons have traditionally had little formal training. Although the goal remains to cure with a minimum of morbidity and mortality, the surgeon must now accept the additional role of ethicist in order to achieve this goal. Doing so typically means sharing the right to make clinical choices with patients, with families, with other physicians, and the owners and managers of necessary resources, while continuing to limit self-interest and represent one's abilities honestly.

This book grew from our conviction as medical educators that surgeons, surgery residents and fellows, and medical students need a reliable scholarly resource to help them chart the shifting terrain of surgical ethics so that they can conduct themselves in a morally responsible fashion in patient care, surgical research, and surgical education. We have therefore designed this textbook to begin with the basics of surgical ethics that are relevant to all surgeons, general and sub-specialty alike: the principles and practices of surgical ethics; informed consent; confidentiality; and advance directives. We have aimed for clinical comprehensiveness by including chapters on the full range of surgical cases: emergency patients; acute, high-risk patients; acute yet non-emergent patients; elective patients; patients who are poor surgical risks; and dying patients. These clinical topics are complemented by a consideration of the distinctive clinical ethical issues that arise when the patient is a family member, friend, colleague, or family member of a colleague. Ethics in surgical research is addressed in a chapter on research and innovation in surgery. We include consideration of intra-professional and inter-professional ethical issues in chapters on preventing and managing unwarranted bias toward patients, on self-regulation in surgical practice and research, on surgery and the other medical specialties, and on obligations of the surgeon to non-physician members of the surgical team. No textbook on surgical ethics would be complete without taking up the economic dimensions of surgery, including managed care. Thus, the book concludes with chapters on financial relationships with patients, conflicts of interest, and relationships with institutions that manage and deliver patient services.

Our decision to compile a volume dedicated to surgeons reflects our sense that the field of bioethics remains incomplete so long as it fails to give sufficient attention to all medical specialties. Scholars and teachers in bioethics will find here a series of analyses and arguments that address comprehensively what is still a relatively new area for bioethics. We hope and expect that this book will stimulate further attention to, and scholarly work on, surgical ethics by the bioethics community.

Finally, this work grew from our conviction as medical educators that the ethical issues arising in surgical practice and research should be addressed in the training of surgery residents and fellows and in the education of medical students during their surgery rotations. As we undertook such teaching ourselves, we found our efforts frustrated by the absence of a single teaching resource to which we could direct our trainees. In preparing *Surgical Ethics*, our intent has been to bring to these future surgeons and physicians an intellectual resource that will serve them well in their practice lives.

To provide the book with scholarly rigor, clinical comprehensiveness, and practical applicability we have invited teams of bioethicists (philosophers and physicians) and surgeons to write the various chapters. Each chapter represents an original, collaborative work of bioethics scholarship and we are proud to be associated with such intellectually and clinically dedicated colleagues.

We are especially pleased and honored that Paul A. Ebert, M.D., F.A.C.S., Director of the American College of Surgeons, has provided the foreword to this book. Much to the credit of Dr. Ebert and its officers, the College has taken an important leadership role in recent years in stimulating interest and debate in surgical ethics. *Surgical Ethics* builds on and advances these strong foundations.

No editors can hope to accomplish the task of assembling a volume like this one without the crucial assistance of others. We want especially to thank Cynthia Cox, Delores Smith, and Joan Jones for their assistance at various stages in the preparation of the book. Bruce Richman provided and stimulated many valuable ideas, as well as excellent editorial support. Many of the ideas in the first two chapters were developed in our teaching of Baylor's surgery residents and medical students and we are grateful for the opportunity to learn from them as we teach. We appreciate also the support of Jeffrey House and his colleagues at Oxford University Press during the preparation of the manuscript and the process of seeing it into the world.

Finally, we could not have completed a project of this size and duration without the unstinting and wonderful support of our wives, for which we are very grateful. We therefore dedicate this book to them.

Baylor College of Medicine   L. B. M.
Houston, Texas   J. W. J.
September, 1997   B. A. B.

Contents

Contributors

MARGARET ALLEN, M.D., is Associate Professor of Surgery at the University of Washington School of Medicine, Seattle, Washington.

ROBERT ARNOLD, M.D., is Associate Professor of Medicine and Associate Director for Education of the Center for Medical Ethics, University of Pittsburgh Medical Center, Pittsburgh, Pennsylvania.

JOHN C. BALDWIN, M.D., is DeBakey-Bard Professor of Surgery and Chairman of the Department of Surgery, Baylor College of Medicine, and Chief of Surgical Services at The Methodist Hospital, Houston, Texas.

BARUCH A. BRODY, Ph.D., is Leon Jaworski Professor of Biomedical Ethics and Director of the Center for Medical Ethics and Health Policy, Baylor College of Medicine, and Professor of Philosophy at Rice University, Houston, Texas.

DONNA A. CANIANO, M.D., is Associate Professor of Surgery and Pediatrics at the Ohio State University College of Medicine and Children's Hospital, and Director of the academic program in the medical humanities for the College of Medicine, Columbus, Ohio.

PAUL A. EBERT, M.D., is Director of the American College of Surgeons, Chicago, Illinois.

H. TRISTRAM ENGELHARDT, JR., Ph.D., M.D., is Professor of Medicine, Obstetrics and Gynecology, and Medical Ethics, in the Center for Medical Ethics and Health Policy, Baylor College of Medicine, and Professor of Philosophy at Rice University, Houston, Texas.

JOHN C. FLETCHER, Ph.D., now retired, was Emily Davie and Joseph S. Kornfeld Professor of Biomedical Ethics and Director of the Center for Biomedical Ethics, University of Virginia School of Medicine, Charlottesville, Virginia.

JOEL E. FRADER, M.D., M.A., is Associate Professor of Pediatrics and of Medical Ethics, Northwestern University Medical School and Children's Memorial Hospital, Chicago, Illinois.

ROBERT R.M. GIFFORD, M.D., is Professor of Surgery at the University of South Carolina School of Medicine, and Program Director, Kidney Transplant Program, Richland Memorial Hospital/University of South Carolina School of Medicine, Columbia, South Carolina.

AMIR HALEVY, M.D., is Assistant Professor of Medicine and Assistant Professor of Medical Ethics in the Center for Medical Ethics and Health Policy, Baylor College of Medicine, Houston, Texas.

ROBERT C. HARLAND, M.D., is Assistant Professor of Surgery and Director of Pancreas and Renal Transplantation Programs at Duke University Medical Center, Durham, North Carolina.

KENNETH V. ISERSON, M.D., M.B.A., is Professor of Surgery and Director of the Arizona Bioethics Program, University of Arizona College of Medicine, Tucson, Arizona.

BRUCE E. JARRELL, M.D., is Professor of Surgery and Head of the Department of Surgery, University of Arizona College of Medicine, Tucson, Arizona.

NANCY S. JECKER, Ph.D., is Associate Professor in the Department of Medical History and Ethics at the University of Washington School of Medicine, Seattle, Washington.

JAMES W. JONES, M.D., Ph.D., is Professor of Surgery and Cell Biology, Professor of Medical Ethics in the Center for Medical Ethics and Health Policy, and Vice-Chairman of the Department of Surgery, Baylor College of Medicine, and Chief of the Surgical Service, Houston Veterans Affairs Medical Center, Houston, Texas.

R. SCOTT JONES, M.D., is Stephen Hurt Watts Professor of Surgery and Chairman of the Department of Surgery, University of Virginia School of Medicine, Charlottesville, Virginia.

GEORGE KHUSHF, Ph.D., is Assistant Professor of Philosophy and Humanities Director of the Center for Bioethics at the University of South Carolina, Columbia, South Carolina.

ARTHUR E. KOPELMAN, M.D., is Professor of Pediatrics and Head of the Section of Neonatology, Department of Pediatrics, East Carolina University School of Medicine, Greenville, North Carolina.

LORETTA M. KOPELMAN, Ph.D., is Professor of Medical Humanities and Chair of the Department of Medical Humanities, East Carolina University School of Medicine, Greenville, North Carolina.

DONALD R. LANNIN, M.D., is Professor of Surgery and Director of the Leo W. Jenkins Cancer Center at East Carolina University School of Medicine, Greenville, North Carolina.

FRANK E. LUCENTE, M.D., is Professor of Otolaryngology and Chairman of the Department of Otolaryngology, and Vice Dean, Graduate Medical Education, at the State University of New York Health Science Center at Brooklyn and Chairman of the Department of Otolaryngology at Long Island College Hospital.

ANDREW LUSTIG, Ph.D., is Academic Director of the Institute of Religion at the Texas Medical Center, Adjunct Associate Professor of Clinical Ethics at M.D. Anderson Cancer Center, and Adjunct Member of the Center for Medical Ethics and Health Policy, Baylor College of Medicine, Houston, Texas.

MARY FAITH MARSHALL, Ph.D., is Assistant Professor of Medicine and Graduate Studies and Director of the Program in Bioethics at the Medical University of South Carolina, Charleston, South Carolina.

KENNETH L. MATTOX, M.D., is Professor of Surgery and Vice Chairman for Interhospital Affairs of the Department of Surgery, Baylor College of Medicine, and Chief of Staff and Chief of Surgery at the Ben Taub General Hospital of the Harris County Hospital District, Houston, Texas.

LAURENCE B. MCCULLOUGH, Ph.D., is Professor of Medicine and Medical Ethics, in the Center for Medical Ethics and Health Policy, Baylor College of Medicine, Houston, Texas, and Adjunct Professor of Ethics in Obstetrics and Gynecology, Cornell University Medical College, New York, New York.

ROBERT MILCH, M.D., is Clinical Associate Professor of Surgery, School of Medicine, State University of New York at Buffalo and Medical Director of Hospice Buffalo, Buffalo, New York.

JONATHAN D. MORENO, Ph.D., is Emily Davie and Joseph S. Kornfeld Professor of Biomedical Ethics and Director of the Center for Biomedical Ethics, University of Virginia School of Medicine, Charlottesville, Virginia. He was formerly

Professor of Pediatrics and of Medicine and Director of the Division of Humanities in Medicine at the State University of New York Health Science Center in Brooklyn, New York.

RUTH PURTILO, Ph.D., is Mabel L. Criss Professor of Medical Ethics and Director of the Center for Health Policy and Ethics, Creighton University School of Medicine, Omaha, Nebraska.

PETER T. SCARDINO, M.D., is Russell and Mary Hugh Scott Professor of Urology and Chairman of the Department of Urology, Baylor College of Medicine, Houston, Texas.

BYERS W. SHAW, M.D., is Musselman Professor of Surgery and Chairman of the Department of Surgery at the University of Nebraska Medical Center, Omaha, Nebraska.

JERRY M. SHUCK, M.D., D.Sc., is Oliver H. Payne Professor of Surgery and Chairman of the Department of Surgery, Case Western Reserve University School of Medicine, and Director of Surgery, University Hospitals of Cleveland, Cleveland, Ohio.

C. D. SMITH, III, M.D., is Associate Professor of Surgery and Pediatrics at the Medical University of South Carolina and Associate Director for Quality at the Medical University Hospital, Charleston, South Carolina.

JEREMY SUGARMAN, M.D., M.P.H., M.A., is Associate Professor of Medicine and Co-Chair of the Ethics Consultation Service at Duke University Medical Center, Durham, North Carolina.

ROBERT WALLACE, M.D., is Professor of Surgery and past Chairman of the Department of Surgery at Georgetown University, Washington, D.C.

STEPHEN WEAR, Ph.D., is Clinical Associate Professor of Medicine, Obstetrics and Gynecology, and Philosophy and Co-Director of the Center for Clinical Ethics and Humanities in Health Care in the School of Medicine, State University of New York at Buffalo and Head, Ethics Consultation Team at the Buffalo Veterans Affairs Medical Center, Buffalo, New York.

WM. LYNN WEAVER, M.D., is Professor of Surgery and Chair of the Department of Surgery at Morehouse School of Medicine, Atlanta, Georgia. He was formerly Professor of Surgery at the School of Medicine, State University of New York at Buffalo and Chief of Surgery at the Buffalo Veterans Affairs Medical Center, Buffalo, New York.

KEVIN WM. WILDES, S.J., Ph.D., is Associate Professor of Philosophy and Senior Research Scholar and Associate Director of the Kennedy Institute of Ethics at Georgetown University, Washington, D.C.

STUART J. YOUNGNER, M.D. is Professor of Medicine, Psychiatry, and Biomedical Ethics at Case Western Reserve University School of Medicine and Director of the Clinical Ethics Program at University Hospitals of Cleveland, Cleveland, Ohio.

Surgical Ethics

1

Principles and Practice of Surgical Ethics

LAURENCE B. MCCULLOUGH
JAMES W. JONES
BARUCH A. BRODY

This book addresses ethical problems that surgeons confront on a daily basis in patient care, surgical research, and surgical education. The topics considered in the chapters that follow range from the fundamentals of surgical ethics—informed consent, confidentiality, advance directives, and the determination of death—through the range of surgical patients, from elective and high-risk patients to poor-risk and dying patients, to intra-professional and inter-professional issues, surgical innovation and research, and the financial aspects of surgical practice, including managed care and the ethical issues that it raises for surgeons.

To our knowledge, this is the first such bioethics volume directed to surgeons and the unique conditions of their work in the medical community. Our goal has been to provide a comprehensive account of surgical ethics by classifying and analyzing most ethical issues that arise in patient care, with other health care professionals, in research and education, in the institutional setting, and with regard to financing and money in surgery. To achieve this goal we invited teams of authors—a surgeon and an ethicist, usually in pairs—to collaborate on each chapter. Leaders in both surgery and bioethics will be found among our contributors.

In their deliberations our contributors have aimed to define the best available ethical position on the issues addressed in their chapters, on the basis of ethical analysis and argument well grounded in surgical experience and reality.

They have taken concrete—and sometimes controversial—positions on particular issues and how surgeons should respond to them in an ethically responsible fashion. We believe they have succeeded in developing a book that will serve as a practical, clinically applicable, reference work for ethically informed and responsible surgical practice, research, and education.

We turn now to the two main tasks of this introductory chapter: first to introduce the reader to the basic concepts and language of surgical ethics and then to provide a method for using the concepts and language of surgical ethics in surgical practice, research, and education.

Basic Concepts

Ethics can be usefully defined as the disciplined study of morality. Morality, in turn, comprises both good and bad character and right and wrong behavior. Ethics asks the general question, "What ought morality to be?" Typically, this general question is broken down into two more concrete questions, "What ought character to be?" and "What ought conduct to be?"

In answering the first question, ethics analyzes characteristics of virtues (habits or traits of character that focus our concern on the interests of others, as well as our own legitimate interests, and motivate us to protect and promote the interests of others as our primary consideration) and vices (habits or traits of character that excessively emphasize self-interest so that it systematically becomes our first and overriding concern) and then develops arguments about the virtues that are required for seeing and routinely fulfilling our obligations and about the vices that put self-interest first and thus undermine our ability to see and do our duty. In answering the second question, ethics analyzes ethical issues about right and wrong action and develops arguments about which actions are ethically defensible, and in this sense "right," and which actions are ethically indefensible and in this sense "wrong."

Surgical ethics, as a sub-discipline of both ethics and surgery, asks, "What ought morality to be in surgery?"—including clinical practice, research, and education. Surgical ethics breaks this general question down into two questions, directed especially to surgery, surgeons, surgical trainees, and other institutional managers, "What ought the character of surgeons to be?" and "What ought the conduct of surgeons to be?"

The Basic Rights of Patients

Surgical ethics is based on a recognition of the rights of patients who require the care of surgeons. Although it is understood that the surgeon is "an authority" in the practice and outcomes of surgery, it is the patient who is "in authority"—that is, the individual in the transaction between caregiver and care-seeker on whom the salient rights devolve.[1] The patient has seven basic rights: three negative rights and four positive rights.[2] The patient has the negative rights not to be killed intentionally or negligently by the surgeon, not to be harmed by intent or negligence of the surgeon, and not to be deceived by the surgeon. The patient has the positive rights to be adequately informed about the risks and benefits of surgery, to be treated by a knowledgeable, competent practitioner, to have his or her health and well-being more highly valued than the surgeon's own economic interest, and to decide whether to accept treatment under the conditions described. The surgeon's ethical behavior and ethical character should be consistent with recognition of these rights.

Character, Virtues, and the Ethical Concept of the Surgeon as Fiduciary of the Patient

Consider the first question in surgical ethics, what ought the character of surgeons to be? This question arises for surgeons, as for physicians generally, especially around issues of payment. The introduction of capitation into the way surgeons are paid creates a strong financial incentive for the surgeon not to do surgery; in contrast, fee-for-service payment creates a strong incentive for the surgeon to perform surgery. Both systems of payment invite the surgeon who is uninformed by ethical analysis and argument to put his or her own economic interests first. The surgeon who does so then loses sight of the patient's interests—whether surgery is indicated in reliable clinical judgment and how the risk-benefits ratio of surgery compares with medical alternatives (see Chapter 18).

Is a surgeon's willingness to put his or her own financial self-interest ahead of the patient's well-being a vice? Putting self-interest systematically first is antithetical to the character traits that the surgeon should develop because doing so violates the expectation that the surgeon will put the patient's interest first, acting as the patient's fiduciary. Systematically granting primacy to self-interest over and above the life and health of the patient is avoided by the ethical surgeon.

The concept of acting as moral fiduciary of the patient is central to virtually all of surgical ethics. The moral character of the conscientious surgeon is therefore one of the central themes addressed in this book. The law provides a useful departure point for understanding this ethical concept. Being a fiduciary is legally understood to be "a person holding the character of trustee, in respect of the trust and confidence involved in it and scrupulous good faith and candor which it requires" and also to be a "person having duty, created by his undertaking, to act primarily for another's benefit in matters connected with such undertaking."[3] The key concept here is that a fiduciary should put aside self-interest, focus primarily on the interest of the person for whom he or she serves as fiduciary, act to protect and promote that individual's interest, and so earn the trust and confidence of that individual. The concept of the surgeon as the patient's moral fiduciary captures these ideas in the following way. The surgeon should make the protection and promotion of the patient's interests the primary consideration in the surgeon-patient relationship and in surgical research and education. This primary commitment holds self-interest in check and makes it a systematically secondary consideration. Self-interest is thus blunted and not permitted to generate the vice of selfishness in the surgeon's professional character. This makes the fiduciary's role morally demanding.

When the surgeon's ethical, fiduciary-based obligations come into conflict with self-interest, the surgeon confronts the ethical issue of conflict of interest. This issue arises, obviously, regarding money, other compensation, and the changing institutional and financial conditions of surgery in the United States and many other countries. Economic conflicts of interest are addressed in Chapters 17, 18, and 19. Furthermore, surgeons also confront threats to their own health in the care of patients, especially from exposure to blood-borne pathogens, creating an even more complex conflict of interest; while the surgeon has an obligation to treat even those with communicable diseases, the surgeon is entitled to protect his or her own health and has an additional legitimate concern for the many future patients who might be helped (see also Chapter 9).

Ethical Principles

The virtues of being the moral fiduciary of the patient permit the surgeon to maintain his role as "an authority" while permitting the patient to maintain his position "in authority."[2] The surgeon's attention to the patient's interests include exercising and explaining his status as an authority, whose knowledge and skill the patient seeks, while protecting the patient's right to expect that the surgeon's authoritative posture is properly based in training, experience, wisdom, and concern for the patient. Honesty becomes the general fiduciary commitment to protect and promote the interests of the patient if surgical ethics is to guide the clinical judgment and practice of surgeons in a comprehensive way. The surgeon must be the expert he or she represents himself or herself to be if he or she is to honor the patient's rights not to be deceived, to be fully informed of risks and benefits, and to be free from avoidable risks. The conceptual tools used by ethicists to provide surgeons with such practical guidance are the ethical principles.[4] Ethical principles guide the surgeon toward concrete actions in the care of patients and the management of their problems.

The ethical principles of beneficence and respect for patient autonomy are directly pertinent to surgical practice, research, and education; they are prominently addressed in the chapters that follow. These two principles apply dual perspectives on the interests of patients to concrete clinical action.

The first perspective is clinical: the well-informed, rigorous clinical judgments of the surgeon about which clinical management strategies can reliably be expected to protect and promote the patient's health-related interests and which strategies can reliably be expected not to do so. This clinical perspective is captured by the ethical principle of beneficence, which instructs the surgeon to act in ways that are reliably expected to result in a greater balance of clinical goods over harms for the patient.

The second perspective is the patient's: on the basis of his or her values and beliefs, the patient evaluates information about medical and surgical alternatives and makes judgments about which alternatives are more or less likely to protect and promote his or her values. This patient-oriented perspective is subsumed by the ethical principle of respect for autonomy, which instructs the surgeon to identify the patient's values and beliefs, to respect their role in the patient's life, and to elicit the patient's preferences from among medical and surgical alternatives supported in beneficence-based clinical judgment.

Consider the refusal of blood products during surgery for religious reasons, an ethical issue surgeons confront in the surgical management of Jehovah's Witnesses. Recent improvements in surgical technique have greatly reduced intraoperative blood loss and new blood-saving technologies have reduced the need for administration of blood products and non-autologous blood. Nonetheless, the use of blood products and whole blood is often "medically indicated." This common surgical term is beneficence-based: if blood products or whole blood are not used, the patient's risk of death, serious disease, or disabling injury may significantly increase. These outcomes can be avoided, given that the risk of infection from blood-borne pathogens is quite low. Otherwise, serious risks are taken with the patient's health, which appear to be inconsistent with beneficence-based clinical care and therefore are ruled out in good surgical practice.

A surgical perspective on the use of blood and blood products during and after surgery, however, is not the whole of the story any longer in surgical ethics; the patient's perspective must also be honored. The religious beliefs of Jehovah's Witnesses are as sincere as the beliefs of any other of this world's religious communities and traditions. The principle of respect for autonomy teaches that the beliefs of Jehovah's Witnesses about the administration of blood products are worthy of the surgeon's respect. Moreover, because beneficence-based clinical judgment is limited to the patient's health-related interests, the surgeon is in no position to judge the merit of such religious beliefs.

The two principles thus seem to generate a conflict. On the one hand, the surgeon has a beneficence-based obligation to avoid intraoperative and postoperative risks that can be prevented with an intervention that is efficacious and—relative to those risks—sufficiently safe. Such an obligation also implements the patient's right to be neither killed nor injured by surgery. On the other hand, the surgeon has an autonomy-based obligation not to interfere with the preferences of the patient, especially when those preferences represent and express deeply held values, matters of substantial moral and religious conviction. Such an obligation implements the patient's right to make decisions about his or her care, and to be in authority. How these apparent ethical conflicts should be analyzed and resolved in surgical practice are addressed in Chapters 7, 8, and 9.

Surgeons and the institutions in which they practice no longer simply take care of patients one at a time; surgeons and institutions are increasingly responsible for the care of populations of patients. While this has been true of the military medical corps, the Public Health Service, the Veterans Affairs medical system, and local public hospitals for many decades, managed care organizations (MCOs) also think of themselves as responsible for populations of patients. In addition, the rapid increase in health care costs that this country experienced during the 1970s and 1980s had become unsustainable, in both the private and public sectors, by the 1990s. Surgery, as well as other medical specialties, has entered the era of limited and often scarce financial resources.

In these constrained circumstances, surgeons—and institutions that support their work—confront a systemic and challenging ethical issue: how to ethically allocate limited resources. The reality of surgical practice is that spending resources for the care of one patient may well mean that there will be insufficient resources to care for other patients, a particularly acute ethical issue in the context of flat, or even declining, institutional budgets. These considerations may obscure the boundaries of who is "an authority" and who is "in authority" in the surgeon-patient relationship as institutions assert their power to control the allocation of resources.

Ethics addresses issues concerning the allocation of resources by using principles of justice. More than two thousand years ago, Aristotle conceptualized justice as the rendering to each individual of what is due to him or her.[5] The key word in this formulation, obviously, is *due*. In the ensuing centuries, there have emerged competing accounts of what is due to someone in the allocation of limited or scarce resources.[6] In the history of Western philosophy, some have argued that such allocation should be based on meeting fundamental human needs, such as for shelter, clothing, and food. Others have argued that such allocation should be based on natural rights, which precede political orders, to life, liberty, and property. Still others have argued for utilitarianism, allocation of scarce resources with the goal of producing the greatest good for the greatest number. Others still have argued that allocation should be based on merit and accomplishment, what people have earned through personal ability, effort, and sacrifice.

This philosophical debate remains unresolved because each of these concepts of justice, as well as other formulations of the concept, is intellectually and practically compelling and captures our different intuitions about what is fair and just in the treatment of people when resources are limited or scarce.

Issues of just distribution of resources become relevant in surgical ethics in transplantation surgery, where organs are scarce and eligible patients are many, and in the financing of surgery, particularly with regard to such third-party payers as public treasuries and private, for-profit insurers. These issues are dealt with in Chapters 6, 17, and 19.

A Surgical Ethics Workup

The reader can use the tools of ethical analysis and argument to address and manage clinical cases in an intellectually rigorous and clinically applicable fashion by following the steps of a surgical ethics workup.[7] We propose a four-step process.

Identifying the Facts of the Case

Ethical analysis and argument, like clinical judgment and decision making, require a solid foundation in the facts of the clinical case. Otherwise, surgical ethics becomes an abstract and irrelevant exercise. To be well grounded in clinical reality, therefore, a surgical ethics workup begins with the history and clinical workup of the patient's chief complaint. There are two key factual considerations on which subsequent ethical analysis and argument vitally depend.

First, all medically and surgically reasonable alternatives, that is, all alternatives that have a positive and at least neutral risk/benefit ratio, should be identified. The alternative of a trial of non-intervention should be carefully evaluated in this respect. Except for emergencies, such a trial is often medically and surgically reasonable.

Second, it is especially important to identify the patient's social history. Such factors as the patient's occupation, the patient's routine of daily life and activities, the patient's support and caregiving network (a crucial consideration for patients with chronic illnesses), the patient's religious beliefs, and the patient's other relevant values and beliefs should be identified. To elicit the patient's values and beliefs it is clinically useful to ask, "What is important to you about your condition?"[8] The surgeon should be attentive to expressions of the patient's values and goals for surgical and medical care.

Ethical Analysis

Ethical analysis should be undertaken by considering four "appeals" that together gather relevant information pertaining to the surgeon as the patient's moral fiduciary and to ethical principles. The first of these appeals addresses the fiduciary role in particular and the remaining three speak to the ethical principles of beneficence, respect for autonomy, and justice.[2] In applying these four appeals to individual clinical cases, the reader should use the methods of ethics analysis and argument, described here and in the chapters to follow.

Appeal to Virtues. The virtues of the surgeon as moral fiduciary relevant to the case should be identified, along with their implications for the surgeon's ethical obligations. What do the relevant virtues require of the surgeon's clinical judgment, decision making, and behavior? To answer this question, the reader should identify the implications, both short-term and long-term, of the virtues of the surgeon as fiduciary of the patient. Compassion, for example, focuses concern on relief of postoperative pain and suffering, as well as on prevention of long-term suffering from added morbidity and decreased quality of life, considerations that loom large in the care of patients who are poor surgical risks (Chapter 9) and patients who are dying (Chapter 10).

Appeal to Consequences. Beneficence-based clinical judgment is concerned with the clinical consequences of reasonable alternatives for managing the patient's problem. The appeal to consequences therefore involves a careful, precise, and thorough identification of both the clinically good consequences (benefit) and the clinically bad consequences (risk) of available alternatives. In beneficence-based clinical judgment, good consequences are the prevention of premature and unnecessary death and the prevention and effective management of disease, injury, and unnecessary pain and suffering. Pain and suffering are necessary in the surgical management of patients only when they cannot be avoided in the effort to reduce mortality and morbidity.

There are two important dimensions of the appeal to consequences. First, it usually results in the identification of a range of alternatives that are acceptable in beneficence-based clinical judgment. An appeal to consequences that identifies only one reasonable alternative in non-emergency cases is probably flawed and, worse, sets up the surgeon and patient for entirely preventable ethical conflict. Second, it sometimes happens that surgical management is inconsistent with beneficence-based clinical judgment, either because the patient is a poor surgical risk (Chapter 9) or is dying (Chapter 10). The limits of beneficence-based judgment should be identified. What do the beneficence-based consequences require of the surgeon's clinical judgment, decision making, and behavior?

Appeal to Rights. The principle of respect for autonomy grounds and generates the rights of patients that surgeons should take into account. In making the appeal to rights, it is crucial to distinguish negative from positive rights.[2] Negative rights involve claims against others to be left alone, unless one is putting others at risk of harm to which they do not consent. As a rule, negative rights, because they do not make strong claims on the resources of others, are very difficult to limit. In contrast, positive rights involve claims against others for access to and use of their resources of time, money, and ability. Positive rights always come with limits; the only debate concerns what those limits should be. Appeals to rights therefore should always distinguish negative from positive rights.

We earlier identified three negative and four positive rights relevant to surgical ethics. The implications and limits of these rights and of the patient's other relevant values and beliefs for the clinical facts of the case should be identified in the making the appeal to rights. What do the autonomy-based rights and values of the patient require of the surgeon's clinical judgment, decision making, and behavior? Consideration of the clinical implications of these seven rights helps to answer this question.

Appeal to Justice and Equality. Issues of justice and equality arise in surgical ethics primarily with regard to the allocation of limited financial, material, and human resources in the care of patients. An appeal to justice and equality, because of the historical and deep philosophical disagreement about principles of justice, is the most controversial of the four appeals. It should therefore be made with care.

Three concepts of justice currently enjoy prominence in contemporary bioethics.[2] The first is an egalitarian concept of justice, which requires that patients be treated as equally as possible. At first, this concept was applied to outcomes of care, but recognition of the biologic variability of disease and of patients' responses to medical and surgical management of their problems has called this concept into question. The emphasis has therefore shifted to a concept of a *process* of care that is, insofar as possible, equal for patients with similar problems. Practice guidelines and clinical pathways implicitly adopt an egalitarian concept of justice.

The second prominent concept of justice in bioethics is redistributive justice. This concept has been deployed in response to the limited access of many Americans to health care and even more limited access of those in less developed countries. These variations are thought to be unfair, some have argued, and so health care resources and income should be redistributed—away from those with considerable access and wealth and toward those with no or little access and wealth. Redistributive justice calls for universal access to medical and surgical services.

The third prominent concept of justice is libertarian. This concept of justice emphasizes private property and respect for marketplace exchanges of private property and other forms of wealth. This concept of justice calls for a level "playing field" by providing patients with adequate information about the quality of medical and surgical care from different providers and allowing patients and providers to make their own, independent decisions. The marketplace will thus sort out a just distribution of health care resources.

The particular concept or principle of justice to which appeal is made should always be clearly identified and its implications for the case made clear. The same two tasks should also be undertaken for competing concepts and principles of justice. The goal of doing so in the appeal to justice and equality is to avoid the unargued introduction of a favored principle of justice.

The Four Appeals Together. The implications of the four appeals together for the surgeon's clinical judgment, decision making, and behavior should be identified. Areas of agreement and areas of conflict should be precisely stated. Ethical conflicts, especially those generated by the principles of beneficence and respect for autonomy and those generated by conflicts of interest, are addressed in the next step of the clinical surgical workup, ethical argument.

Ethical Argument

Ethical argument requires the surgeon to present clearly stated premises that *together* support a conclusion about what the surgeon's clinical judgment, decision making, and behavior ought to be in the case under consideration. Argument does not start with a "gut feeling" about what the conclusion ought to be, followed by a search for friendly premises. This is flawed ethical reasoning and should be avoided in responsible surgical practice, research, and education.

Instead, the reader should marshal clearly stated reasons about why one or more of the four appeals should guide the surgeon's clinical judgment, decision making, and behavior in the case at hand. The goal is to follow one's reasons, and therefore argument, where they lead. In this way, one submits one's thought processes to the intellectual discipline of ethics and thus achieves an intellectually disciplined study of what the morality of surgeons ought to be.

Once having made an argument, one should invite the critical evaluation of one's colleagues. One should ask the following sorts of questions and address the deficiencies that they identify.

1. Are the reasons clearly stated? If not, return to the stage of ethical analysis, because lack of clarity in the formulation of reasons is usually the function of lack of clarity and completeness in the four appeals.
2. Do the reasons connect to each other? Argument should not proceed in a shotgun style, with a disintegrated approach that simply lists appeals and asserts a priority among them. Reasons should clearly connect to each other and *together* support the conclusion.
3. Are there other conclusions that could follow? Reasonable people working with the same ethical analysis and argument can reach different conclusions when they interpret clinical facts differently.

4. What clear and coherent opposing reasons could be offered? The goal here is to be open to the well-made ethical analysis and arguments of others.

By making arguments based on thorough ethical analysis that incorporates the four appeals and by subjecting those arguments to critical scrutiny, one is typically assured of an ethically sound conclusion.

Issues of Authority and Power

Ethical analysis and argument can help to address issues of authority and power in the surgeon-patient relationship. These are especially important in surgical ethics because the surgeon is in charge of intraoperative and immediate post-operative care; the patient is in an especially passive role in these time periods, in contrast to the patient's role in most other medical specialties. In undertaking ethical analysis and argument the reader should, therefore, carefully distinguish the surgeon as someone who is "an authority" from someone who is "in authority,"[1] as we noted earlier. The surgeon is surely an intellectual authority about matters of clinical judgment and decision making. Patients therefore expect surgeons to be knowledgeable in these matters and tend to treat surgeons as authorities—that is, as individuals qualified by training and experience to identify and protect, through competent surgical management, the patient's clinical, beneficence-based interests.

To be in authority is different. This involves the power to act on clinical, beneficence-based judgment. The principle of respect for autonomy indicates that this power resides in the competent, adult patient or the surrogate of patients who lack decision-making capacity, either by reason of disease or developmental stage (roughly associated with age in children). The reader should therefore *not* conclude that because the surgeon is *an* authority about clinical matters, the surgeon is therefore also *in* authority to decide whether surgical management will actually occur. The latter consideration becomes especially important in the care of emergency patients (Chapter 5), patients who are poor surgical risks (Chapter 9), and dying patients (Chapter 10).

Conclusion

The discussions in this volume will, we expect and hope, provoke serious thought and lively controversy by raising ethical issues that are pertinent to surgical practice, research, education, and management. As surgery becomes more technologically advanced, as unanticipated surgical therapies are developed and become commonplace (as transplantation has), and as public policies, such as limitations on specialty training programs and cost reimbursement, impose themselves on surgical practice, new ethical questions will arise. It has been our goal, in assembling this book with the contributions of our colleagues in bioethics and surgery, to establish a sufficiently sturdy base on which present and future clinical surgical ethical questions may be laid with some sense of stability and confidence that the good of patients, medical institutions, surgery and medicine, and society will be served.

References

1. H. Tristram Engelhardt, Jr., *The Foundations of Bioethics*, 2nd ed. New York: Oxford University Press, 1996.
2. Baruch A. Brody and H. Tristram Engelhardt, Jr., "The Major Moral Considerations," in *Bioethics: Readings and Cases*, Baruch A. Brody and H. Tristram Engelhardt, Jr., eds. Englewood Cliffs, NJ: Prentice-Hall, Inc., 1987, pp. 3–33.
3. Henry Campbell Black, *Black's Law Dictionary*. St Paul, MN: West Publishing Co., 1979, p. 563.
4. Tom L. Beauchamp and James F. Childress, *Principles of Biomedical Ethics*, 4th ed. New York: Oxford University Press, 1994.
5. Aristotle, *Nichomachean Ethics*, in *The Complete Works of Aristotle*, Jonathan Barnes, ed. Princeton, NJ: Princeton University Press, 1985, pp. 1729–1867.
6. James P. Sterba, "Justice," in *Encyclopedia of Bioethics*, 2nd ed., Warren Thomas Reich, ed. New York: Macmillan, 1995, pp. 1308–1315.
7. Laurence B. McCullough and Carol M. Ashton, "A Methodology for Teaching Ethics in the Clinical Setting: A Clinical Handbook for Medical Ethics," *Theoretical Medicine* 15 (1994): 39–52.
8. Laurence B. McCullough, Nancy L. Wilson, Thomas A. Teasdale, et al., "Mapping Personal, Familial, and Professional Values in Long-Term Care Decisions," *The Gerontologist* 33 (1993): 324–332.

2

Informed Consent: Autonomous Decision Making of the Surgical Patient

LAURENCE B. MCCULLOUGH
JAMES W. JONES
BARUCH A. BRODY

The clinical skills required in the informed consent process tend not to be taught to fellows, residents, and medical students within the formal curriculum. Furthermore, surgical residents are seldom supervised during their communication with patients. As a result, faculty and trainees alike forgo an opportunity to identify, evaluate, and address weaknesses in the resident's interpersonal skills with patients generally, and during the informed consent dialogue in particular. Surgical practice is distinctive in that the surgical patient plays a more passive role than patients of other medical specialties once anesthesia is induced. The patient then becomes incapable of participatory intraoperative decision making; the surgeon has full control of the decision-making process at this point. As a result, surgeons may have a less fully developed sense of an active physician-patient partnership in the work of healing than colleagues in other specialties, and this can affect their approach to the informed consent process. The surgeon may also assume that the referring physician has already made the necessary intellectual and emotional preparations and effectively has obtained the patient's consent for surgical resolution of the clinical problem. In combination, these factors can lead the unwitting surgeon to underestimate the capacity and willingness of the patient to participate in the informed consent process that should precede induction of anesthesia. As a consequence, the surgeon can lose the opportunity to form an effective therapeutic alliance with the patient.

Our approach to informed consent in this chapter responds to these ethical challenges and opportunities. We consider informed consent a morally essential course of action that the surgeon should utilize to form a strong therapeutic alliance with the patient. Our evaluation of the informed consent process in surgical practice will include assessment of how the process should occur under both uncomplicated and adverse conditions to ensure the mutual rights and responsibilities of all involved parties.

We first provide an ethical analysis of the concept of informed consent. We then discuss its implementation in typical and atypical circumstances, and describe the most commonly encountered problems in the process, as well as proposals for their effective management. Our emphasis is on a preventive ethics approach, that is, clinical strategies designed to prevent ethical dilemmas. We close with clinical conclusions intended to guide the reader's continuing self-evaluation and improvement, as well as serve as a resource for teaching.

Ethical Analysis of the Informed Consent Process: Its Three Elements

Surgeons should conceptualize and practice informed consent as a continuing process, rather than a static event. Properly utilized, informed consent provides the basis for a strong and enduring therapeutic alliance between the surgeon and patient, with shared responsibility for decision making. Thus understood, informed consent is not simply the signature on the authorization form. This is part of documentation, and although documentation is important in satisfying the legal component of the consent process, documentation does not constitute the most important ethical element of informed consent. The patient's signature on the informed consent form is far less crucial than the process that it serves to document.

The concept of informed consent includes three elements, each of which presumes and builds on its predecessor.[1] The first is disclosure by the surgeon to the patient of adequate, clear information about the patient's diagnosis; the alternatives available to manage the patient's problem, including surgical and nonsurgical management; the benefits and risks of each alternative, including non-intervention (i.e., allowing the natural history of the disease to continue); and a frank explanation of those factors about which the medical profession, and the individual surgeon in particular, are uncertain and cannot provide guarantees. This disclosure should be individually tailored in its presentation to the intellectual and emotional capacity of each patient to understand, absorb, and retain information and make decisions. The second of the three elements is the patient's understanding of this clinical information. The third element is the patient's process of decision, based not only on what the surgeon has told him, but information he or she has been exposed to from other sources, including other physicians, family and friends, perhaps an acquaintance who has had a similar procedure, what he or she has read in independently researching the problem, and his or her own emotional response to illness and all that it changes in one's life. We now consider the ethical requirements of each of these three elements in greater clinical detail.

The Physician's Disclosure Obligation

The history of medical ethics before the twentieth century was marked by a debate between physicians who held the view that the patient should be told little or nothing about his condition and physicians who held the view that the physician should be more forthcoming.[1] Both sides of this debate based their ethical arguments on the physician's beneficence-based obligation to avoid unduly harming the patient. Beneficence obligates the physician to seek for the patient the greater balance of goods over harms, as those goods and harms are understood and balanced from a rigorous clinical perspective.[2]

This traditional debate was transformed by the ethical and legal analysis in several important legal cases. We therefore take as a starting point the common law of informed consent as a patient's right, which is a twentieth-century concept with origins in nineteenth-century case law and resultant common law pertaining to medical malpractice. A number of the landmark cases involved surgical treatment. Two key features of the legal history of informed consent are relevant here: simple consent and informed consent.[1]

Simple consent involves one question, "Did the patient agree to be treated?" If the answer was yes, then the conditions of consent were thought to be satisfied. If the answer was no, then the conditions were not satisfied and the surgeon could not operate. In 1914 Judge Benjamin Cardozo wrote a landmark opinion in the case *Schloendorff v. The Society of New York Hospital* that legally defined simple consent and changed the history of American medical ethics.[3]

In 1908, Mrs. Schloendorff, with a complaint of abdominal pain, had consented to an examination under anesthesia but stipulated that there was to be no surgical operation. When the surgeons identified an abdominal mass during the exam they excised it, exercising their beneficence-based clinical judgment that it is in any patient's medical interest to have a potentially life-threatening tumor removed without exposure to a second, unnecessary, and dangerous anesthesia episode. Mrs. Schloendorff developed complications and sued, citing her stated refusal to have surgery. Cardozo stated, "Every human being of adult years and sound mind has a right to determine what shall be done with his body; and a surgeon who performs an operation without his patient's consent commits an assault, for which he is liable in damages, . . . except in cases of emergency, where the patient is unconscious, and where it is necessary to operate before consent can be obtained."[3] In other words, beneficence-based clinical judgment was no longer the sole legitimate basis for the physician's obligations to the patient; respect for the patient's autonomy was at least equally important. Respect for autonomy obligates the physician to seek for the patient the greater balance of goods over harms, as those goods and harms are understood and balanced from the patient's perspective.[2]

Two major clinical implications followed from this decision. First, the surgeon retained the authority to make beneficence-based clinical judgments about how to manage a patient's condition. Second, the surgeon no longer possessed authority to *act unilaterally* on such clinical judgments. This settled at least one aspect of the historical debate about the physician's disclosure obligations: permission must explicitly be obtained from the patient for medical interventions. The power to authorize action based upon the surgeon's beneficent clinical judgments and recommendations now vests in the patient "of adult years and sound mind," the competent adult patient.

Simple consent shaped the common law of informed consent for four decades. The concept of simple consent addresses only whether the physician had obtained explicit permission from the patient, not the quality of the information upon which that permission was based. The subsequent legal history of informed consent focused on the nature and quality of the physician's disclosure and obligation. Instead of one question, two questions must be asked: "Did the physician provide the patient with an adequate amount of information?" and "On the basis of this information, did the patient consent?" As the common law developed from the late 1950s through the early 1970s, two standards of adequacy emerged.

The first is the *professional community* or *professional practice standard*.[1,4] Under this physician-oriented standard of disclosure, the patient should be told what an appropriately experienced physician would tell the patient about the patient's condition, alternatives available for managing the condition, and the benefits and risks of each alternative. By definition, normative behavior under this standard of disclosure is determined entirely by how surgeons tacitly or specifically have reached consensus on how to conduct themselves.

The courts gradually came to regard the professional community standard as inadequate, largely because of growing skepticism about the adequacy for patients' decision making of a solely physician-based standard. A major event in the development of an alternative standard was the case of *Canterbury v. Spence*, decided in 1972 but occurring in 1958.[5] Canterbury, then a legal minor, was diagnosed with a " filling defect " in the region of the fourth thoracic vertebra. This problem had been diagnosed with the help of a myelogram. A laminectomy was recommended to repair a suspected ruptured disk. Surgeon Spence responded to the inquiry of the patient's mother about potential risks by saying that a laminectomy held no more risk than other surgical procedures. Mrs. Canterbury then consented to the procedure, which was completed without complications. The patient suffered paralysis from a postoperative fall and claimed that had he been aware of this risk of the surgery, he would not have consented to it.

The court therefore focused on the adequacy of Dr. Spence's disclosure regarding the risks of a laminectomy. This court rejected the professional community standard as inadequate and, following other courts that had already gone in this direction,[1] replaced it with *the reasonable person standard*. Informed consent involves meeting the needs of the "reasonable patient." This legal construct means that the informational needs of a patient should be identified on the basis of what a reasonable patient, not a particular patient in a particular, subjective circumstance, would need to know in order to make a meaningful decision. The patient needs to know material information, that is, what the layman patient would be unlikely to encounter in daily life. In practical terms, physicians need not detail abstract concepts without genuine clinical application, but must provide clinically pertinent information, such as benefits, potential risks, possible discomfort, and limits of the treatment's effectiveness, which a reasonable patient would find sufficient as the basis for a decision to accept or refuse what the physician has recommended.

> The discussion need not be a disquisition, and surely the physician is not compelled to give his patient a short medical education; the disclosure role summons the physician only to a reasonable explanation. This means generally informing the patient in non-technical terms as to what is at stake: the therapy alternatives open to him, the goals expectably to be achieved, and the risks that may ensue from particular treatment and no treatment. So informing the patient hardly taxes the physician, and it must be the exceptional patient who cannot comprehend such an explanation at least in a rough way.[5]

The "reasonable person" standard is ethically preferable to the professional community standard because it places appropriate control in the hands of the patient and implies a division of responsibility between surgeon and patient for determining the shape of the informed consent process. A personal, rather than purely utilitarian, relationship with patients requires that the patient's informational needs should be met to the extent reasonably possible. At its most basic level, this means that the patient should be able to reconstruct in lay, practical terms the surgeon's clinical judgments about the patient's condition; management options, including a trial of nonsurgical management; and the benefits and risks of each alternative. For example, the Wisconsin Supreme Court recently considered the issue of whether the reasonable person requirement that significant potential risks and the availability of alternatives be disclosed creates an obligation for the surgeon to disclose comparative information about success rates. The Court's decision extends the reasonable person standard to create an obligation to make such disclosure when "different physicians have substantially different success rates with the same procedure and a reasonable person in the patient's position would consider such information material . . ."[6] Such information would be material to the layperson of average sophistication because he or she might elect to have surgery from the more successful surgeon and thus significantly lower the risks of surgery, an especially pertinent consideration when nonsurgical management is less risky than surgical management.

While the courts seem satisfied when the patient is educated to the point that he or she has a "rough understanding" of what is being proposed,[5] as a matter of ethics the conscientious surgeon should not be. Patients may need, and will often welcome, an offer to help think through their options. Because the decisions often involve subtle trade-offs that are best understood and judged only by the patient, the surgeon should monitor himself against coercing the patient, overtly or subtly. The surgeon may, and should, present the best case for surgical treatment if he or she believes it is the safest and most effective course, but the surgeon should not exaggerate the detriments of other alternatives or the benefits of surgery. In explaining the risks and discomforts attendant to any course, the surgeon should be wary of making these sound so frightening that the patient will reject all varieties of crucial treatment. To the extent that the patient is inclined to trust the advice and competence of the surgeon and exercise a measure of denial to help himself or herself prepare for the ordeal ahead, the surgeon's zeal to fully disclose should not attempt to breach these emotional defense mechanisms and deprive the patient of his or her comfort. In these ways, the surgeon can help the patient to think through his or her clinical options. Doing so provides a valuable ethical service while strengthening the bond of trust and rapport that is so important in a successful surgeon-patient relationship.

In summary, in addition to the obligation to obtain consent, the patient's "yes" or "no" to intervention, the reasonable person standard includes an affirmative duty (i.e., a duty to provide information without first being asked questions by the patient) of the surgeon to explain clinical judgments and recommendations that will enable the patient to make an independent, informed decision. The patient's perspective on his or her own interests should be respected by the surgeon. The ethical principle of respect for autonomy captures what is at stake clinically. The surgeon should acknowledge and accept the integrity of the competent patient's values and beliefs, whether or not the surgeon agrees with them, and should provide the patient with an adequate amount of information. A surgeon's disclosure is adequate when it includes the salient features of the surgeon's clinical thinking in arriving at the recommended therapy and explains to the patient the basic thought process that brought the surgeon to the conclusion that surgical management is a reasonable course of therapeutic action for this patient in this case.[7] The patient's preference should be carried out unless there are ethically compelling reasons to the contrary. Adult patients should be presumed to be autonomous and capable of making their own decisions and are therefore in authority over themselves.

The Patient's Understanding of What the Surgeon Has Disclosed

The law emphasizes the surgeon's role in the informed consent process. This is not surprising; patients bring tort actions against surgeons, not vice versa. The courts have not been asked to address the patient's role in the informed consent process. Ethics takes a balanced approach and therefore addresses both the surgeon's and the patient's roles and responsibilities in the informed consent transaction. Ethical consideration therefore goes on to evaluate what the surgeon has explained and what the patient has understood, the second substantive element in informed consent. Patients need to understand what surgeons tell them about a proposed surgical procedure.

Patients need, first, to attend to what the surgeon is saying. Patients can sometimes become distracted or concerned by something that the surgeon has said and pay little or no attention to what is subsequently said. Some patients, for example, may become anxious or fearful when they hear a diagnosis of cancer or details of surgery such as stopping the heart during a coronary artery bypass operation. The surgeon should be alert to changes in the patient's level of attention and invite the patient to stop the discussion and ask questions and to express concern or anxiety at any time without embarrassment.

Patients also need to absorb, retain, and recall what the surgeon has said. This need can be effectively met by using a vocabulary level not above the tenth grade, adjusted lower as necessary. The pace of disclosure can sometimes impede the patient's ability to absorb and retain what the surgeon says. For patients who exhibit difficulty in these tasks, mental status examinations can be used to identify where the patient is having difficulty. The appropriate response to patients with reduced decision making capacity is discussed below.

More substantively, patients need to understand that they are being asked to authorize surgical management. Faden and Beauchamp point out that this means that the patient needs to grasp that, by consenting to surgical management, the patient authorizes the surgeon and surgical team to perform the procedure that the surgeon has described to the patient. The patient needs to understand that the surgery cannot proceed without the patient's permission.[1]

Finally, the patient needs to understand what he or she is authorizing.[1] The patient needs to grasp the nature of the procedure, its goals, its expected duration, and what can be expected during both near- and short-term recovery. Sequelae of surgery, particularly functional changes such as those that affect job performance, valued activities, or sexuality, and significant aesthetic changes, such as the length and appearance of scar tissue, need to be understood.

It is important for the surgeon to have confidence that the patient does indeed reliably understand what the surgeon has said in the disclosure aspect of the informed consent process. At the same time, it is difficult to know for certain when patients have developed an adequate understanding. This is a matter of clinical judgment that each surgeon learns to develop.

Patients may find it embarrassing or even demeaning to be subjected to tests or quizzes of their understanding. Thus, despite what others propose in this volume, we do not advocate a strategy of asking the patient to repeat what has been said. Instead, we suggest that a well-crafted informed consent form can be a valuable clinical aid to both the surgeon and the patient. After the disclosure aspect of the informed consent process has been completed, the surgeon can use the informed consent form to reinforce and evaluate the patient's understanding. Written at no more than a tenth-grade language level, the consent form should include a statement of the patient's diagnosis, the name of the procedure and a translation of that name into lay terms, the goal of the procedure, the major aspects or steps of the procedure, the length of time that the procedure is expected to take, the benefits and risks of the procedure, and what to expect in both near- and long-term recovery. The form should state that the patient authorizes the surgeon and surgical team to perform the procedure. The contents of the consent form should be reviewed with the patient and the patient encouraged to identify what is still unclear or confusing to the patient, so that these matters can be addressed.

The Patient's Process of Deciding

The process of making an explicit decision by the patient with the surgeon is importantly placed as the third and culminating element of the informed consent process. In making their decisions about surgery, patients need to appreciate that present conditions and actions have future consequences. The patient should be able to reason from present events to future consequences and to have an adequately developed sense of the probabilities that these consequences may indeed occur. This is called cognitive understanding.[8] The surgeon's important role in the development of cognitive understanding includes correcting errors in the patient's fund of knowledge, helping to augment the patient's fund of knowledge, and helping the patient grasp the nature and likelihood of the future consequences attendant upon each of the therapeutic choices available.

This approach to the informed consent process helps to strengthen the patient's decision-making capacity. In addition, this approach aids the surgeon in determining how much the patient wants to participate in the decision-making process and emphasizes the surgeon's responsibility to ensure that the patient does develop an adequate cognitive understanding of his or her condition and the alternatives available for managing it.

In response to the patient who desires very little role in the decision-making process but wants surgical management of his or her problem, the surgeon should nonetheless provide a brief explanation of the surgical procedure by reviewing with the patient the consent form, as described above. The surgeon should also prepare the patient for the immediate postoperative period with a brief explanation of what this will entail so that the patient will not be surprised or alarmed when he or she wakes up in the recovery area or surgical intensive care unit. Finally, the surgeon should point out risks that can occur.

Patients considering surgery also need to evaluate benefits and risks of the alternatives available to them. These are value judgments and concern how much worth or importance to attach to potential favorable and unfavorable outcomes associated with each available option. Making such value judgments involves evaluative understanding,[8] a clinical ethical consideration overlooked altogether in the law governing informed consent. In making decisions about surgery, each patient needs to make value judgments about the benefits, risks, and discomforts of surgery, of other available medical interventions, and whether surgery or other intervention is less dire than living with the risks and discomforts of untreated illness. Evaluative understanding is thus just as essential to the patient's decision making as cognitive understanding.

The surgeon can assist the patient to develop evaluative understanding of available alternatives. Asking a patient, "What is important to you as you consider . . . ?", with the ellipsis completed with each alternative, is effective in eliciting the patient's values.[9] The surgeon should attempt to discern patterns of values in conversation with the patient and identify them for the patient who is struggling to articulate what is important to himself or herself. Patients do not make decisions on the basis of isolated values and helping patients to connect otherwise unarticulated concerns promotes individual autonomy. Their values can make reference to job performance, sexual activity, mental function, physical appearance, and particularly important hobbies. For example, it would not respect the patient's values to place a pacemaker on the side of the chest from which the patient fires a shotgun while dove hunting. Such assistance also directs the surgeon's relationship to the patient's most fundamental values and beliefs as they give meaning to the alternative possible futures the patient must contemplate.

The surgeon should initially take a nondirective approach in helping the patient to develop evaluative understanding. After all, the patient is entitled to make a decision on the basis of his or her values and beliefs, which can sometimes differ sharply from those of the surgeon. Once the patient has identified his or her relevant values and evaluated the alternatives on this basis, the surgeon may wish to offer a recommendation.

Respect for the autonomy of the patient means that the patient's decision should be free of controlling influences.[1,2] The surgeon should therefore make a recommendation only after the patient has developed evaluative understanding without fear of bringing undue influence to bear on the patient's autonomy in the decision-making process. Most patients highly value the surgeon's recommendation as they struggle to reach their own decisions. Appropriately timed recommendations therefore play an important role in the informed consent process and may even support the independent nature of the patient's decision.

Summary

The ethics of the informed consent process emphasizes the role of this process in developing solid rapport with the patient. Such a rapport has a number of clinical advantages. First, the surgeon does not function as a disinterested unbiased fund of information, consulted as one might consult a book as a noninteractive source. Instead, the surgeon has important experiences and opinions with which to assist the patient in the decision-making process, as well as the technical information and knowledge of the patient's personal medical history that constitute important data in the decision-making process. Failure by the surgeon to provide the patient with the full range of his or her knowledge for fear of violating the patient's autonomy could reduce the patient's capacity to become genuinely informed and ultimately defeat the high-minded principle the surgeon is seeking to guard on behalf of the patient. Ultimately, no one knows more or is more intimately concerned about the details of the patient's surgical treatment than the surgeon and the patient, which makes their mutually respectful cooperation essential to the process of genuine informed consent. Second, forming a therapeutic alliance with the patient through the informed consent process will result in a more-informed, better-prepared patient, who has developed a sense of his or her own responsibility. In other words, patient compliance may increase, leading to a smoother, more effective postoperative course. In an era of managed care, this outcome will help to promote the valued goal of the more economically efficient use of expensive medical resources such as surgery. Third, the open and honest two-way communication called for by the ethics of the informed consent process should increase the patient's confidence and trust in the surgeon. This will go a long way to establishing good rapport with patients, which makes the practice of surgery more rewarding in human terms for both surgeon and patient.

Formed by this ethical analysis, the informed consent process becomes a process of mutual decision making. The surgeon and the patient both have active and important roles to play in this process and responsibilities to discharge, as well. The surgeon, as the patient's fiduciary, should share beneficence-based clinical judgment with the patient. As the patient's fiduciary (i.e., as someone who acts primarily to protect the patient's interests), the surgeon should also be committed to doing the right thing for the patient, but the ultimate decision about what is right for the patient rests with the patient. For this reason, the ethics of the informed consent process places strong emphasis on the surgeon's respect for the patient's autonomy.

Clinical Topics: Putting the Consent Process into Clinical Practice

Responding to the Patient's Questions

In initiating the informed consent process, the surgeon's conversation with the patient should stress that decisions will be made jointly by the surgeon and patient after information is exchanged between them. The surgeon will usually make recommendations, and the patient needs to understand and evaluate those recommendations. The patient must also be assured that he or she is encouraged to express any concerns and ask any questions without fear or embarrassment.

The first question of many patients is often, "How long will this operation take?" and, of course, the surgeon should respond with an estimate of the customary range of time it has taken him or her to complete this procedure in the past. The surgeon should also understand that the real question being asked usually is, "When should my family begin to worry that things aren't going well?" To help the patient with questions he or she may have difficulty articulating, the surgeon should direct the conversation to questions that prior patients have asked about this procedure, and invite the patient to discuss these questions in the context of his personal concerns. The patient frequently becomes relaxed enough to start asking his or her own questions and genuinely begin to seek information about the operation.

Where the Consent Process Should Occur

Initiation of the consent process in the surgical holding area just before the operation is scheduled to begin should be avoided in all but the most urgent or most minor procedures. Instead, the discussion should be initiated well in advance of surgery because decisions should be made without added tension, and with the time appropriate to what may be a major life decision. The patient's outpatient visits for preoperative workup provide an ideal opportunity to engage in the informed consent process.

A Seven-Step Clinical Process

The consent process can be organized around seven practical steps. *First*, tell the patient, and if the patient agrees, his or her attendants briefly, about the process of informed consent. This may take no more than a sentence or two, to amiably introduce the process and the patient's role in it. *Second*, elicit the patient's understanding of his or her problem and the alternatives for managing it. The surgeon should listen for inaccurate or incomplete information and respectfully supply needed corrective information. *Third*, the surgeon should elaborate on the patient's condition and options for treatment, aiming for a reasonable person standard of disclosure. This should involve reviewing with the patient information already discussed by the referring physician. *Fourth*, the surgeon should assist the patient in developing cognitive understanding of his or her situation, with regard to both short-term and long-term consequences of choices made now. The surgeon should explain his or her own limitations with respect to predicting and controlling outcome and the idiosyncratic responses of individual patients to the same or similar procedures. *Fifth*, to guide the patient's development of evaluative understanding, the surgeon should then assist the patient in evaluating the alternatives available. The technique just discussed of asking patients what is important to them about each alternative helps the patient to identify and express values. *Sixth*, the surgeon should offer a recommendation. This recommendation should include an acknowledgment that no single therapy is clearly optimal or superior if such is the case, and that the surgeon is willing to abide by the patient's decision. When surgical management is clearly superior, the surgeon should so state and proceed to recommend it. It is important to wait until the process has developed to this later stage before offering a recommendation, to respect the patient's autonomy and minimize the possibility that the surgeon has intentionally or unintentionally introduced a coercive influence to the process. *Seventh*, the patient articulates a decision for or against surgery.

The seven-step informed consent process should be described, dated, and timed in the patient's medical record as part of the preoperative workup. After the surgeon and patient complete this process and after the consent form has been reviewed with the patient, as described above, a nurse or other member of the surgical team can obtain the patient's signature on a consent form or operative permit constituting the formal record of consent.

This seven-step process will address two questions that surgeons have before any surgery: "Is the patient competent to make a decision?" and "How much control of the decision-making process does the patient prefer or desire?" The answers to these questions cannot be given *a priori*, because they depend on the individual capacities and preferences of each patient. As the seven-step process advances, the surgeon will develop a more reliable, clinical basis for judgments about the patient's capacity for decision making and desires regarding degree of control. The informed consent process can readily be adjusted in response to the first factor; most hospitals are prepared to provide for a psychiatric evaluation when there are questions of diminished competence for decision making. This process will be discussed shortly.

How Much Influence Should the Surgeon Exert?

We noted in the first part of this section that the surgeon's recommendations have a proper role in the informed consent process. Most patients value their surgeon's recommendations and customarily give them considerable weight in their own decision-making process about whether to accept surgical management of their condition. In principle, therefore, surgeons exercise permissible influence through their recommendations.

Altering the frame of reference in an attempt to influence the patient's decision by excessively emphasizing either benefits or risks, a process termed "framing,"[1] poses clinical ethical challenges. Framing is inconsistent both with the surgeon's fiduciary role and with respect for patient autonomy and therefore should be avoided. For example, the surgeon may describe the risk of surgery as routine, which it may seem to the surgeon, and the benefits as a great boon and as a certainty. These factual descriptions may be correct in terms of the individual surgeon's experiences, but they are incorrect in terms of predicting the outcome for the specific operative patient and therefore are deceptive. Inadvertently, a surgeon may seek to reassure a patient by making such statements as "I can't remember the last time we lost a patient from this operation." Framing in this manner before the patient decides to have surgery is ethically very suspect because the surgeon can seriously impair the development of the patient's evaluative understanding by such framing.

Surgeons should also avoid a particularly corrupt and common type of framing commonly called crepe hanging. This involves exaggerating the gravity of the patient's situation and of the operation in an effort to increase the patient's estimation of and gratitude toward the surgeon when things go well, as they were expected to by the surgeon in the first place. Should the surgery have a poor outcome, the surgeon has only to say that this is as he predicted and the patient nevertheless agreed to proceed.

Surgeons should be especially aware of subtle framing effects that can occur when substituting descriptive terms for quantitative terms, especially in the characterization of risks. For example, the surgeon might tell the patient facing surgery for glaucoma, "You will lose your eyesight without the procedure." However, the more truthful statement would be that a certain percentage of people in this circumstance, perhaps 15% in this hypothetical case, would lose eyesight without the corrective procedure. Surgeons should adhere to quantitative descriptions whenever possible in the early steps of the informed consent process and then help the patient to evaluate this information in the steps concerned with cognitive and evaluative understanding.

Managing Conflicting Opinions Among Professionals

Patients occasionally encounter conflicting opinions among surgeons or between the referring physician and the referral surgeon (see Chapter 15). Everyone in the medical profession understands, but may not readily acknowledge, that clinical judgment can vary widely among the specialties and even among practitioners within the same specialty. For example, the referring physician may focus on the operation's morbidity risks, whereas the surgeon may be most concerned about reducing disease-related mortality and so may discount, to some extent, the inconvenience, cost, morbidity, and discomfort of the procedure. Mentions of pain and possible major inconveniences, such as not being able to drive a car or stoop, were not clearly mentioned in a study of patients undergoing hip replacements.[10] The guiding principle when differences of judgment occur was articulated two centuries ago by the Scottish physician John Gregory (1724–1773). He emphasized that surgeons and physicians should manage such disagreements with a view always toward protecting the interests of the patient. [11]

In the twentieth century, this means educating the patient when physicians have honest disagreements in their clinical judgments and recommendations. The surgeon's goal should be to strengthen the patient's autonomy in the decision-making process. By asking the patient questions, the surgeon can assess the patient's understanding and perceptions about the physicians' disagreement. The surgeon can then assist the patient to identify and consider the merits and possible criticisms of each view. In purely elective situations, the passage of time will often be helpful. In some cases, with especially difficult choices, a meeting with the patient and the disagreeing physicians may be beneficial (see Chapter 15).

Multiple Surgeons and Other Physicians in the Consent Process

The typical surgical patient receives ongoing care from physicians in several specialties, including surgery, before, during, and after procedures. The tendency exists in these team contexts to assume that others have already spoken with the patient, have explained what is happening, and have taken the patient through the informed consent process. This assumption can lead to a defective informed consent process, especially regarding the surgical procedure being contemplated. The operating surgeon should take a preventive ethics approach to this potential problem by accepting responsibility for taking the patient through the consent process for the operation. The anesthesiologist should participate in this process with reference to the alternatives, benefits, and effects of types of anesthesia. All physicians, especially those in training, should avoid giving answers to questions outside their specialty and about which they are uncertain.

When multiple surgeons are involved, the surgical specialist who performs the most essential and most complication-prone parts of the operation has the greatest responsibility regarding informed consent. This surgeon should tell the patient who the other participants will be and what their roles will be in the patient's care. This preventive ethics approach minimizes the chance that the patient will become confused or concerned about the involvement of multiple surgeons.

Involvement of Trainees

Surgeons are ethically obligated to reveal to patients all the individuals who will be involved in their surgery, particularly trainees. The surgeon should not presume that the patient knows how a teaching hospital functions, or that trainees provide patient care in a hospital that may or may not incorporate the word "university" in its name. The patient's consent to trainee involvement should never be presumed. We decry covert two-tiered systems and emphasize the right of the patient to know who is in charge and who is performing what service, because these are essential to the patient's authorization of the procedure.[1]

At the outset, the surgeon should describe generally to the patient the types and roles of trainees who will be involved. The attending surgeon may explain, "Dr. X is a senior level resident in our training program and will be performing portions of your operation; I will be assisting and supervising Dr. X throughout." This is a straightforward, honest approach. A statement such as "Dr. X and I will be performing your operation under my supervision" is deceptive, even though true, because it omits a description of Dr. X's status as a trainee and the surgeon's role as assistant and supervisor. In the case of surgery by a resident without participatory supervision (i.e., without the attending surgeon scrubbing in), we agree with the Council on Ethical and Judicial Affairs of the American Medical Association: "If a resident or other physician is to perform the operation under non-participatory supervision, it is necessary to make a full disclosure of this fact to the patient, and this should be evidenced by an appropriate statement contained in the consent. Under these circumstances, it is the resident or other physician who becomes the operating surgeon."[12] Also, the American College of Surgeons' policy states, "If a resident is to operate and take care of the patient, under the general supervision of an attending surgeon who will not participate actively, the patient should be so informed and consent thereto."[13]

The surgical certification boards state clearly that to receive credit as surgeon for a particular procedure, the resident must meet a number of requirements, including having "either performed or been responsibly involved in performing critical portions of the operative procedure."[14] Therefore, when the surgery resident is to be listed as the operating surgeon, full disclosure is obligatory. The gradual assumption of responsibility by residents to whatever degree the supervising surgeon allows should be frankly explained to the patient/patient's surrogate, as well as the surgeon's role in both assisting in a procedure and in supervising residents. The role and responsibility of medical students should also be made explicit.

When Patients Are Undecided or Refuse Surgery

The patient may refuse a surgical procedure after an adequate informed consent process because he or she is in a state of indecision. If the consent process has gone well, this indecision usually results from the patient's ambivalence about similarly attractive alternatives. The patient may often also be frightened about having an operation and understandably may resolve his or her indecision in favor of nonsurgical management of his or her condition.

In this case the surgeon should explain that the patient has caused no offense by being undecided. Such a decision, after all, does not preclude a decision for surgery later. In elective surgeries, the patient should be encouraged to think matters through and to determine if the decision will become more apparent with time (see Chapter 8). The surgeon should explain, however, that the postponement of surgical treatment, as in the case of cancers, may change the nature of benefits and risks. If the surgeon decides to remain on such a patient's case, the patient should be so informed and told that the surgeon will discuss the patient's decision at any time. The canons of medical ethics and common courtesy are violated if the surgeon vocalizes disappointment or anger toward the patient, or threatens to refuse future treatment for not affirming trust in the consulting surgeon.

Use of blood products poses a particular challenge. It is well known that members of the Jehovah's Witnesses faith community and others with concern about blood-borne pathogens will not accept blood products. The management of this problem in the practice of surgery is discussed at length elsewhere in this volume (see Chapters 7, 8, and 9).

Refusal of Indicated Operations

A patient's refusal to have indicated surgery is not itself evidence of the patient's diminished decision-making capacity. The seven-step process described above is designed to focus the surgeon's attention on the decision-making process and on how such factors as cognitive impairment may affect the patient's ability to complete the steps of the informed consent process. Nonetheless, refusal when surgery is clearly indicated does raise a red flag and prompts any thoughtful surgeon to question the patient's decision-making capacity, especially in potentially life-threatening circumstances. A patient who refuses such surgery without attaching importance to mortality, morbidity, or reduced quality of life causes a surgeon frustration and concern.

Recent studies of noncompliance underscore that failure in communication can result in the refusal of the physician's recommendation or the patient's noncooperation with a treatment plan.[15,16] The surgeon's first response to refusal of surgery is to review with the patient the patient's understanding of the patient's condition, the nature of the surgical procedure, and its benefits and risks. The patient's cognitive understanding may be incomplete, resulting in a refusal that the patient may reconsider when more complete understanding has been achieved. The surgeon's second response should be to explore the patient's evaluative understanding. Of particular concern should be possible mistrust of physicians based on past experience (which may be valid), pressing obligations, or psychological factors such as anxiety, depression, or fear. The surgeon's third response should be to acknowledge value conflicts, when they do occur, and work with the patient to identify a management plan that accords with the patient's values. If the surgeon believes that the patient's values will be supported by surgery, the surgeon should point this out and ask the patient to reconsider. In summary, the preventive ethics approach to refusal of surgery should be respectful exploration of the patient's reasoning, on the assumption that the patient, by his or her own lights, has good reason for refusal but may, with additional information and reflection, reconsider and accept surgery, and not on the assumption that the patient's competence is somehow diminished or compromised.

One very helpful response to refusals when surgery's value in preventing mortality is clear is to offer the patient the alternative of a trial of nonsurgical management—for example, when a patient refuses surgical management of stenotic carotid arteries. Nonsurgical management may be supported by the patient's values that emerge during the consent process. The patient should be informed of this possibility and a mutual plan developed to monitor the nonsurgical trial of management. The goal should be to identify mutually acceptable criteria for evaluating the nonsurgical management and for reconsidering surgery. Should a patient be disinclined to accept surgery or any other invasive management as the first option, the surgeon could propose a trial of medical management and agree with the patient on the conditions under which the surgeon would initiate surgical management. Such circumstances could include recurrent and worsening pathology, even on a regular schedule of medication, unacceptable side effects of medication, or increasing risk of mortality.

Problems with the Patient's Decision-Making Capacity

Some patients may still experience difficulty making decisions, regardless of how ethically, astutely, and carefully the surgeon has attended to the informed consent process. The hospital's consultation-liaison psychiatrist, a physician who has the expertise to evaluate patients' decision-making capacity, can be a valuable adviser and ally. The patient should be told of the role of the psychiatrist to the extent that this is possible. The surgeon should make the following request. First, the psychiatrist should evaluate the patient for a formal cognitive or objective disorder or other psychiatric problem that might significantly affect the patient's ability to make decisions and whether such a disorder will be susceptible to treatment. Second, the psychiatrist and the surgeon should agree on a clear delineation of boundaries in their treatment of the patient. Each should understand what the other will do to attempt to restore the patient's decision-making capacity and cooperate. Third, the psychiatrist and surgeon should develop a plan for improving the patient's decision-making capacity, to the extent at which the patient is able to participate in the informed consent process. In all cases, the surgeon should eschew the strategy of using consultation-liaison psychiatry simply to declare a patient incompetent,[17] thereby enabling others to make decisions for the patient, or discharging the patient to the management of other specialties. Patients with waxing and waning decisional capacity often experience periods of lucidity and may choose to provide informed consent for surgery during such a period, specifying that statements he or she may subsequently make while confused should not supersede his or her decision made during a period of enlightenment. These have been called "Ulysses contracts" in the bioethics literature.[18]

Surrogate Decision Making for Patients with Irreversibly Diminished Decision-Making Capacity

Working up the patient who exhibits problems with decision-making capacity with the aid of consultation-liaison psychiatry should lead to the reliable identification of patients who have irreversibly lost the capacity to participate in the decision-making process. By tradition and now in many states with legal sanction, family members are asked to make decisions for such patients.[19] There is a stable consensus in the bioethics literature for how this process should occur.[18]

Family members should not be asked, "What would you do?" or "What do you want to do?" because these questions invite family members to inadvertently mix up their own concerns and values with those of the patient. Instead, the process should begin with the first four steps of the informed consent process. Step 5 should involve questioning family members about what they believe would be important to the patient at this time and in these circumstances. The goal is to try to construct what the patient's evaluative understanding would be as closely as humanly possible. On this basis the remaining steps of the consent process should be completed. This leads to what is known as "substituted judgment."[18]

Sometimes, for a variety of reasons, family members cannot achieve substituted judgment. In such case they should be asked to make the decision that in their view protects and promotes their loved one's interests. This is called the best interests standard of surrogate decision making.[18]

The best way to assist family members in these circumstances is to encourage patients to take a preventive ethics approach on their own. All patients in their geriatric years, those with chronic diseases (e.g., all cancers, chronic obstructive lung disease), and those in the early stages of dementia should be encouraged to express their values and preferences in advance. Advance directives have legal standing in many states. Various adjuncts to these instruments have been proposed, including the Medical Directive[20] and the Values History.[21] See Chapters 4 and 10 for more detail on advance-directive decision making.

Religiously Based Refusal

Usually some degree of flexibility is inherent in any particular religion's teachings regarding surgery. The surgeon should therefore not assume that the patient's interpretation is necessarily the only one with authority in the patient's faith community. Well-informed hospital chaplains or local religious leaders can help the surgeon to explore a faith tradition for flexibility. The chaplain can also help the surgeon to explain matters to the patient's religious advisers (with the patient's consent beforehand, of course, to protect confidentiality). Religious advisers who have had the opportunity to inform themselves, see the patient in the hospital, and to reflect on the teachings, traditions, holy books, or written theology of a faith community may reach the conclusion that the patient's refusal is not the only posture supported in the patient's faith community. Should these matters remain unresolved, as in the case of Jehovah's Witnesses, the patient's care should be turned over to a surgeon who is comfortable meeting the necessary constraints imposed.

Informed Consent in Pediatric Surgery

Pediatric surgeons confront conceptual and clinical challenges regarding informed consent. Adolescent patients, particularly those with chronic diseases about which the patient has become quite knowledgeable and mature, may be able to complete the steps of the informed consent process as well as adults. When this is the case, the patient's autonomy should be respected by the surgeon and by the adolescent's parents. In these circumstances the surgeon's responsibilities include pointing out to the parents that their child is capable of making an adult decision that deserves respect. When there are differences between parent and child, the surgeon should offer his or her services as a good-faith negotiator. The goal should be to reach a commonly accepted decision rather than to decide whose decision wins.

Not all adolescents can complete the informed consent process, nor can younger children. Nonetheless, children are capable of understanding to a degree appropriate to their age and emotional development the information that they have a disease, what parts of the body the disease involves, and that surgery can help. These matters should be explained to the patient, when the goal is not so much to obtain the patient's consent as to provide information about the clinical course to which the patient's parents have already consented. This concept has led to such practices as familiarizing children with the hospital, including operative and postoperative areas, before elective surgery.[22]

Consent for Innovation and Research

Consent for research and innovation is imperative because the patient's interests are put at additional risk by the investigational or innovative nature of the surgical procedure being offered. The long and disturbing history of abuse of research subjects has led to an oversight apparatus, the Institutional Review Board, to regulate research with human subjects.[1] Chapter 12 provides a detailed discussion of the challenges of informed consent for research and innovation in surgery.

Time Requirements

We have called here for an informed consent process that follows from the ethical analysis that we provided in the first section of the chapter. This process will increase marginally the time needed for the care of surgical patients. This may seem an unrealistic demand in an era when time is money in surgical and medical practices run by giant insurance company plans and acted out in hospital chains across the nation.

These changes are not unique to managed care, but they are epitomized by it. The new managed practice of medicine in all its forms is based on the management concept of quality control, known variously as Total Quality Management and Continuous Quality Improvement.[23] This concept leads to the examination of every medical and surgical process to determine if each of its steps is necessary for achieving a goal and if each necessary step is being performed in the most economically efficient manner. The assumption is that improvements in quality of each necessary step lead to economic efficiency and therefore savings for surgeons and payers.

There is another assumption of total quality management and continuous quality improvement that is gaining increased importance in medical and surgical practice, namely, that every increase in quality adds value.[23] Informed consent increases quality by increasing the participation of patients in the clinical decision-making process and by humanizing the surgeon-patient relationship. The informed consent process that we have described in this chapter adds the value of putting respect for autonomy into everyday surgical practice at a much higher level than that of the bureaucratic model of informed consent. We believe that informed consent is an area of medicine that adds value justifiably in the form of time required and therefore should be considered as an essential element of quality. Surgeons should become vigorous advocates for the management concept that the time required for the informed consent process is an essential and value-adding business cost in managed care settings.

Postponement of Discussion of Adverse Events

Legal provision is made for informed consent to be waived when it can be shown that the process with high probability is likely to be harmful to the patient. This *very rare* exception is called "therapeutic privilege."[1] The seriously ill patient who is very emotionally labile or individuals with paranoid delusions may be harmed by the informed consent process. The suspension of participatory decision making should be very rare and treated very cautiously. It is a more a legal rather than an ethical exception and therefore has a very restricted role in clinical practice.

Overprotective Family Members

Family members are an important social support for patients and will be affected to varying degrees by the outcome of decisions to operate. The role of the family in the informed consent process will vary according to the structure and history of the family. The surgeon should be guided by the patient regarding the role that the family should play. There is no basis whatever for the occasional requests to withhold undesirable information during the informed consent process or postoperatively from the patient who remains capable of understanding. Conversely, there is every moral reason on the basis of confidentiality to honor requests to withhold information from family or friends if requested by the patient (see Chapter 3).

Clinical Conclusions

Informed consent should be understood and put into practice as a clinical process, rather than a signed operative permit or consent form. The informed consent process can be put into practice in seven practical steps that help to build enduring therapeutic alliances with patients and respect their autonomy and thus serve as a powerful antidote to the tendency toward bureaucratization of the informed consent process and to the litigious practice environment. Surgeons should take an active role against this trend of the depersonalization of the surgeon-patient relationship in which the surgeon becomes a technocratic automaton and the patient an object to be manipulated through bureaucratic requirements.

As a matter of ethics, as well as of law, adult patients should be assumed capable of completing the informed consent process. Patients who experience difficulty with the steps of the informed consent process should not be labeled incompetent but assisted, with consultation-liaison psychiatry as necessary, to complete the process.

Patients who experience irreversible difficulty with the steps of the informed consent process require surrogate decision makers, usually family members. Surrogate decision makers should be guided by the principle of substituted judgment, making decisions based as much as possible on the patient's values and beliefs, and, when this is not possible, on the basis of a thoughtful, informed judgment about what is in the patient's best interest.

In teaching environments, explicit description of the residents' and students' role in the case must be provided and documented. Some adolescents may be able to participate in the informed consent process, especially those with chronic illness for which surgical management is considered. These patients should be treated as adults and their parents asked to support them in their decision making. Adolescents and younger children who cannot complete the steps of the consent process should be provided information at a level appropriate to their age and development, with their parents providing surrogate consent on the basis of their assessment of what is in their child's best interest.

When patients or their surrogates refuse surgery, the surgeon should neither take offense nor simply acquiesce. Instead, the surgeon should take the opportunity to work up the refusal and invite the patient or the patient's surrogate to reconsider. The surgeon should be open to negotiated solutions—for example, bloodless surgery for patients with religious objections to the use of blood products, or trial of nonsurgical management.

The informed consent process should be documented in the patient's chart. The signed consent form or operative permit is part of this record but not equivalent to the consent process itself.

The informed consent process takes time. The informed consent process also adds value to the physician-patient relationship. The concepts of Total Quality Management and Continuous Quality Improvement accept the idea that additions of value to patient care justify added costs. Surgeons should thus be vigorous advocates for a true, rather than bureaucratic, informed consent process in the new era of the managed care settings.

References

1. Ruth R. Faden and Tom L. Beauchamp, *A History and Theory of Informed Consent*. New York: Oxford University Press, 1986.
2. Tom L. Beauchamp and James F. Childress, *Principles of Biomedical Ethics*, 4th ed. New York: Oxford University Press, 1994.

3. *Schloendorff v. Society of New York Hospital*, 211 N.Y. 125, 126, 105 N.E. 92, 93 (1914).

4. F. Rosovsky, *Consent to Treatment: A Practical Guide*. Boston: Little, Brown, 1984.

5. *Canterbury v. Spence* 464 F. 2nd 772, 785 (D.C. Cir. 1972).

6. *Johnson v. Kokemoor* 199 Wis.2d 615. 545 N.E. 2d 495 (1996).

7. Stephen Wear, *Informed Consent: Patient Autonomy and Physician Beneficence with Clinical Medicine*. Dordrecht, The Netherlands: Kluwer Academic Publishers, 1993.

8. Becky Cox White, *Competence to Consent*. Washington, D.C.: Georgetown University Press, 1994.

9. Laurence B. McCullough, Nancy L. Wilson, Thomas A. Teasdale, et al., "Mapping Personal, Familial, and Professional Values in Long-term Care Decisions," *The Gerontologist* 33 (1993): 324–332.

10. F. J. Dodd, H. A. Donegan, W. G. Kernohan, R. V. Geary, and R. A. B. Mollan, "Consensus In Medical Communication," *Social Science and Medicine* 37 (1993): 565–569.

11. John Gregory, *Lectures on the Duties and Qualifications of a Physician*. London: W. Strahan and T. Cadell, 1772. Reprinted in *John Gregory's Writings on Medical Ethics and Philosophy of Medicine*, Laurence B. McCullough, ed. Dordrecht, The Netherlands: Kluwer Academic Publishers, 1998.

12. American Medical Association, Council on Ethical and Judicial Affairs, "Substitution of Surgeon without Patient's Knowledge or Consent," in Council on Ethical and Judicial Affairs, *Code of Medical Ethics: Current Opinions with Annotations*. Chicago, IL: American Medical Association, 1994, pp. 121–122.

13. American College of Surgeons, *Statement on Principles*. Chicago, IL: American College of Surgeons, 1989.

14. American Board of Surgery, *Booklet of Information, July 1996–June 1997*. Chicago, IL: American Board of Surgery, 1996.

15. Paul Applebaum and Loren Roth, "Patients who Refuse Treatment in Medical Hospitals," *Journal of the American Medical Association* 250 (1983): 1296–1301.

16. Julia Connelly and Courtney Campbell, "Patients Who Refuse Treatment in Medical Offices," *Archives of Internal Medicine* 147 (1987): 1829–1833.

17. Mark Perl and Earl E. Shelp, "Psychiatric Consultation Masking Moral Dilemmas in Medicine, "*New England Journal of Medicine* 307 (1982): 618–621.

18. Allen E. Buchanan and Dan W. Brock, *Deciding for Others: The Ethics of Surrogate Decision-Making*. New York: Cambridge University Press, 1989.

19. Judith Areen, "The Legal Status of Consent Obtained from Families of Adult Patients to Withhold or Withdraw Treatment," *Journal of the American Medical Association* 258 (1987): 229–235.

20. Linda Emanuel and Ezekiel J. Emanuel, "The Medical Directive: A New Comprehensive Advance Care Document," *Journal of the American Medical Association* 261 (1989): 3288–3293.

21. David J. Doukas and Laurence B. McCullough, "The Values History: The Evaluation of the Patient's Values and Advance Directives," *The Journal of Family Practice* 32 (1991):145–151.

22. American Academy of Pediatrics, Committee on Bioethics, "Informed Consent. Parental Permission and Assent in Pediatric Practice," *Pediatrics* 95 (1995): 314–317.

23. Ellen J. Gaucher and Richard J. Coffey, *Total Quality in Health Care: From Theory to Practice*. San Francisco: Jossey-Bass Publishers, 1993.

3

Confidentiality in Surgical Practice

MARY FAITH MARSHALL
C. D. SMITH III

A famous actor was recently admitted to a university teaching hospital following a tragic and traumatic accident. Once the injury was surgically stabilized, the patient was transferred to the surgical intensive care unit in serious condition. From the outset, it was clear that the patient would undergo a lengthy hospitalization. The actor's popularity and the dramatic nature of the injury fostered immediate worldwide attention. Concern for the patient's privacy was focused both externally, on the news media, and internally, on medical center personnel. The medical center's public relations office galvanized itself for an intense and protracted relationship with the news media. Disclosure of information would be guided by the preferences of the patient and family. The patient's surgeon would be the sole spokesperson for the medical center.

The patient was assigned an alias in keeping with medical center procedure for protecting the privacy of well-known patients. Acknowledging that even this safeguard may not guarantee the privacy of the electronic medical record, hospital administrators activated their recently purchased security audit system. They registered every instance of electronic access to the patient's electronic record.

Each person who accessed the record subsequently received a letter from the medical center's chief administrator asking for a rationale for that person's "need to know" information about the patient. Most instances of access were legitimate. Some were not. Clearly, medical center staff and faculty had pried into the patient's record. The excuse "my computer access code must have been compromised" was heard so frequently that it lost credibility. Some readily admitted to compromising the patient's privacy; most were embarrassed and humiliated.

Their shame was well founded. Unwarranted access of any patient's medical record is a deliberate invasion of privacy, whether the motivation is curiosity or malice. Those who were caught by the security audit knew that they had committed an egregious wrong. Surely none of them would have wanted his or her privacy compromised under similar circumstances.

Ethical Analysis of the Obligation of Confidentiality

Privacy and Confidentiality

Privacy is best thought of as the condition of inaccessibility. This means limited access by others to one's body, feelings, or thoughts, or to information about oneself or one's intimate relationships. Privacy is a state of being. One is either private (no access by others) or not private (access by others). In legal theory, the concept of privacy limits the power that other individuals, third parties, or the government have over each of us.[1]

The right to control physical or intellectual access by others is based on the ethical principle of respect for persons. This means respecting others' autonomy (their right to be self-directed) and treating them beneficently. To be truly autonomous, a person must be free from outside influences as well as from personal limitations.[2]

Confidentiality is an outgrowth of the concept of privacy. Confidentiality pertains to the sharing of personal information, and depends on a trusting relationship between two people. An individual who shares personal information that is considered confidential trusts the receiver of the information not to disclose it to anyone else without the giver's permission. Within a confidential relationship, one could think of personal information as the giver's moral property. In some states, medical information is also the patient's legal property.

The primary reason for honoring a confidence is respect for another person's right to choose which aspects of himself or herself to share with others. A second reason is to foster and maintain a relationship of good faith, or fidelity, with another person. Relationships between surgeons and patients are fiduciary. They are based on trust and mutual respect and depend on mutual obligations such as keeping promises and honoring one's commitments. Intimacy between professionals and their clients (patients and surgeons, clients and attorneys, penitents and clergy) is impossible without a certain level of trust. Real intimacy between persons involves the voluntary sacrifice of privacy. In the relationship between a patient and a surgeon, this sacrifice is unilateral on the patient's part.[3]

A third reason to honor a confidence is to advance social utility. Social utility means maximizing benefits and minimizing harms on a social, rather than an individual, scale. By this criterion, maintaining patient confidences is important because it fosters public trust in the institution of medicine. Without trust in the medical profession, public welfare would suffer. Consider the social consequences if persons with contagious diseases, substance abuse problems, or mental illness did not seek treatment because they mistrusted physicians.

The Patient-Surgeon Relationship

The relationship between a patient and his or her surgeon is often based on unspoken assumptions and implicit promises. The patient shares personal information with his or her surgeon because he or she assumes that his or her disclosures will be held in confidence. This assumption is based on the surgeon's implicit promise to honor the patient's privacy. The surgeon then rightly assumes that the patient will not withhold any information that is necessary in determining the plan of care.

Unwarranted breaches of confidentiality quickly undermine this critical relationship. Once lost, trust can be nearly impossible to reestablish. One of the few studies investigating patients' responses to hypothetical breaches of confidentiality showed that patients prize confidentiality very highly. In this study, thirty psychiatric inpatients said that they would be angry and upset (and some would even leave treatment), if verbal or written information was released without their permission.[4] A similar study of 58 psychiatric outpatients found that these patients would take formal action, such as complaints or legal suits, if their confidentiality was compromised.[5]

While the obligation to maintain confidentiality is not absolute, limits to privacy and confidentiality must be clear from the outset. Understanding and negotiating the bounds of privacy and confidentiality should be part of the ongoing informed consent process described in Chapter 2.

Dissemination of Medical Information

Most patients (and their surgeons) have no idea how widely their medical information is disseminated. Patients often wrongly assume that only their surgeons have access to their medical records. Surgeons often wrongly assume that legal and institutional safeguards will protect their patients' medical records from external (or internal) incursions. Unfortunately, no safeguard against breach of privacy is ever totally effective because too many people have too many avenues of access to patient information. Legitimate users of medical information include insurance companies, government service payers, researchers, welfare agencies, professional accrediting agencies and review boards, employers, public health agencies, credit reporting agencies, law enforcement agencies, computerized registries and data banks, licensing agencies, and institutions such as colleges, prisons, or the armed services.[6] A study by the Institute of Medicine showed 33 representative users of medical records and 50 primary and secondary users.[7]

Patient authorization for surgeons or other physicians to release medical information is not always voluntary. The coercive element is not the surgeon, but the patient's employer or insurance carrier. Patients often have no choice but to authorize disclosure when they are seeking employment, admission to educational institutions, insurance eligibility, or legal protection in the case of rape, paternity, or driving under the influence.[8] At least one study shows that patients often feel coerced into authorizing disclosure. A review of two hundred requests for release of information about psychiatric patients found that 81% of the patients felt they had no choice but to release their records to receive medical or financial help; only 56% of the patients had an accurate knowledge of the content of their medical records; only 34% knew which individuals had access to their medical records; and only 16% had knowledge of legal protections of confidentiality.[8]

Illegitimate access to the medical record occurs by way of unprotected written documents (a chart left open for casual perusal, papers left on a conference room table, a computer screen with a patient's record not erased before the surgeon leaves the computer station), uncontrolled access to the electronic record or to billing information (by hackers, terminated employees, or curious staff), verbal indiscretions (conversations overheard in the elevator or at cocktail parties),[9] visual observation (the patient in the next bed), and personnel errors that release or lose information (an incorrectly addressed fax or e-mail).[10]

In a classic paper on the limits of confidentiality, Siegler tells the story of a patient who complained when he observed a respiratory therapist reading his chart. When Siegler investigated the situation, he found that over seventy-five clinicians or hospital personnel had legitimate access to the patient's medical record. Siegler thus concluded that:

> Medical confidentiality as it has traditionally been understood by patients and doctors no longer exists. This ancient medical principle, which has been included in every physician's oath and code of ethics since Hippocratic times, has become old, worn out, and useless; it is a decrepit concept. [11]

What most patients fear, and what might prevent surgeons (or their families) from receiving their own health care in their home institutions, is the wanton indiscretion. Siegler observes that:

> Somehow, privacy is violated and a sense of shame is heightened when intimate secrets are revealed to people one knows or is close to—friends, neighbors, acquaintances, or hospital roommates—rather than when they are disclosed to an

anonymous bureaucrat sitting at a computer terminal in a distant city or to a health care professional who is acting in an official capacity. . . . I suspect that the principles of medical confidentiality, particularly those reflected in most medical codes of ethics, were designed principally to prevent just this sort of embarrassing personal indiscretion rather than to maintain (for social, political, or economic reasons) the absolute secrecy of doctor-patient communications.[11]

Legal Background

Given that common law in the United States has found physicians liable for both breaching and failing to breach confidentiality, surgeons are best advised to follow ethical guidelines and to act in their patients' best interest when considering issues of patient confidentiality. Practicing defensive medicine leaves the surgeon in a vulnerable posture in the courtroom. Judges and juries are justifiably more sympathetic toward a surgeon whose motivation was to do his or her best for the patient than they are toward a surgeon who claims, "I was afraid that I would be sued."

Under the common law, surgeons and other physicians who have breached confidentiality have been found liable for defamation, invasion of privacy, and breach of an implied contract.[12] They have also been found liable for *not* breaching confidentiality when harm to a third party occurred as a result of their failure to warn. Successful causes of action have been brought for failing to warn third parties about a patient's seizures,[13] murderous intentions,[14] contagious diseases,[15] and of the danger of infection from a patient's wound.[16]

Limits on and Exceptions to the Obligation of Confidentiality

Individual Well-Being and Public Welfare. The obligation of confidentiality is far from absolute. Limits to confidentiality are justified when either the well-being of an individual (the patient or an identifiable third party) or the public welfare is in danger. The *Statement on Principles* of the American College of Surgeons recognizes the boundaries of the surgeon's obligation of confidentiality. It holds that "the surgeon should maintain the confidentiality of information from and about the patient, except as such information must be communicated for the patient's proper care or as is required by law,"[17] which is consistent with the AMA *Principles of Medical Ethics.*[18]

Public health policy is grounded in balancing the privacy rights of individuals against the public good. Legitimate exceptions to privacy in the public health sphere include requiring vaccination for admission to public school, mandatory reporting of epileptic seizures to the department of motor vehicles, mandatory reporting of certain infectious diseases, identifying and notifying contacts at risk of infection from sexually transmitted diseases, reporting child abuse and neglect, and reporting gunshot and knife wounds.

The Duty to Warn. The physician's duty to warn an endangered third party has been most clearly identified within the scope of mental health treatment. This duty was articulated in the precedent-setting case of *Tarasoff v. Regents of the University of California* in 1976. In this case, Prosenjit Poddar, a graduate student at the University of California, disclosed his plans to murder his former girlfriend, Tatiana Tarasoff, to his psychologist. After consulting with his colleagues, the psychologist decided not to commit Poddar for inpatient therapy. The psychologist did not warn Ms.Tarasoff's family that she was at risk of harm (Ms. Tarasoff was in Brazil at the time). Shortly after returning from her visit abroad, Ms. Tarasoff was murdered by Prosenjit Poddar.

Ms. Poddar's parents sued the University of California for "failure to warn of a dangerous patient." In finding that the psychologist did indeed have a duty to warn Ms. Tarasoff or her parents of the impending danger, the judges stated in their majority opinion that "the protective privilege ends where the public peril begins."[14]

The requirements for a duty to warn are much less narrowly defined for surgeons and other physicians than for psychotherapists. One study shows that in the case of legally mandated breaches of confidentiality, such as reporting gunshot wounds, child abuse, and contagious diseases, no evidence exists of a harmful effect on the physician-patient relationship or of a decrease in patient use of the medical system.[4]

When Ethical Obligations Conflict. In some situations, the surgeon may be faced with a difficult ethical dilemma when he or she feels that the legal requirement to breach a patient's confidentiality could harm the patient. Surgeons, like other citizens, are obligated to uphold the law. This duty, however (just like the duty to maintain confidentiality), is *prima facie*; this means that the duty "must be fulfilled unless it conflicts on a particular occasion with an equal or stronger obligation."[2] Thus, breaking the law may be justified if the surgeon feels a greater responsibility to the patient. The third principle of the AMA Principles of Medical Ethics enjoins physicians to respect the law, but also to "recognize a responsibility to seek changes in those requirements which are contrary to the best interests of the patient."[18] Beauchamp and Childress concur and advise that "difficult moral dilemmas cannot be resolved merely because a law requires disclosure, and if a code of medical ethics were formulated only by reference to legal rules, that code would be inadequate."[2]

Testimonial Privilege and Tort Law. While over forty states have statutory provisions for testimonial privilege, these laws operate within a narrow context; they apply only in a court of law, where they prevent the surgeon from disclosing medical information without the patient's consent. Although the patient, not the surgeon, holds the privilege, it is the surgeon who must exercise that privilege on the patient's behalf if subpoenaed to release medical records or to testify in court. Many surgeons wrongly interpret a subpoena as a court order mandating disclosure of medical information. In some jurisdictions, the court may not have ruled on protective privilege in a particular case. The surgeon's initial response to a subpoena for medical information should be to notify the patient or the patient's attorney so that the patient may register a protest with the court.

Testimonial privilege does not apply in certain types of legal proceedings, such as criminal trials, or in civil actions where medical facts are pertinent to the case (this may also be true for testimony before a workers' compensation board). Pertinent civil actions might include personal injury cases, malpractice suits, divorce or custody proceedings, and commitment hearings. In these cases, however, tort law allows the patient a cause of action for harms due to unauthorized disclosures of medical information.

Testimonial privilege also does not govern cases in federal courts. The Federal Rules of Evidence allow only for a psychotherapist-patient privilege, not for a general physician-patient privilege. In federal court, disclosures of medical information or patient-physician communications are required at the court's discretion.[6]

The Patient's Record

Paper-Based Record. Because of the many faults inherent in the traditional paper-based record keeping system, the trend in medical information management is toward a totally electronic record. Paper-based systems are often poorly organized and incomplete; they must be physically transported from place to place; they do not lend themselves to research activities; and they are passive (cannot recognize abnormal test results and warn users).[19] As a result of these shortcomings, most cases of harm arising from confidentiality breaches involve paper-based, not electronic, records.[20]

The Electronic Record. In 1991 the Institute of Medicine recognized the computer-based, or electronic, medical record as "an essential technology for healthcare" and recommended its widespread adoption for information management.[7] While superior to the paper-based record in many ways, the electronic record raises new confidentiality issues. There are two reasons for this. First, the electronic record lends itself to greater abuse than the traditional paper-based system because it is more accessible. Not only is the information in a computerized record or database easily accessed from a remote location, it is also easily transported; information downloaded onto a disk is readily concealed and carried. Second, the electronic patient record is developing toward a longitudinal (or life-long) record, and the amount of information that is available will be much greater than with the traditional system where paper-based records are stored and maintained in physically separate locations by different clinical disciplines.

> Consider that computerized patient records contain obviously sensitive data, such as information about mental health, sexually transmitted diseases, and sexual behavior. Such records also contain information about birth control and pregnancy status; cosmetic and reconstructive surgery (including computerized images); genetic test results with family histories and prognoses, which may limit employability or increase an employer's insurance burden; substance dependence and treatment information; and prescriptions of a variety of drugs and diagnostic tests from which one might make inferences about the patient's behavior. When compiled into massive databases, such items are attractive to those seeking information about a person, as well as to "hackers," sensation seekers, and the merely curious.[21]

Unauthorized users, unauthorized access by hackers or masqueraders, unprotected downloaded files, and the use of "Trojan horses" (see below) pose the most common threats to the security of the electronic record.[22] Data integrity is most often violated by employees or former employees either through error in data entry or by unknowingly introducing a computer virus into the system.[23] Intentional breaches of privacy may be perpetrated by disgruntled employees who plant viruses or corrupt data.[24]

Hackers usually find their way into computer systems by appropriating valid passwords. This is accomplished through the use of "demon programs" that use sequential word combinations to identify authentic passwords. Multiple unexplained log-on attempts may thus indicate the presence of a hacker. Casual hackers can be discouraged by programs that limit the number of log-on attempts by a particular user within a specific time frame.[23]

The "Trojan horse" is another device used by hackers to break into a computer system and obtain confidential data. A Trojan horse is a program that disguises itself as an authorized program while it surreptitiously carries out a second function, such as copying files to an unprotected area of the computer system to which the hacker has access.

Privacy may also be compromised when data are downloaded from a protected environment, such as a mainframe or other host computer, to a microcomputer or local area network. Security measures are often less stringent in local area networks than they are in mainframe systems, and data are easily loaded onto diskettes which can be smuggled out and shared or sold.

Information Security. A combination of methods should be used to safeguard the electronic record. Failure to institute thorough security measures is not only an act of bad faith toward a surgeon's patients but increases that surgeon's legal liability.

The first and most important method of preventing confidentiality breaches is strong employee endorsement of patients' rights to privacy and confidentiality. This includes all levels of employees, from attending surgeons (who often feel entitled to information that they have no need to know) to clerical staff (who are frequently curious) and students (who usually want to know everything!). Personnel contracts should condition initial and continued employment on compliance with an institutional confidentiality policy. Student matriculation should depend on compliance with institutional confidentiality policies. Formal educational programs should ensure that employees and students understand the confidentiality policy and that consequences of noncompliance range from a written warning to a formal citation to termination of employment. Mandatory retraining (including review of the written policy) should occur annually. Sanctions should be imposed against *any* employee who breaches patient confidentiality. A cavalier or undemocratic approach to enforcement of confidentiality policies sends the message to patients and employees that confidentiality breaches may occur with impunity.

Technical security methods include ways of restricting access to databases, individual computers, and networks through the use of access codes, data encryption, immediate loss of access to terminated employees, and restriction of access on a "need to know " basis. Methods of monitoring include continual or frequent audits to detect entries into patient records, evaluations of whether confidentiality policies are being adhered to and whether or not they are effective, and employing a computer consultant "hacker" to break into the computer system. Large institutions may hire an Information Safety Officer whose job is to monitor, evaluate and upgrade security systems.

Physical security methods include the use of badges to access computer terminals and locking diskette files.[21] Special care should be used when destroying electronic medical records. The process involves more than deleting magnetic files; all backup and remote copies must also be destroyed.

Patient identifiers should be carefully evaluated for the degree of privacy protection that they offer. Use of the patient's social security number provides little protection. Physical identifiers such as fingerprints, retinal scans, or voice prints guarantee the highest degree of security, but are often prohibitively expensive or inefficient for large scale use. A unique patient code or patient number may be the best compromise among security, affordability, and efficiency.

Clinical Topics

The Emergency Encounter

Maintaining privacy and confidentiality are among the special challenges that the emergency patient presents to the surgeon (see also Chapter 5). Surgical emergencies often demand a high degree of judgment and sensitivity on the surgeon's part to balance the patient's need for privacy with the family's need for information. The emergency patient has less than usual control over himself or herself and his or her privacy and special safeguards may be necessary to avoid breaches of confidentiality. The crisis atmosphere that often attends surgical emergencies, especially traumatic injury, may heighten needs of family members and loved ones for information and reassurance. Surgeons, however, should not allow the exigencies of an emergency situation to undermine traditional privacy safeguards.

If the patient's decisional capacity and clinical status permit, the surgeon should determine the patient's preferences for disclosure of medical information. The surgeon should seek permission to give a concise status report of the patient's condition to the immediate family. More detailed information can be disclosed to the legal surrogate if the patient has diminished capacity or is incapable of participating in decision making. In this case, all information necessary for informed consent and refusal of treatment should be disclosed to the surrogate. The surrogate can then use substituted judgment (determining what the patient would want) or a best-interest assessment (weighing the benefits and burdens of treatment) to arrive at an appropriate treatment decision (see Chapter 2).

When the patient is incapacitated, the surgeon should disclose information only to the patient's surrogate, who has a legitimate "need to know" the patient's medical status. Otherwise, family members and friends are not entitled to access to patient information, unless the patient has given prior consent for this. The surgeon should explain to the family that in order to protect the patient's privacy, the surgeon will discuss the patient's situation in depth only with the surrogate decision maker. The surgeon should counsel the surrogate to consider the patient's privacy preferences and needs when discussing the patient's case with others.

Conversations with surrogate decision makers and family members should occur in a setting that ensures both visual and auditory privacy. This precludes conversations in hallways or crowded waiting rooms. A private conference room or waiting area is the best setting for discussing the patient's situation and for sharing the family's concerns. Surgeons should remember that other waiting room occupants are no more entitled to overhear auditory information about a patient whom they don't know than they are entitled to read the patient's chart or scan the patient's computer record.

While patient stabilization and management is the paramount concern in the emergency setting, the patient's need for privacy should be honored to the fullest extent possible. Patients in extremis are often disheveled, fully or partially unclothed, frightened, anxious, and in pain. Lack of privacy may exacerbate their distress. They depend on others to control their immediate environment and to secure their privacy. Emergency rooms, trauma centers, surgical suites and intensive care units are designed in ways that enhance visualization and allow efficient traffic flow. Achieving visual and auditory privacy may be extremely difficult, or even impossible, in such environments. When possible, visual privacy can be obtained through the use of curtains, screens, or closed doors. Auditory privacy may be achieved through the use of private rooms or alcoves, or simply by speaking in a manner that is difficult for others to overhear.

The HIV-Infected Patient

Although the social stigma associated with AIDS is declining, real threats to patients' welfare still hinge on disclosure of the diagnosis. A pertinent example is the case of William Behringer, an otolaryngologist and plastic surgeon who contracted HIV. In June of 1987, Dr. Behringer was voluntarily admitted to the hospital in which he practiced, the Medical Center at Princeton, for treatment of an acute pulmonary illness. He was diagnosed as having *Pneumocystis carinii* infection and subsequently tested positive for HIV. Existing mechanisms to safeguard the laboratory results failed, in spite of attempts by Dr. Behringer and his physician to forestall their entry into the medical record. In a further attempt to maintain his privacy, Dr. Behringer insisted on being discharged immediately from the hospital to his home, where his fiancée would care for him.

Within hours of returning home, the couple began receiving sympathy calls from surgeons and other physician colleagues at the Medical Center. These physicians clearly knew Dr. Behringer's condition, although none of them had participated in his care.

Patients and referring physicians soon began calling Dr. Behringer's office with inquiries. His practice dwindled as appointments were canceled and referrals diminished. Dr. Behringer's surgical privileges at the Medical Center were suspended within weeks of his diagnosis. He subsequently sued the Medical Center at Princeton for breach of the institution's (and certain employees') "duty to maintain the confidentiality of his diagnosis and test results." The court found in his favor, stating that:

> The confidentiality breached in the present case is simply grist for a gossip mill with little concern for the impact of disclosure on the patient. While one can legitimately question the good judgement of a practicing physician choosing to undergo HIV testing or a bronchoscopy procedure at the same hospital where he practices, this apparent error in judgement does not relieve the medical center of its underlying obligation to protect its patients against the dissemination of confidential information. It makes little difference to identify those who "spread the news." The information was too easily available, too titillating to disregard. All that was required was a glance at the chart and the written words became whispers, and the whispers became roars. And common sense told all that this would happen . . . while the medical center argues that the decision regarding charting is one for the physicians to make, the medical center cannot avoid liability on that basis.

It is not the charting per se that generates the issue; it is the easy accessibility to the charts and the lack of any meaningful medical center policy or procedure to limit access that causes the breach to occur. Where the impact of such accessibility is so clearly foreseeable, it is incumbent on the medical center, as the custodian of the charts, to take such reasonable measures as necessary to insure that confidentiality. Failure to take such steps is negligence.[25]

The Behringer case raises a separate confidentiality issue: that of the HIV-infected surgeon and whether his patients have the right to know his diagnosis. Public opinion is clearly for mandatory reporting of HIV-positivity. A 1991 Gallup poll asked a sample of adults "which kinds of health care workers should be required to tell patients if they are infected with the HIV virus?" The response was: surgeons 95%; all physicians 94%; dentists 94%; all health care workers 90%.[26] Although survey respondents made no distinction between invasive and noninvasive procedures, the evolving professional guideline is that all health care professionals who are involved in invasive procedures should have themselves tested for HIV and should notify their patients of their status.

In a similar vein, patients who are scheduled to undergo invasive procedures should also have themselves tested and should notify their surgeons (or other clinicians) of their status.[26] In the above-mentioned Gallup poll, 97% of respondents stated that HIV-infected patients should tell their health care workers that they are infected. The data, however, argue against routine preoperative screening for HIV. CDC data from mid-1991 show that of 6,453 cases of AIDS among health care workers (720 cases among physicians), only 40 cases were attributable to their occupations.[26] Hagen and his colleagues argue that:

> If the risks of sexual and surgical contact are of the same order of magnitude, why should we eschew screening in low-risk heterosexual populations but recommend it for low-risk patients awaiting surgery? Arguing that we should screen low-risk patients before surgery implies that preventing HIV infection in a physician, a nurse, or a technician is more important than preventing the infection in others. Is that argument either rational or ethical?[12]

Occasionally the surgeon faces the troubling question of whether to warn a spouse, sexual partner, or person otherwise at risk of contracting HIV from a surgical patient who is HIV-positive. State statutes may protect the surgeon from legal risk of making such a disclosure, but they rarely require the disclosure, leaving the decision up to the surgeon. The authors propose the following guidelines for warning a person at risk: (1) confirm the HIV test; (2) encourage the patient to make the disclosure himself; (3) try to ascertain that the third party is at risk; and (4) consider ethics consultation if the patient refuses to make the disclosure. If, upon consultation and careful consideration, the surgeon chooses to override the patient's refusal to disclose, the surgeon should minimize the breach of confidentiality when making the disclosure.[27]

Domestic Violence

In the United States, the family has traditionally been viewed as a sacrosanct, inviolable entity. Physicians' beliefs about the nature of the family, that it should function privately as a discrete social unit, have fostered support for such important rights as birth control and other reproductive freedoms. Ironically, these same beliefs may enable abusive and violent relationships in dysfunctional families to continue unchecked.

Sexual and physical abuse are epidemic in our society. Most violence occurs within the confines of close relationships. Most of it is directed by men against women; it takes the shape of assault, battery, rape, and murder. Physical abuse is among the leading causes of injury for women who seek treatment in the emergency setting.[28] Women are more often the victims of current or former male partners than of all other assailants combined.[29]

Surgeons and other physicians who see evidence of physical abuse are often reluctant to voice their suspicions to patients for fear of violating the integrity of the family. A recent survey of primary care physicians showed support for making inquiries about sexual and physical abuse routine. However, the vast majority of those surveyed never made inquiries about sexual or physical abuse during initial or annual visits.[28] Other studies support this finding:

> Stark et al reported that when physicians said one among 35 of their patients was battered, a more accurate approximation was one in four; when they acknowledged that one injury among 20 resulted from domestic abuse, the actual figure approached one in four; and what they described as a rare occurrence was in reality of "epidemic proportions." Similarly, Kurz found that in 40% of emergency department staff interactions with battered women, staff made no response to abuse. Finally, Warshaw examined the medical records of encounters among medical staff (nurses and physicians) and women whose injuries were highly indicative of abuse, and found nondetection, nonintervention, and nonreceptiveness to be the norm.[29]

Patients support inquiries about domestic violence, and patients and surgeons believe that surgeons and other clinicians can help their patients with problems of violence and abuse. The initial response to the discovery of abuse is referral for support and counseling, which does not entail a breach of patient confidentiality. When required by law to report suspected abuse or neglect of the patient, the surgeon should do so.

The High-Profile Patient

Do celebrities or public figures have the same rights to privacy and confidentiality that other patients have, or does the public have a "right to know" clinical information about them? National debate about this issue arose recently in the case of liver transplant recipient Mickey Mantle. At Mantle's request, officials at Baylor University Medical Center in Dallas withheld his cancer diagnosis (made during the transplant surgery) from the news media. With the family's permission, the diagnosis was disclosed only after Mantle's death. This disclosure fueled an already contentious debate over whether Mantle should have received a liver transplant given his history of substance abuse. Foreknowledge of the cancer would have precluded transplantation.

The public's claim to medical information has greater strength when the patient is a public figure (either a public official or a person who uses public funds) than when the patient is simply a celebrity.[30] Fame and curiosity about celebrities who are not public figures do not entitle the news media, the general public, or most hospital staff to information about a patient's medical condition.

On the other hand, because the decision-making capacity of public figures can be affected by diseases or injuries, as well as by surgical management of them, more than mere curiosity is involved. The public may legitimately be entitled to information about public figures when such disclosure is determined to be for the "public good." Inadequate or incomplete disclosure of medical information about important public figures may undermine the public's trust in its government and may fuel unnecessary fears. These sorts of decisions generally involve highly placed government leaders, such as the president, and disclosure is guided by preestablished protocols.

Disclosure of medical information about celebrity patients should follow standard guidelines for disclosure and should be articulated in a hospital policy; medical information may be released only with the patient's permission. This obtains for release of information to family members, friends, third-party payers, the news media, and members of the clinical staff.

Surgeons should have a working knowledge of their institutional policies for maintaining the privacy of high-profile patients. When warranted, the hospital's public relations experts should train surgeons so that they will be prepared for interviews by the news media. When the high-profile patient has asked for privacy, the appropriate response to queries by the news media is, "The patient has asked me not to discuss this."[30]

Disclosing Information to the Immediate Family

Surgeons should not assume that the patient will want all information about himself or herself disclosed to family members. The patient may wish to withhold certain information or may wish to impart it himself or herself. Therefore, these preferences should usually be discussed prior to surgical procedures. There may, however, be cases in which the family dynamics clearly support disclosing information when such discussion has not taken place. Ways of meeting the family's needs for postoperative (or intraoperative) status reports should be discussed with the patient and agreed upon early in the course of treatment. The patient may wish to appoint a family spokesperson to share information with extended family and friends. If the patient is decisionally incapacitated, the legal surrogate should assume this role. These disclosures should be authorized by the patient.

Inquiries by the Patient's Employer

Requiring new employees to provide comprehensive medical information authorizing release of medical records by their physicians is a troubling and growing practice. In some circumstances, employees are required to fill out extensive medical histories and to undergo physical examinations by company physicians. Large corporations generally have access to insurance company databases or to other mechanisms of information redisclosure. Often, copies of insurance records or medical histories become part of employees' personnel records. When this occurs, employees are in jeopardy of privacy invasions by coworkers and of having medical information used for personnel decisions such as promotion.

Disclosures of medical information to employers should follow the same guidelines as disclosures in other contexts: no disclosure should occur without the patient's permission unless required by and consistent with the law, especially the Americans with Disabilities Act.[31] This includes workers' compensation claims, which are generally covered by patient waiver.

Documentation for Payment

Rarely do patients pay out of pocket for health care services. When they do it is generally because they want to keep their medical treatment private. Third-party payers, such as employers, insurers, and governments, all require access to the patient's record in order to verify treatment and process payments. Indeed, the quantity of data collected by third party payers is so vast that the insurance industry has established its own databank called the Medical Information Bureau.[6]

Patients are entitled to know the contents of their medical records so that they can give informed authorization to release of information. They are also entitled to set limits or specify what type of information should be released to a third-party payer. Surgeons should disclose only that information that has been authorized by the patient. In some instances, as a result, the patient may have to pay the bill rather than have billing information disclosed to the third-party payer.

Use of Audiovisual Materials

Most hospitals require separate consent documentation for taking photographs or making videotapes of patients. These materials are subject to the same confidentiality obligations as other forms of patient information. They should not be disclosed without the patient's explicit permission. This includes use of visual images in making professional presentations, in telemedicine, in publications, in the teaching context, and in presentations to the general public. In *Vassiliades v. Garfinkles Brooks Bros.*, a patient justifiably and successfully sued her plastic surgeon for unauthorized use of before-and-after photographs of her plastic surgery in a department store display.[32]

Clinical Conclusions

Two guiding principles govern access to and disclosure of medical information: (1) the patient's permission is required for access and disclosure and (2) access is given only on a "need-to-know" basis. Discussion of the patient's preferences for release of information should be part of the ongoing process of informed consent. Documentation of consent for release of information should be specific and separate from consent for treatment. Included in consent for release of medical information should be the patient's name and signature, the names and signatures of those releasing and receiving information, the purpose of the disclosure, the type of information to be released, the date, prohibitions on redisclosure, a six-month expiration date, and a clause allowing the patient to revoke the consent at any time.[33]

A statement of the institution's commitment to patient confidentiality should be articulated in a comprehensive confidentiality policy. This policy should cover personnel rules, enforcement and disciplinary rules, access, security features, accountability, limits to confidentiality, methods of risk assessment, and responsibilities of agents and contractors.[21]

Limits to confidentiality must be discussed with the patient as part of the informed consent process. These may include threats to the well-being of the patient or an identifiable third party, or threats to the public welfare. Many exceptions to the obligation of confidentiality are established in case law or by legislation. On rare occasions, these requirements may conflict with the surgeon's responsibility not to harm the patient. Resolving the dilemma will depend on the surgeon's judgment and professional values.

The surgeon is responsible for using a combination of effective methods for safeguarding patient information. These include annual educational programs, technical and physical security methods, and the use of appropriate patient identifiers. When destroying electronic records, care should be taken that all backup and remote copies are also destroyed.

The patient's wishes should be followed when disclosing information to family members, friends, or the news media. No one other than the patient or the patient's surrogate is entitled to medical information about the patient. In an emergency situation, attempts should be made to safeguard the patient's privacy and confidentiality to the fullest extent possible. Care should be taken to maximize auditory and visual privacy.

To decrease the risk of transmission of the HIV virus, all health care providers who perform invasive procedures should know their HIV status and should disclose this information to their patients. Likewise, patients scheduled to undergo invasive procedures should ascertain their HIV status and should disclose it to their surgeons. When the surgeon is faced with the problem of notifying a third party who is at risk for HIV transmission, he or she should first confirm the HIV test, then encourage the patient to make the disclosure himself. If the patient refuses, the surgeon should then determine whether the third party is clearly at risk, and should minimize the breach of confidentiality when making the disclosure.

Surgeons who suspect domestic violence should raise the issue with their patients and should refer them for appropriate support and counseling. Privacy concerns should not override concern for the patient's physical well-being.

Disclosure of information about high-profile patients should be driven by the patient's preferences and should follow hospital policy. Surgeons should turn to their institutional public relations staff for guidance in these situations. Audiovisual materials such as photographs and videotapes should enjoy the same security safeguards as other types of patient information. They should not be shared without the patient's clear understanding of their use.

Care should be taken to disclose only necessary information to employers and third party payers. The patient must give consent to this disclosure and generally has the right to limit the disclosure in any way.

In sum, obligations of confidentiality should be informed by common sense and good judgment. The surgeon should demonstrate the same sensitivity to and appreciation of the patient's need for privacy and confidentiality that one would, in turn, want for oneself. The patient-surgeon relationship is anchored by this fundamental building block.

References

1. Ian G. Barbour, *Ethics in an Age of Technology*. San Francisco: Harper San Francisco, 1993.
2. Tom L. Beauchamp and James F. Childress, *Principles of Biomedical Ethics*, 4th ed. New York: Oxford University Press, 1994.
3. John C. Fletcher, Charles A. Hite, Paul A. Lombardo, and Mary Faith Marshall, *Introduction to Clinical Ethics*. Frederick, MD: University Publishing Group, Inc., 1995.
4. Kenneth Appelbaum and Paul S. Appelbaum, "The HIV Antibody-Positive Patient," in *Confidentiality Versus the Duty to Protect: Foreseeable Harm in the Practice of Psychiatry*, ed. James C. Beck. Washington, D.C.: American Psychiatry Press, Inc., 1990.

5. Paul S. Appelbaum et al., "Confidentiality: An Empirical Test of the Utilitarian Perspective," *Bulletin of the American Academy of Psychiatry and the Law* 12 (1984):109–116.

6. Evan Hendricks, Trudy Hayden, and Jack D. Novik, *Your Right to Privacy: A Basic Guide to Legal Rights in an Information Society*, 2nd ed. Carbondale and Edwardsville, Southern Illinois University Press, 1990.

7. Richard Dick and Elaine Steen, eds., *The Computer-Based Patient Record* (Washington D.C., National Academy of Sciences, I.O.M., 1991) in Tom L. Beauchamp and James F. Childress, *Principles of Biomedical Ethics*, 4th ed. New York: Oxford University Press, 1994, p. 408.

8. Jo Anne Czecowski Bruce, *Privacy and Confidentiality of Health Care Information.* 2nd ed. Chicago, IL: American Hospital Publishing, Inc., 1988.

9. Peter A. Ubel, Margaret M. Zell, David J. Miller, et al., "Elevator Talk: Observational Study of Inappropriate Comments in a Public Space," *American Journal of Medicine* 99 (1995):190–194.

10. Marion J. Ball and Morris F. Collen, eds. *Aspects of the Computer-based Patient Record.* New York: Springer-Verlag, 1992.

11. Mark Siegler, "Confidentiality in Medicine—A Decrepit Concept," *New England Journal of Medicine* 307(1982):1518–1521.

12. Michael D. Hagen, Klemens B.Meyer, and Steven J. Pauker, "Routine Preoperative Screening for HIV: Does the Risk to the Surgeon Outweigh the Risk to the Patient? *Journal of the American Medical Association* 259 (1988):1357–1359.

13. *Lemmon v. Freese* 210 NW 2d 576, Iowa (1973).

14. *Tarasoff v. Regents of the University of California* 551 P2d 334 (1976) Calif Supreme Court.

15. *Skillings v. Allen* 173 NW 663Minn (1919); *Davis v Rodman* 147 Ark 385, 391, 227 SW 612, 614 (1921); *Jones v Stanko* 118 Ohio St 147 (1928).

16. *Edwards v. Lamb* 69 NH 559, 45 A 480 (1899).

17. American College of Surgeons. *Statement on Principles.* Chicago, Il: American College of Surgeons, 1989.

18. American Medical Association. Principles of Medical Ethics, *Code of Medical Ethics: Current Opinions with Annotations*, Chicago, Il: American Medical Association, 1994.

19. Gina Pruitt, "Securing and Controlling Computer Based Patient Records," *Prescriptions for Success.* Nashville, TN: Deliotte and Touche LLP, Computer Assurance Services, 1997.

20. Alan Westin, "Designing Privacy in Computerized Health Care Information," as cited in Larry Lawrence, "Safeguarding the Confidentiality of Automated Medical Information." (See Ref. 21)

21. Larry M. Lawrence, "Safeguarding the Confidentiality of Automated Medical Information," *Journal of Quality Improvement* 20 (1994):639–646.

22. Merida L. Johns, *Information Management for Health Professions.* Albany, NY: Delmar Publishers, 1997.

23. Larry O. Gostin, et al., "Privacy and Security of Health Information and Security of Health Information in the Emerging Health System," *Health Matrix* 5 (1995): 1–36.

24. Diana J. P. McKenzie, "Medical Records Networking: Banking on Security," *InfoCare* May/June (1996):35–39.

25. *Estate of William Behrenger, MD v. the Medical Center at Princeton, Dennis Doody, and Leung Lee, M.D.* 249 N.J. Super. 597, 592 A 2d 1251 (1991).

26. Gerald R. Stine, *Acquired Immune Deficiency Syndrome: Biological, Medical, Social, and Legal Issues.* Engelwood Cliffs, NJ: Prentice-Hall, 1993.

27. Mark A. Hall and Ira Mark Ellman, *Health Care Law and Ethics.* St. Paul, MN: West Publishing Co., 1990.

28. Lawrence S. Friedman, Jeffery H. Samet, Mark S. Roberts, Margaret Hudlin and Paul Hans, "Inquiry About Victimization Experiences," *Archives of Internal Medicine* 152 (1992):1186–1190.

29. Nancy S. Jecker, "Privacy Beliefs and the Violent Family," *Journal of the American Medical Association* 269 (1993):776–780.

30. "Assuring the Celebrity Patient's Right to Privacy," *Medical Ethics Advisor* (1995) 126–127.

31. The Americans with Disabilities Act of 1990, 42 USC § 1202 *et. seq.*

32. *Vassiliades v. Garfinkel's Brooks Bros.*, 492 A.2d 580 (D.C. App. 1985).

33. Gregory L. Larkin, John Moskop, Arthur Sanders, et al., "The Emergency Physician and Patient Confidentiality: A Review" *Annals of Emergency Medicine* 24 (1994): 1161–1167.

4

Advance Directives
and the Determination of Death

STUART J. YOUNGNER
JERRY M. SHUCK

The introduction and extensive development of life-sustaining technology three decades ago has brought wonders to humankind only dreamed of in previous times. Like all technology, however, medical technology is a two-edged sword. On one hand, it enhances life by extending its length and improving its quality. On the other, it creates complex moral choices where none existed before. In this chapter we discuss two situations in which medical technology has created difficult moral choices: decisions to limit life-sustaining treatment, including the introduction of advance directives, and the determination of death.

Experience has taught surgeons and patients that the application of this technology does not, in all instances, serve the wishes and best interests of patients. This realization has confronted surgeons, patients, and families with hard choices about when it is appropriate to withhold or even withdraw aggressive interventions such as intensive care, mechanical ventilation, hemodialysis, and cardiopulmonary resuscitation. In fact, a legal, ethical, and clinical consensus has emerged that mere extension of biological life need not be the only goal of medicine—that comfort and dignity are entirely appropriate goals when cure is no longer possible. This rejection of an absolute vitalism has been complemented by an equally important legal and ethical principle: that decisions about end-of-life care rest primarily with the patient. The issues addressed in this chapter arise for surgeons particularly when the surgical patient is doing poorly in the intraoperative or postoperative periods. We will therefore explore the application of this principle in the acute care surgical setting, with attention to a full range of treatment limitation options, including the controversial issue of do-not-resuscitate orders during the perioperative period. We will emphasize the importance of timely communication about treatment planning and goals, with special emphasis on the use of advance directives.

Until the invention and application of the mechanical ventilator and the modern intensive care unit, death was a relatively uncomplicated matter. Severe failure of any one of the body's vital subsystems (cardiac, pulmonary, central nervous system) led immediately to failure of them all. Today, by substitution and support, surgeons can maintain some life functions after the natural capacity for others has been irretrievably lost. Thus, surgeons must decide when, in the presence of some signs of life, the patient has died. Aside from its biomedical parameters, a determination of death also has tremendous social, psychological, religious, and legal implications. As we will see, the effort to redefine death, through the introduction of neurological criteria, has been successful to some degree but has introduced still another series of concerns and debates.

Advance Directives

Ethical Analysis

While there is an impressive consensus in our society that competent adults have a right to make treatment decisions, including the right to refuse life-sustaining treatment, decision making for incompetent adults is much more problematic. Courts and ethicists have identified two general approaches to making decisions for patients who are no longer capable of making them on their own.

The first approach is to try to determine what is in the best interest of the patient, that is, some assessment of the relative proportion of good and harm that would result from a given treatment decision (see Chapter 2). The problem with the "best interests" standard is that the proportionality of goods versus harms is a value judgment about which reasonable people can often disagree. For this reason, a consensus has emerged that the competent patient is in the best position to make such value judgments for himself or herself.

The second approach attempts to carry competent patients' wishes into a future in which they are no longer competent by the use of *advance directives*. Advance directives comprise a variety of mechanisms by which competent patients make their wishes about treatment known ahead of time. With an advance directive, theoretically at least, an incompetent patient can be treated or not treated according to her own wishes and values rather than those of others trying to interpret what is best *for* her. The second approach, when possible, is the one preferred by courts and ethicists alike—precisely because it approximates the standard of promoting autonomy, by following the wishes of the competent patient in the informed consent process (see Chapter 2).

Types of Advance Directives

Advance directives may be formal or informal. Examples of *informal* advance directives include conversations with family, friends, or health professionals. Advance directives become more *formal* as they are written down, standardized, and recognized by policy or law. There is often a misconception that only formal advance directives are useful. Conversations and "unofficial" documents can provide health professionals, hospital ethics committees, or even courts of law excellent evidence of the patient's wishes. In fact, one of the problems with formal advance directives is that patients too often fail to discuss them with key persons. When advance directives appear suddenly in a crisis, surgeons and family members may have trouble accepting them.

It is also useful to distinguish the *living wills* or instructional form in which the patient has stated his or her specific treatment/nontreatment preferences,[1-3] from the *durable power of attorney for health care* by which the patient appoints a proxy who has legal authority to make treatment decisions for the patient.[2,3] Both the living will and durable power of attorney become operative only when the patient is determined to be unable to participate in decisions about his or her clinical treatment. This determination can be made by clinicians and, unless formally challenged, does not require active participation by the legal system. Living wills are usually used to limit end-of-life treatment, although some allow a provision for requesting it. Durable power of attorney for health care allows the patient to appoint an agent of his or her choice to act as surrogate decision maker in the event the patient loses decision-making capacity. Some states have laws recognizing a hierarchy of family members who have legal authority to make end-of-life decisions for "non-declarants"—patients who have not executed a living will or durable power of attorney. This priority list of family members (that usually goes in the order of spouse, adult children, parents, siblings) may be the best reason for a patient to appoint a durable power of attorney—that is, if the "default" person at the top of the list is not the person the patient would prefer to make decisions.

A third form of advance directive, used much less commonly, is called the *values statement* or *values history*. Rather than give specific instructions or appoint a proxy to make decisions, the values statement attempts to represent the patient's general values (such as religious beliefs, quality of life preferences, etc.) with which treatment decisions should be consistent.[4]

There has been great enthusiasm for advance directives. All but two states have adopted legislation recognizing living wills and durable power of attorney arrangements. In 1991 the Congress of the United States passed the Patient Self-Determination Act (PSDA).[3,5] This statute requires that all hospitals, nursing homes, skilled-nursing facilities, hospices, home health care agencies, and health maintenance organizations must, upon admission of each adult patient, provide written information about (1) the patient's right under state law to make medical decisions, including the right to refuse life-sustaining medical interventions to have an advance directive, and (2) the institution's policy about life-sustaining treatment and advance directives. Institutions must document that they have so informed each patient and any advance directives must be documented in the patient's medical record. Care cannot be made conditional upon whether or not a patient has an advance directive.

Hospitals have used admitting clerks, social workers, or admitting nurses to conduct the required PSDA "intervention." Some have included a special section in the patient's chart to include documentation about whether the patient has or desires to have an advance directive and in which to place any advance directives brought with the patient. It is important that the surgeon familiarize him or herself with both state law and institutional policy with regard to advance directives.

Problems with Advance Directives

Despite the PSDA and widespread educational efforts and publicity, relatively few patients admitted to the hospital claim to have filled out formal advance directives.[6] Even fewer bring their advance directives to the hospital on admission. Why? It is possible that the public has not yet absorbed the information necessary to plan and execute an advance directive. It is equally likely that many persons (including surgeons) simply do not want to think about the tragic choices they may have to face at a later date. Some studies indicate that most patients want to talk about advance directives but are waiting for their physician to bring it up.[7] Many people have urged that the outpatient setting is the optimum time and place for physicians to discuss advance directives with their patients. The advantages of this approach include a greater chance that the physician and patient know each other, a non-crisis atmosphere, and an opportunity to discuss this complicated issue over time. Because many surgical patients are seen in the ambulatory setting, before admission and especially after discharge, this provides an excellent opportunity for the surgeon to bring up and discuss advance directives.

Living wills are too often vague in the direction they give for both the event not to be treated and the level of treatment desired.[6] So, for example, most state advance directive statutes suggest or require living wills that allow only the option, "When I am terminally ill, I do not want heroic [or life-sustaining] treatment." The word *terminal* is itself sometimes vaguely defined, giving health professionals and family members alike great latitude (and responsibility) for interpretation. In response to this problem, some persons have suggested more specific living wills that specify both health state scenarios (such as permanent vegetative state or far-advanced dementia) as well as specific choices about treatment options (such as ventilators, dialysis, and artificially provided fluids and nutrition).[1] Although most states' advance directive laws require that patients be terminally ill before their living wills can go into effect, some legal scholars have pointed out that the U.S. Constitution gives patients the right to make their own decisions about treatment whether they are terminally ill or not.[8] Therefore, while living wills that speak to non-terminal situations (e.g., severe dementia) do not have the formal protection of state law, they are entirely consistent with constitutional and common law rights as interpreted by the courts.

Some have argued for the advantage of the durable power of attorney for health care, which gives a designated proxy the legal right to make decisions and "interpret" any vague aspects about the advance directive[9,10] (see also Chapter 10). However, many studies indicate that surrogates have a far less than perfect knowledge of the end-of-life preferences of patients.[11-14]

There is growing evidence that families and health professionals often ignore the wishes expressed in patients' living wills.[15] At first glance, these findings may be alarming, implying perhaps that physicians and family members are running roughshod over patients' rights. However, closer scrutiny of the data reveals two compelling reasons why this apparent disregard of patients' wishes may be quite acceptable under some circumstances. First, as we discussed earlier, living wills go into effect when the patient is no longer able to speak for himself or herself. Thus, a currently incompetent patient who said in an advance directive that he or she would not want surgery if he or she were in a severely demented state might be in that state but develop a painful bowel obstruction that could be easily relieved by surgery. Under these circumstances, the surgeon and family might decide that the ratio of harms to benefits for this now incompetent patient would clearly be served by surgery. Similarly, a patient who had requested, when competent, that "everything" be done to extend his or her life might be suffering terribly because those things were being done (e.g., postoperative dialysis, in response to which the now-incompetent patient screamed in pain and begged "no more)." In this case, the surgeon and family might well choose to forgo the aggressive interventions. It is worth noting that in one study 61% of dialysis patients would give surrogates at least some leeway in overriding their advance directive for reasons similar to the those just cited.[16] Another problem is that patients and physicians too often use advance directives as a way to bypass rather than enhance face-to-face discussion about end-of-life care. Each party may be uncertain about how to discuss the possibility or even probability of death or find the topic anxiety-provoking. Too often patients and surgeons think about advance directives in the reductionistic terms discussed earlier in this chapter.

The patient fears that producing an advance directive is tantamount to saying, "I am ready to die." Such thinking leads patients to keep advance directives at home when they enter the hospital, or surgeons to be put off by advance directives produced by patients who are coming into the hospital for aggressive treatment.

Advance directives are a useful adjunct to planning for end-of-life decisions, especially when they stimulate conversation with family members and health professionals. Surgeons should read advance directives produced by competent patients and discuss their implications in light of current conditions and choices, with an emphasis on clarifying the patient's goals for surgical management of problems. Patients should be encouraged to discuss their advance directives with family members. When patients do not have advance directives, surgeons should encourage them to anticipate and think about the choices that will likely face them if their current condition worsens (e.g., after high-risk surgery for intracranial tumors that may leave the patient unresponsive in the SICU) (see Chapters 9 and 10).

Do-Not-Resuscitate (DNR) Decisions

Because cardiopulmonary arrest is the final event in every death, every patient is subject to cardiopulmonary resuscitation (CPR). Therefore, a decision about whether or not to use CPR must be made in every case. And in every case, the patient's wishes should, ideally, guide the decision. In the course of the debate about life-sustaining treatment, decisions not to apply cardiopulmonary resuscitation (CPR) became a paradigm for decisions to limit a spectrum of life-sustaining interventions.[17] There are several reasons to explain this phenomenon. First, CPR is a dramatic intervention. Cardiopulmonary arrest is the last event in the dying process in every death no matter what the cause (with the exception of brain death which we will consider at the end of this chapter). Failure to act results in certain death. Second, because cardiopulmonary arrest is the last event before death, successful CPR represents a great triumph, snatching life from the jaws of death. Third, because of the finality of untreated cardiopulmonary arrest and the necessity to act immediately if it is to be reversed, it is performed routinely as the "default mode" in hospitals and nursing homes. That is, without a physician's order to the contrary, CPR must be administered when a patient arrests. This approach is based on every patient's right to receive prompt and appropriate response to life-threatening events.

CPR also represents the "down" side of aggressive intervention. It is rarely successful. Multiple studies have demonstrated that only 15% of persons who receive CPR in the hospital live to leave the hospital.[18] In some subpopulations the results are much better—for example, for otherwise healthy patients with sudden witnessed cardiac arrest or patients who arrest during the heavily controlled conditions of surgery. For others, such as those with multiple organ system failure or metastatic cancer, the figures are worse.[17,18] Moreover, CPR is a particularly invasive and undignified intervention. Common complications include rib fractures and pneumothorax.

Because of these unique characteristics and problems, various guidelines have been suggested for DNR orders. The Joint Commission for the Accreditation of Healthcare Organizations (JCAHO) requires that hospitals and nursing homes have such guidelines. Written guidelines promote accountability, allow evaluation and revision, can educate the hospital community including health professionals, patients, and families, and improve risk management. Guidelines share several common themes:

1. DNR orders are like any other treatment order. They must be documented in writing in the physicians' orders.
2. DNR orders should specify the exact nature of the treatment to be withheld and the pathophysiologic event (e.g., cardiopulmonary arrest) for which it should be withheld.
3. Patients, when they are able, and families must participate in DNR decisions.
4. The rationale for the DNR decision, along with the nature of the discussions with patient and family, should be documented in writing in the progress notes.
5. DNR decisions should be discussed with other members of the health care team caring for the patient.
6. DNR status should be reviewed on a regular basis.
7. DNR is not equivalent to the medical or psychological abandonment of the patient and can be logically and morally consistent with other forms of aggressive care, including transfer to an intensive care unit.

Problems with DNR Orders. Despite widespread adoption of guidelines and recognition of the importance of patient and family involvement, significant problems remain. A recent study of nearly 10,000 seriously ill patients in both surgical and medical settings (overall 6-month mortality rate of 47%) at five major teaching hospitals revealed that "only 41% of patients in the study reported talking to their physicians about prognosis or about cardiopulmonary resuscitation (CPR)."[19] Physicians misunderstood patients' preferences regarding CPR in 80% of cases. Furthermore, physicians did not implement patients' refusals of interventions. When patients wanted CPR withheld, a DNR order was never written in about 50% of cases."[20]

The SUPPORT Study also found that nearly one half of DNR orders were written within two days of death, that nearly 40% of patients who died spent at least 10 days in surgical or medical intensive care, and that nearly one half of patients who died received mechanical ventilation within three days of death. An intensive intervention to provide better prognostic information and facilitate communication and advance planning failed to improve care or patient outcomes.[19]

The results of the SUPPORT Study are discouraging. They suggest deep-seated problems of communication and decision-making at the end of life, including some involving surgery. There are likely several explanations. Exploration of the possible problems that remain will suggest possible ways to improve the situation.

The False Dichotomy of Treat/Don't Treat. Patients, families, and health professionals tend to conceptualize treatment limitation dichotomously—either we go all out to save the patient or we let the patient die. This binary approach is even more common among surgeons. In most cases, this is a mistakenly reductionistic view. True, one can envision cases at the two extremes of the spectrum. At one end is the patient who wants to be maintained alive as long as possible and is willing to endure any and all invasive treatment no matter how unlikely it is to succeed. At the other end is the patient who is unequivocally ready to die. This patient is concerned only with comfort and dignity and wants death to be allowed to come as soon as possible. These two extremes do not, in fact, describe most patients as they near the end of their life course. Most patients today die of chronic illness. As their disease or diseases progress and their quality of life deteriorates, they begin thinking that there can be things worse than death.

Such thoughts do not mean that the patient no longer wants to live, only that he or she begins to conceive of situations where that might be so. For example, a patient with chronic obstructive lung disease lives a very restricted, but satisfactory, life at home but, having undergone aggressive hospital care in the past, decides that should he develop pneumonia and progressive respiratory failure, he is unwilling to endure endotracheal intubation, mechanical ventilation, and intensive care unit (ICU) admission to achieve what his physicians have told him is a 20% chance of returning home. This patient might well accept intravenous antibiotics at home for his pneumonia or even outpatient surgery to drain a painful abscess or repair an uncomfortable inguinal hernia. He may also accept a chest tube for a sudden pneumothorax. Such a patient might well refuse CPR in the event of an arrest, but clearly wish to go on living so long as the conditions that lead to arrest do not develop. In fact, studies have shown that up to 60% of patients designated DNR in the hospital never arrest and are alive at discharge.[21]

Such fine tuning is entirely logical, ethical, and consistent with excellent medical and surgical care, but it forces everyone to ask and answer difficult questions about what is an acceptable quality of life, what degree of invasive treatment is one willing to put up with to achieve it, and what is a chance worth taking to achieve it. For surgeons, such discussions may put them into the uncomfortable position of having to refrain from performing interventions that they believe would prolong their patients' lives. Under such circumstances, surgeons may feel powerless or derelict in their responsibilities. The all-or-nothing approach may be procedurally and emotionally simpler for persons not interested in dealing with subtleties. It runs the risk, however, of violating patients' rights and causing avoidable harms.

Distinguishing DNR Orders from Other Treatment Limitation. If the notion that treatment limitation is not always an all-or-nothing proposition is acceptable, then surgeons must learn to communicate with patients, families, and other health professionals about the options. To do this surgeons must clearly define, for example, exactly what we mean by DNR, specifically what intervention is to be withheld and under what circumstances it is to be withheld.

When Uhlmann and his colleagues studied the charts of 56 patients who had received DNR orders, 43% of them "contained no documentation of treatment limitation plans beyond the no-code order."[22] When cross-covering physicians were questioned about their interpretations of specific DNR orders, both "the intention and interpretation of the orders were characterized by variability, and the interpretation of the orders was characterized by uncertainty as well."[22] The authors wrote, " This potential for misinterpretation of a no-code order increases with the number of physicians, nurses, and other personnel who may become responsible for patient care when the primary physician is not available, a common situation in large teaching hospitals and in urgent care situations."[22]

Problems in communication about treatment limitation result, in part, from confusion about the meaning of the term "resuscitate," which may be used to describe responses to a variety of life-threatening conditions and situations.[23] "Thus, DNR, by not specifying the clinical condition under which it applies, the exact treatment to be forgone, or the rationale for the decision, may encourage health professionals, patients, and families to think in reductionistic terms about treatment planning. . . ."[23] For example, it might lead patients or families to reject a DNR because they assume it means that no effort will be made to extend the patient's life, or, conversely, it might lead surgeons to eschew some life-sustaining interventions wanted by a patient who has accepted DNR status.

It is most useful to think of DNR as a decision to withhold cardiopulmonary resuscitation, that is, advanced cardiac life support (ACLS), from a patient in the event of cardiac, pulmonary, or cardiopulmonary arrest.[23] But a DNR order, even specifically defined, does not give instruction about what to do or not to do in the event of life-threatening events short of full arrest.

It is useful to conceptualize the progression from health to disease as a journey down a funnel.[17] At the widest part, the top, one finds a variety of disease processes. As one progresses down the funnel toward death, the slope becomes steeper and the patient sicker as the disease process affects more and more of the patient's vital organ systems. At the most narrow portion of the funnel, there is a final pathophysiological "common pathway" of death, characterized by a limited number of conditions. So, for example, whether a patient has lung cancer due to cigarette smoking, multiple organ system failure, extensive burns, or severe head injury, the final stages before death will invariably involve the failure of one or more vital body systems. The last point in the dying process, at the bottom of the funnel, is cardiopulmonary arrest.

While nonmedical values may compete with the goal of maximizing longevity at the top of the funnel (e.g., a patient decides she wants to continue smoking cigarettes after bypass surgery), decisions contrary to that goal are most often reversible and have statistical, rather than immediate, clinical consequences. As one nears the bottom of the funnel, the consequences of nontreatment are much more likely to be immediate and irreversible.

When patients are critically ill and unstable, a DNR order tells health care professionals not to institute CPR in the event of an arrest, but it does not tell them about the management of other life-threatening conditions such as hypotension, arrhythmia, respiratory distress, or renal failure that might occur higher up in the funnel. For the surgeon who is covering a patient in the SICU and is called in the middle of the night, a simple DNR order leaves many important questions unanswered. Should the DNR patient be given vasopressors or blood products? Should he or she be cardioverted, intubated, or placed on hemodialysis? Without thinking and planning for these decisions ahead of time, with clear identification and documentation of treatment goals, the answers to these questions may be left to surmise, impulse, or personal inclination.

The Importance of Identifying Treatment Goals

Too often surgeons, patients, and families focus on specific treatments rather than the goals those treatments might or might not serve.[24–26] By considering individual treatments first, we run the risk of (1) giving false expectations about prognosis, (2) encouraging reductionistic thinking about treatment limitation, (3) failing to identify the outcome desired by the patient, and (4) increasing the likelihood of conflict or uncertainty later on. Let us examine each of these problems in turn.

First, by starting out with a question such as "Would you like us to try to start your heart if it stops?" or "Would you want to be put on a breathing machine?" or (in our opinion, the worst of all questions) "Do you want us to do everything?" surgeons too often give the impression that any of these interventions can or will be successful in saving the patient's life and, perhaps, even in curing the patient. Sometimes, of course, these goals are possible. But when they are not, starting out by offering them implies to the patient or family that they are. Why else would they be offered? In irreversibly dying patients, the first job is to help the patient and/or family come to grips with this unhappy reality. Offering futile treatment before compassionately assisting people to give up unrealistic goals is not helpful. Second, by focusing first on specific treatments, patients may wrongly infer that a refusal of one treatment means a commitment to no treatment.

Finally, treatment interventions can serve multiple goals. By offering interventions before clarifying goals, the surgeon may have goals in mind different from those of the patient, family, or other health professionals. This may lead to confusion, misunderstanding and potential conflict down the line. Consider, for example, an elderly female patient with a bad heart and chronic renal failure on dialysis, who becomes septic four days after an appendectomy. The patient is increasingly unstable and may require critical care. Under these circumstances, the conversation with the patient begins, "You are becoming very ill. We think you have a blood infection. We think you should go to the surgical intensive care unit." So far so good, but then comes the question, "Would you want us to intubate you and put you on a mechanical ventilator if that became necessary?" This question, asked without a clarification of goals, could easily cause confusion in two directions. On one hand, a patient who wants a chance at returning home with her family—but is fearful of dying attached to machines—might refuse SICU admission and intubation altogether, thereby missing an opportunity to meet her goal of returning home. On the other hand, such a patient might agree to the aggressive intervention but once transferred to the SICU decompensate. When it becomes clear that the patient will never leave the SICU, the question of withdrawing aggressive support is likely to be raised, but without the clarification of goals—that the patient did not want to die on machines—the patient may well be doomed to the high-tech death she feared.

Patients may have a variety of goals in mind when they accept or refuse treatments that are offered. In addition to the goals at the extremes—continued biological life at any cost and being allowed to die as quickly and comfortably as possible, a variety of goals are both possible and reasonable. Some patients may want treatment only if it can return them home. Others may be satisfied with life in a chronic care facility, but only if they are able to recognize and interact with family members. Still others want treatment only if it is likely to restore function they have lost or keep them from losing yet more function. Of course, once treatment goals are identified, patients may be willing to put up with some but not other interventions to achieve them. So, for example, a patient whose goal is to return home might be willing to put up with surgery, but not chronic hemodialysis, to achieve it.

DNR in the Operating Room (OR)

Nowhere is the DNR order more confusing and potentially divisive than in the operating room; and nowhere are good communication, identification of goals, and documentation more important. At first glance, DNR in the operating room seems paradoxical.[27] Why would a patient who wants to be allowed to die if he or she arrests want surgery in the first place? In fact, surgery in the DNR patient can be quite reasonable and entirely consistent with the patient's goals. Even in patients with terminal illness, surgery may be necessary for palliation. Examples include relieving a painful bowel obstruction in a patient with colon cancer, setting a pathological fracture in a patient with metastatic cancer, putting in a central line for the administration of pain medication, and the creation of a tracheotomy. Patients who are not dying may also have DNR orders because of the low probability of successful resuscitation should they arrest.

The usual practice is for all preoperative orders to be suspended during the perioperative period. A new set of orders is written postoperatively. During surgery, orders are given verbally and recorded in the operative record. Thus, preoperative DNR orders are normally suspended during the perioperative period. Surgeons and anesthesiologists are uncomfortable with the idea of DNR in the OR for a variety of reasons.

First, death in the operating room is viewed as a bad outcome.[28] "Because surgery, more than any other activity, involves physicians doing things to patients, any death associated with surgery quickly raises the suspicion of human error and the specter of malpractice."[27] In a time of open economic competition and heightened attention to quality assurance, bad outcomes can reflect poorly on individual surgeons, departments, or entire hospitals.

Second, as Walker has suggested, "The operating room is a powerful stronghold of pure physician authority. In the OR there is a strict hierarchy of personnel, with the surgeon in command. Allowing a patient's directives to influence protocol in this structured environment threatens this last vestige . . . [of physician authority and power]."[28] Third, because patients are so carefully monitored in the operating room, the cause of arrest is usually apparent and is much more often reversible than in the regular hospital ward or even the medical or surgical intensive care unit.[28,29]

Fourth, patients may choose an operative procedure with the specific intent of exposing themselves to the possibility of death. As such they intentionally use the surgeon and anesthesiologist as unwilling and unwitting agents in their suicide.

Each of these reasons for opposition to DNR in the OR can be countered. Deaths in the OR resulting from either the informed decision of a surgeon to operate on a high-risk patient to palliate the patient's suffering, or the informed decision of a patient to undergo surgery but forgo resuscitation in the perioperative period, should not be classified as bad outcomes.[27] There is a place for surgeon authority in the operating room, but it is difficult to defend the notion that this authority overrides a patient's right to accept or refuse certain kinds of interventions. Next, although resuscitation is more successful in the operating room, patients must consent to treatment no matter how successful it might be. Finally, it is doubtful that many patients would choose surgery as the easiest way out.

The most credible argument in favor of suspending DNR orders in the OR is that surgery and general anesthesia sometimes induce conditions that without resuscitation would mean the death of the patient. The most extreme and absurd example would be to ask for general anesthesia but refuse intubation and mechanical ventilation. Other examples are less dramatic but are, nonetheless, troublesome to conscientious health professionals.

> For example, mesenteric stimulation by the surgeon occasionally leads to vagal responses and sometimes long asystoles. Here, the treatment might be cessation of stimulation and the injection of adrenergic or anticholinergic drugs that restore homeostasis. Spinal anesthetics are not infrequently followed by hypotension, occasionally severe, as a response to the sympathetic blockade caused by the anesthetic. Timely treatment with vasopressors and fluids restores homeostasis. Other examples include the proper control of blood loss by clamping or cauterizing bleeding vessels and fluid replacement during surgery to remove bowel obstruction.[27]

As Walker has pointed out, there is a useful distinction between maintaining homeostasis and resuscitating the patient.[28] It seems reasonable that many OR personnel would be willing to forgo only resuscitation. "To demand otherwise would be an unreasonable intrusion and distortion of practices that form the very core of the professional identity of surgeons and anesthesiologists. Failure to respond to easily·correctable disruptions in homeostasis would engender a greater sense of agency in causing the patient's death."[27] Sometimes, of course, it is impossible to draw a clear line between restoring homeostasis and resuscitation. At other times, it may seem reasonable to cease resuscitative efforts when they seem a direct extension of the disease, for example, uncontrollable bleeding that develops "in a patient with cirrhosis and encephalopathy who is undergoing portacaval shunting."[29]

Both patients and OR personnel have important interests at stake in these decisions. Walker and others have suggested guidelines for resolving this complicated issue.[28] These guidelines stress that:

1. Surgery may be entirely appropriate for DNR patients.
2. Patients' rights do not end at the doors to the operating room.
3. Surgeons and anesthesiologists may reasonably insist on reversing disruptions in homeostasis caused by their actions during the perioperative period.
4. The surgeon and anesthesiologist must speak directly with the patient or surrogate to clarify the patient's goals and the reason for the DNR order and explain their own intended behavior in the OR and its rationale.
5. In most instances, frank and respectful communication can resolve the issue. If the patient refuses to accept the perioperative limitations to the

DNR order, the surgeon or anesthesiologist may either decide to agree with the patient or respectfully withdraw from his or her care.

6. When DNR orders are suspended during surgery, they should be re-instituted following the perioperative period, including withdrawal of life support if that no longer serves the preoperative goals of a patient who has irreversibly deteriorated during or immediately following surgery.

7. If resuscitative measures are withheld or terminated and intraoperative death occurs, such deaths should be classified as "expected."

Defining Death

Ethical Analysis

In 1968 an ad hoc committee at Harvard Medical School published a seminal paper in which they called for a new definition of death based on neurological rather than the traditional cardiovascular criteria.[30] These neurological criteria, the irreversible loss of all brain function, gained rapid and widespread consensus throughout the United States. Today they are recognized by specific law or court decision in every jurisdiction in our country. Most states recognize death as determined either by neurological or cardiovascular criteria. The Uniform Determination of Death Act, which served as a model for most state statutes, reads:

> An individual who has sustained either (1) irreversible cessation of circulatory and respiratory functions, or (2) irreversible cessation of all functions of the entire brain, including the brain stem, is dead. A determination of death must be made in accordance with accepted medical standards.[31]

The rapid acceptance of the neurological criteria, often referred to as "brain death," was influenced by three factors. First, when determined by competent clinicians, the diagnosis of brain death is practical and entirely reliable. Second, the prognosis of patients who meet this criteria is entirely predictable and dismal. No patient meeting the criteria has ever awakened and, until recently at least, these patients were extremely unstable, suffering asystole within hours or days despite maximum efforts. Finally, these patients, so-called heart-beating cadavers, were excellent sources for solid organs.

After nearly three decades of experience with brain death, several problems and challenges have emerged. While none of them has seriously threatened widespread social acceptance of brain death, they illustrate some of the scientific, conceptual, and cultural difficulties of defining death in an age of sophisticated medical technology.

The Conceptual Basis for Declaring Death

The conceptual basis of brain death has never been uniformly or completely accepted. Any formulation of death must have three components: a concept or definition of death; operational criteria for determining that death has occurred; and, finally, specific medical tests, demonstrating whether or not the criteria have been fulfilled.[32,33] The definition of death is at the conceptual level and asks the question, "What quality is so essentially significant to a living entity that its loss constitutes the death of that entity?" This is a philosophical question that can not be answered alone by science.

The ad hoc Harvard Committee did not in fact give a philosophical rationale for the choice of neurological criteria for death and it was not until thirteen years later that one was provided.[34] In 1981 Bernat and his colleagues argued that brain-dead patients were dead because they had lost the brain's integrative function, without which the organism could no longer function as a whole.[33] Others, however, argued that if brain-dead patients were dead, it was because they had lost the capacity for consciousness and cognition.[32,35-37]

A study of health professionals (ICU physicians, neurosurgeons, anesthesiologists, and ICU and OR nurses) likely to be involved in the care of brain-dead patients found considerable variation in the conceptual basis for their acceptance.[38] While 25% cited the brain's integrative capacity, 36% said these patients were dead because they had lost the capacity for consciousness and cognition. Most surprising (and revealing), fully 32% of respondents gave answers indicating that although they had said brain-dead patients were dead, they did not really believe it. When asked what exactly made a brain-dead individual dead, they answered either that the patient's quality of life is unacceptable or that, no matter what was done, the patient would soon die.

These two last answers are logically incompatible with the patient being dead and indicate that many persons believe that brain-dead patients are nearly dead or as good as dead, but not actually dead. This finding confirms the observation that the persistence of the term "brain death" itself is an indication that it represents a state different from traditional death. Phenomenologically this is true. When a patient suffers cardiovascular arrest, the body and its organs come quickly and quietly to rest. Visible signs of life, such as respirations, consciousness, and electronic tracings on machines that monitor vital signs disappear, more or less, at once. Brain-dead patients do not look or feel dead. True, they are comatose, but their hearts continue to beat red, oxygenated blood throughout their bodies to kidneys, livers, pancreases, and lungs that continue to function normally (which is, of course, what makes brain-dead patients such desirable sources of organs). Brain-dead women have gestated living fetuses for weeks, giving birth to healthy babies.

Under these circumstances, it is not surprising that the term "brain death" persists, or that health professionals and journalists continue to describe brain-dead patients as "being kept alive on life support" or "dying when life support was withdrawn"—despite admonitions from the transplant community that such comments do not make sense.[39-41]

A minority of persons rejects the notion of brain death on religious grounds, leading the state of New Jersey to allow by law a religious objection that vetoes a diagnosis of death by neurological criteria.[42] Some commentators have called for uniform legal recognition of conscientious objection to brain death.[43]

Clinical Issues

Widespread experience reveals that many patients who have been declared brain-dead by commonly used tests do, in fact, retain brain functions. The criteria for brain death have always rejected the notion that every cell must be dead or that all electrical activity must cease for a declaration of death to occur. The criteria have centered on *function* rather than *activity*, as reflected in the Uniform Determination of Death Act mentioned earlier. While the law and institutional policies insist on irreversible loss of *all* brain function, the tests commonly employed do not look for the presence or absence of some brain functions. So for example, many patients who are declared dead by brain-death criteria continue to demonstrate the presence of certain brain functions, including the production of argenine vasopressin and auditory evoked potentials.[26,44] It is difficult to dismiss these as mere "activities," especially the production of vasopressin, which helps maintain homeostasis by preventing the development of diabetes insipidus.[44] The British deal with this problem by rejecting whole-brain death, relying instead on the notion of brain-stem death.[44]

As mentioned above, one of the reasons for acceptance of brain death has been the clinical reality that such patients suffer asystole very quickly despite maximum efforts. However, with the advancement of technology and clinical experience, brain-dead patients have been maintained for weeks and even months. Efforts to extend care have been motivated by the wish to allow fetuses to mature to extra-uterine viability. However, there have been reported cases where physicians and hospitals have accepted requests by family members to maintain intensive care of dead patients. Dead patients have even been discharged home on ventilators, where their bodies have been maintained for months. This extended "life-in-death" inevitably attenuates some of the appeal of brain death.

New Methods for Obtaining Organs
Stretch the Boundaries Between Life and Death

As transplantation becomes the treatment of choice for more diseases, and as the number of brain-dead organ donors remains constant, the number of people waiting for, and dying waiting for, organs rises each year (see Chapter 6). The organ shortage has bred an almost desperate attempt to increase the potential organ donor pool. One method is the use of so-called non-heart-beating cadavers (NHBCs), persons who have died traditional cardiopulmonary deaths. This method puts the premium on taking organs as close as possible to the time of death in order to protect them from warm ischemia.[45] This has raised questions never before considered important about (1) how precisely to determine the time of death following cardiopulmonary arrest, (2) the exact meaning of the term "irreversible," and (3) whether neurological criteria are more important than those that rely on loss of cardiopulmonary function.

By declaring death two minutes after measurable asystole and immediately removing organs, the University of Pittsburgh Medical Center Protocol assumes not only that auto resuscitation will not take place, but also that a decision not to resuscitate (at a time when CPR might well get the heart beating again) is equivalent to saying that the loss is irreversible.[46,47] Many persons still believe that irreversible means one cannot start the heart, not that one has chosen not to do so. Moreover, the Pittsburgh Protocol relies strictly on cardiac function without any attention to the central nervous system. Is brain function irreversibly lost two minutes after asystole? This question is never addressed.

Should We Uncouple a Diagnosis of Death from Behavior Usually Reserved for the Dead?

Some authors have raised the question of whether it might be better in the long run for public policy to recognize that organs can be taken from persons who are almost dead, probably dead, and as-good-as-dead, rather than to continue to manipulate the line between life and death in order to increase the organ donor pool.[48,49] These commentators argue that some severely brain-damaged, but technically still-living patients are beyond harm and that if they or their surrogates want to give organs, they should be allowed to do so. By dealing with the issues of "beyond harm" and patient autonomy directly, rather than constantly gerrymandering the line between life and death, public trust will be enhanced rather than undermined.

None of the problems discussed here has risen to the level of a public policy debate. In most ways, brain death has been an effective scientific, philosophical, and social compromise. How long the compromise will hold remains to be seen.

Clinical Conclusions

Medical technology has brought our society many benefits and challenges. Its ability to extend life has forced us to make complex decisions about life's quality. After nearly three decades of debate and discussion, our society has rejected an absolute vitalism in favor of letting its citizens make their own choices about the application of life-sustaining technology. Because these decisions are best made in partnership with the surgeon, good communication and planning are essential. Good communication involves timely setting of goals that are consistent with surgical reality and the particular values and preferences of the patients. Advance directives have been introduced as a way to plan for the very likely possibility that some end-of-life decisions will be made when the patient no longer has decision-making capacity.

An essential ingredient of good planning is the recognition that decisions near the end of life more often represent a nuanced rather than artificially dichotomous approach to limiting aggressive care. The surgeon has a responsibility not only to work with the patient or family to construct an individually tailored plan, but to adequately communicate this plan to the other members of the health care team so that they will know how to respond to life-threatening events. This approach is particularly important for patients with do-not-resuscitate orders who come to the operating room. Here, a carefully made plan should be negotiated prospectively regarding intraoperative and postoperative events. Deaths subsequent to planned treatment limitation would be classified as such, so that they do not reflect on a surgeon's mortality ratings.

Brain death has been recognized by law in every state as a legal criterion for the determination of death. The diagnosis of brain death is straightforward clinically and the prognosis as certain as anything in medicine: patients who fulfill its criterion never recover. However, brain-dead patients who are maintained on ventilators in intensive care units present a phenomenological paradox. While legally and clinically dead, they retain considerable signs of life. This paradox makes them both ideal organ donors and emotionally confusing to many families and health professionals. Surgeons must be patient in helping grieving families to come to terms with the paradox of so much apparent life in a dead person.

While new controversies about the philosophical, cultural, and even clinical legitimacy of brain death have raged in academic circles, it is unclear whether they will ever reach the level of public debate or clinical controversy.

References

1. Linda L. Emanuel and Ezekiel J. Emanuel, " The Medical Directive: A New Comprehensive Advance-Care Document," *Journal of the American Medical Association* 261 (1989): 3288–3293.
2. David Orentlicher, "Advance Medical Directives," *Journal of the American Medical Association* 263 (1990): 2365–2367.
3. Susan Wolf, Brian Boyle, Daniel Callahan, et al., "Sources of Concern About the Patient Self Determination Act," *New England Journal of Medicine* 325 (1991): 1666–1671.

4. David J. Doukas and Daniel W. Gorenflo, "Analyzing the Values History: An Evaluation of Patient Medical Values and Advance Directives," *The Journal of Clinical Ethics* 4 (1993): 41–45.

5. Omnibus Reconciliation Act 1990. Title IV. Section 4206. Congressional Record. October 26, 1990: 12638.

6. Ezekiel J. Emanuel, D. S. Weinberg, R. Gonin, et al., "How Well is the Patient Self-Determination Act Working? An Early Assessment," *The American Journal of Medicine* 95 (1993): 619–628.

7. L. L. Emanuel, M. J. Barry, J. D. Stoeckle, et al., "Advance Directives for Medical Care—A Case for Greater Use," *New England Journal of Medicine* 324 (1991): 889–895.

8. Alan Meisel, *The Right to Die*. New York: Wiley Law Publications 1994, cumulative supplement No.2.

9. J. Cohen-Mansfield, B. A. Rabinovich, S. Lipson, et al., "The Decision to Execute a Durable Power of Attorney for Health Care and Preferences Regarding the Utilization of Life-Sustaining Treatments in Nursing Home Residents," *Archives of Internal Medicine* 151 (1991): 289–294.

10. Dallas M. High, "Why Are Elderly People Not Using Advance Directives?" *Journal of Aging and Health* 5 (1993): 497–515.

11. Ezekiel J. Emanuel and Linda L. Emanuel, "Proxy Decision Making for Incompetent Patients: An Ethical and Empirical Analysis," *Journal of the American Medical Association* 267 (1992): 2067–2071.

12. J. Hare, C. Pratt, and C. Nelson, "Agreement Between Patients and Their Self-Selected Surrogates on Difficult Medical Decisions," *Archives of Internal Medicine* 152 (1992): 1049–1054.

13. Robert A. Pearlman, R. F. Uhlmann, and Nancy S. Jecker, "Spousal Understanding of Patient Quality of Life: Implications for Surrogate Decisions," *Journal of Clinical Ethics* 3 (1992): 114–121.

14. J. Suhl, P. Simons, T. Reedy, et al., "Myth of Substituted Judgement: Surrogate Decision Making Regarding Life Support Is Unreliable," *Archives of Internal Medicine* 154 (1994): 90–96.

15. Marian Danis, L. I. Sutherland, J. M. Garrett, et al., "A Prospective Study of Advance Directives for Life Sustaining Care," *New England Journal of Medicine* 324 (1991): 882–887.

16. Ashwini Sehgal, A. Galbraith, M. Chesney, et al., "How Strictly Do Dialyisis Patients Want Their Advance Directives Followed?" *Journal of the American Medical Association* 267 (1992): 59–68.

17. Stuart J. Youngner, "Do-Not-Resuscitate Orders: No Longer Secret, but Still a Problem," *Hastings Center Report* 17 (1987): 23–33.

18. M. Saklayen, H. Liss, R. Markert, "In-Hospital Cardiopulmonary Resuscitation: Survival In 1 Hospital and Literature Review," *Medicine* 74 (1995): 163–175.

19. SUPPORT Principal Investigators, "A Controlled Trial to Improve Care for Seriously Ill Hospitalized Patients: The Study to Understand Prognoses and Preference for Outcomes and Risks of Treatments (SUPPORT)," *Journal of the American Medical Association* 274 (1995):1591–1596.

20. Bernard Lo, "Improving Care Near the End of Life: Why Is It So Hard?" *Journal of the American Medical Association* 274 (1995) 1634–1636. (editorial)

21. Cynthia J. Stolman, John J. Gregory, D. Dunn, et al., "Evaluation of Patient, Physician, Nurse, and Family Attitudes Toward Do-Not-Resuscitate Orders," *Archives of Internal Medicine* 150 (1990): 653–658.

22. R. F. Uhlmann, C. K. Cassel, and W. J. McDonald, " Some Treatment-Withholding Implications of No-Code In An Academic Hospital," *Critical Care Medicine* 12 (1984): 879–881.

23. Elizabeth E. O'Toole, Stuart J. Youngner, Barbara Juknialis, et al., "Evaluation of a Treatment Limitation Policy with a Specific Treatment-Limiting Order," *Archives of Internal Medicine* 154 (1994): 425–432.

24. Tom Tomlinson and Howard Brody, "Sounding Board: Ethics and Communication in Do-Not-Resuscitate Orders," *New England Journal of Medicine* 318 (1988):43–46.

25. Stuart J. Youngner, "Applying Futility: Saying No Is Not Enough," *Journal of the American Geriatrics Society* 42 (1994): 887–889.

26. Robert D. Truog, "Is It Time to Abandon Brain Death?" *Hastings Center Report* 27 (1997): 29–37.

27. Stuart J. Youngner, Helmut F. Cascorbi, and Jerry M. Shuck, "DNR in the Operating Room: Not Really a Paradox," *Journal of the American Medical Association* 266 (1991): 2433–2434.

28. R. M. Walker, "DNR in the OR: Resuscitation as an Operative Risk," *Journal of the American Medical Association* 266 (1991): 2407–2412.

29. Cynthia B. Cohen and P. J. Cohen, "Do-Not-Resuscitate Orders in the Operating Room," *New England Journal of Medicine* 325 (1991): 1879–1892.

30. Ad Hoc Committee of the Harvard Medical School to Examine the Definition of Brain Death, "A Definition of Irreversible Coma," *Journal of the American Medical Association* 205 (1968): 337–340.

31. Uniform Determination of Death Act. 12 Uniform Laws Annotated 320 (1990 Supp.)

32. Edward T. Bartlett and Stuart J. Youngner, "Human Death and Destruction of the Neocortex," in: *Death: Beyond Whole-Brain Criteria*, Richard M. Zaner, ed. Dordrecht, The Netherlands: D. Reidel Publishing Co. 1988, pp. 199–216.

33. James L. Bernat, Charles M. Culver, and Bernard Gert, "On the Definition and Criterion of Death," *Annals of Internal Medicine* 94 (1981): 389–394.

34. President's Commission for the Study of Ethical Problems in Medicine and Biomedical and Behavioral Research, *Defining Death*. Washington DC: U.S. Government Printing Office; 1981.

35. Karen G. Gervais, *Redefining Death*. New Haven CT: Yale University Press, 1986.

36. Michael B. Green and Daniel Wikler, "Brain Death and Personal Identity," *Philosophy and Public Affairs* 9 (1980): 105–133.

37. R. Pucetti, "Does Anyone Survive Neocortical Death?" in *Death: Beyond Whole-Brain Criteria*, Richard M. Zaner, ed. Dordrecht, The Netherlands: Kluwer Academic Publishers, 1988: pp. 77–90.

38. Stuart J. Youngner, Charles S. Landefeld, Claudia J. Coulton, et al, " 'Brain Death' and Organ Retrieval: A Cross-Sectional Survey of Knowledge and Concepts Among Health Professionals," *Journal of the American Medical Association* 261 (1989): 2205–2210.

39. Daniel Wikler and Alan J. Weisbard, "Appropriate Confusion Over 'Brain Death,'" *Journal of the American Medical Association* 261 (1989) 2246.

40. Stuart J. Youngner, "Some Must Die," in *Organ Transplantation: Meanings and Realities*, Stuart J. Youngner, Renée C. Fox, and Lawrence J. O'Connell, eds. University of Wisconsin Press, 1996, pp. 32–55.

41. Stuart J. Youngner, "Defining Death. A Superficial and Fragile Consensus," *Archives of Neurology* 49 (1992): 570–572.

42. NJH Declaration of Death Act, 1991(West), New Jersey Statutes Annotated title 26: sections 6A1–6A8.

43. Robert M. Veatch, "The Impending Collapse of the Whole-Brain Definition of Death," *Hasting Center Report* 3 (1993): 18–24.

44. Amir Halevy and Baruch Brody, "Brain Death: Reconciling Definitions, Criteria and Tests," *Annals of Internal Medicine* 119 (1993): 519–525.

45. Stuart J. Youngner and Robert M. Arnold, "Ethical, Psychosocial, and Public Policy Implications of Procuring Organs From Non-Heart Beating Cadaver Donors," *Journal of the American Medical Association* 269 (1993): 2769–2774.

46. Robert M. Arnold, Stuart J. Youngner, Renie Schapiro, et al., eds., *Procuring Organs for Transplantation: The Debate Over Non-Heartbeating Cadaver Protocols.* Baltimore: Johns Hopkins University Press, 1995.

47. "University of Pittsburgh Medical Center Policy and Procedure Manual: Management of Terminally Ill Patients Who May Become Organ Donors after Death," *Kennedy Institute of Ethics Journal* 3 (1993): A1–A15.

48. Robert M. Arnold, Stuart J.Youngner, "The Dead Donor Rule: Should We Stretch It, Bend It or Abandon It?" *Kennedy Institute on Ethics Journal* 3 (1983): 718–732.

49. Norman Fost, "The New Body Snatchers: On Scott's 'The Body as Property,'" *American Bar Foundation Research Journal* 3 (1983): 718–732.

5

Emergency Patients:
Serious Moral Choices with Limited Time,
Information, and Patient Participation

KENNETH L. MATTOX
H. TRISTRAM ENGELHARDT, JR.

Emergency surgical patients are those who appear to require immediate or nearly immediate intervention to save life, limb, or major health interests. A traditional assumption in surgical practice has been that emergency surgical patients should be provided rapid management at whatever level of intervention the surgeon reasonably thinks is required to preserve their lives or protect them from a serious compromise to their prior health status. This assumption is based on three further considerations: (1) the general life-preserving orientation of medicine, (2) the belief that most patients would want their lives and health protected when they are in emergency situations in which there also is no time for an adequate consent process, and (3) reductions in mortality and the protection of significant health interests are generally worth the risk of compromises to health or quality of life that may result from aggressive surgical management. The actual moral content of these assumptions can only be fleshed out in particular communities within particular societies and will under different circumstances have different expressions in law and policy.[1] This chapter explores these assumptions, selecting moral themes generally salient in American health care law, public policy, and medical ethics.

The context of treatment is framed by the assumption that time really is of the essence, such that when the patient is not clearly competent, the surgeon is justified in acting promptly on the traditional assumption in favor of life and health preservation without risks of a delay occasioned by searching for surrogate decision makers. The traditional assumption in favor of aggressive response to surgical emergencies is balanced by an equally traditional concern that aggressive surgical management is sometimes limited in its effectiveness and that reliable clinical judgment predicts that the likelihood of success in saving the patient's life or health may at times be very low or even nonexistent. Moreover, aggressive surgical management of some physiologically compromised patients may result in iatrogenic harms that may outweigh possible benefits. Finally, some emergency surgical patients may indeed be capable of consent[2] or may beforehand have made decisions, which are available during an emergency, to refuse aggressive surgical management of emergencies. In this chapter we address these ethical challenges of emergency surgical patients. We begin with a consideration of limits to the traditional assumption that favors aggressive surgical response to the emergency patient and then turn to a consideration of the challenges surrounding the consent process.

Ethical Analysis: Limits on the Traditional Assumption in Favor of Aggressive Surgical Management of the Emergency Patient

Clinical Decision Making under Intense Time Constraints

At best, surgical decision making is undertaken with a database derived from historical, examination, laboratory, and radiographic information. The database is virtually always incomplete. Decisions must be made taking into account the likely costs of both under- and overtreating.[3] In the situation of emergency care, the incompleteness is accentuated: up to 50% of the data is inconclusive or frankly incorrect. Both society and the medical associates of the surgeon assume that time constraints create a sense of overbearing urgency, thereby further morally clouding decision making. This has strengthened the impression that evaluation and treatment must precede within "the golden hour." Ambulances with red lights and sirens as well as air ambulance systems give an often false perception that more speedy retrieval and treatment will always significantly increase the quality of outcome for the emergency surgical patient. As a consequence, urgent evaluation centers have emerged in civilian and military environments. Although some urgent surgical conditions exist whereby drainage of a subdural hematoma, establishment of an airway, or staunching the bleeding from a major exsanguinating source are required, such conditions represent less than 1% of the entire emergency surgical caseload in any emergency surgery center. Surgical decision making is usually straightforward and simple.

Though branch-chain algorithmic decision making is offered as a model by many textbooks, actual decision making is made by surgeons in a cluster mode. By means of a cluster logic, a volume of widely derived information frequently encountered during the initial survey of a surgical patient in the emergency department results in a "go" or "no-go" decision for admission or an operation. Should a secondary volume of information be required, a second cluster is ordered. This second cluster may involve even more observation time. Surgeons are usually very adept at providing surgical treatment or observatory treatment for their patients, though they are generally intervention-oriented. The roles of both observer and intervener involve a careful analysis of data. Such decisions are rarely significantly time constrained. It is the extraneous environment, such as the hospital laboratory, the speed of the ECT scanner, or the availability of operative sites, and so on, that logistically frustrate the surgeon, creating conflict among the critical hospital pathways and between different clinical standards of practice or practice guidelines. Clinical ethical decision making requires the courage to work honestly and compassionately through these conflicts.

Challenges to the Traditional Assumption in Favor of Aggressive Surgical Management of Life-Threatening Emergencies

Emergency surgeons see patients for whom treatment will likely be very costly, success very unlikely, the length of life to be secured brief, and the quality of life to be achieved marginal. These conditions create concerns as to when treatment should be characterized as futile, inappropriate, or marginally useful.[4,5] Characterizations of interventions as futile or inappropriate incorporate complex clinical ethical judgments regarding how much expense must be invested to save a life, how certain one must be about success, how long a postponement of death must be in order to be significant, and what quality of life justifies what level of intervention.[6]

To determine that treatment is futile, inappropriate, or marginally useful is not just to describe reality, but to place a state of affairs within a web of explanations and evaluations. Such determinations create social reality. Such determinations are performative somewhat as the declaration of a sheriff, "You are under arrest." Just as a physician's determination that a patient is partially or totally disabled will have impact on various welfare rights, so, too, if a surgeon determines that treatment is futile and inappropriate, the duty to provide such treatment may be ended. Similarly, when treatment can be characterized as marginally useful, the obligation to offer it can be qualified. Such determinations establish warrant to treat, to treat in a particular fashion, or not to treat. Surgeons therefore look for ways of characterizing emergency patients. These will either warrant further curative interventions or warrant instead providing comfort care.

Emergency Patients for Whom Surgery Survival Is Unprecedented. Surgeons responding to emergency patients who are most assuredly "going," who in highest probability will very shortly die, are torn between rapid full-steam-ahead aggressive
resuscitative measures (because that is the way surgeons have been trained to
react) and the recognition that interventions may succeed only in increasing the
potential misery to the patient and the family, as well as the financial burdens.
Such circumstances are represented by the 100% third- and fourth-degree burn
in an elderly patient, the final admission for a patient with terminal metastatic
cancer, and some victims of trauma whose survival is unprecedented, such as
persons with prolonged pre-hospital CPR following trauma and irreversible
metabolic acidosis. Burns from various causes such as scald, flame, and elec-
tricity affect mainly the patients at the extremes of the ages, the very young and
the elderly, although patients of all ages are at risk. The patient with a major
third-degree burn has a mortality rate roughly equivalent to the patient's age
plus the percent of total body burn. Although significant advances have been
made in the control of burn wound sepsis and the development of skin coverage, it is often the case that aggressive surgical management achieves only a
delayed death following much expense, operative intervention, pain, and suffering, instead of an early death. Though there is often some time to reflect on
the decision to treat aggressively, it is usually necessary to begin the process of
reflection regarding an appropriate decision as early as possible. Surgeons should
aid patients and surrogate decision makers in confronting these difficult decisions about patients for whom survival is unprecedented and for whom, in this
sense, aggressive surgical management is futile.

The more secure surgeons are in their ability to resuscitate patients effectively
with complex surgical problems, the easier it is to reach the decision not to initiate or even to terminate curative care in a patient who has an emergency surgical condition for which treatment is futile in the sense that it is not reliably
expected to prevent death. The decision to attempt to do everything possible in
all circumstances is most often made by surgeons who are insecure, inexperienced, fearful of their own inabilities, or fearful of sanctions by the hospital or
the medical-legal community. A commitment to resuscitation at all costs usually
creates logarithmically more moral problems for subsequent health providers
and increases the moral as well as medical-legal complications.

Emergency Patients for Whom Survival with Severe Central Nervous System Injury is a
High Probability. Surgeons and surgical specialists can be significantly frustrated
when confronted with emergency surgical conditions that they cannot immediately attack and repair. The patient with either an isolated central nervous system injury, a central nervous system surgical diagnosis, or such a diagnosis with
other secondary conditions presents complex and difficult ethical challenges.
Should a patient with a transected aorta from blunt injury die during an appro-

priately expeditious evaluation followed by an operative treatment, surgeons are rarely sanctioned. However, if the same patient undergoes an emergent complex operative repair and sustains a paralysis, there is at least a 25% chance that the same surgeon and hospital treating team will be subject to extensive and very expensive legal tort action. A trial of treatment will therefore be discouraged when the risk of malpractice action is greater from action rather than from inaction. Under such circumstances, surgeons are advised to consult liberally their neurological colleagues about the extent and reversibility of head and spinal cord surgical conditions.

Because of numerous "miraculous reversals" of central nervous system injuries and continuing advances made in the treatment of these conditions, the surgeon facing such conditions should be wary of considering a central nervous system injury a trustworthy signal for non-response. Even when patients have enacted effective and available advance directives that exclude treatment in the face of the expectation of serious central nervous system injury, it may initially be difficult to establish such an expectation with a useful degree of certainty.[7]

Rather than take an "either/or" approach, the surgeon should undertake aggressive management of such patients as a trial of intervention. The traditional assumption in favor of aggressive response to emergency surgical patients justifies the surgeon in continuing the intervention, so long as the prognosis for the recovery of some degree of significant central nervous system function remains positive, even guardedly so. However, especially in the postoperative period, if the most reliable prognosis is that the patient is not expected to recover to a cognitive, sapient existence (i.e., some reasonable degree of central nervous system function that allows the patient to interact with his environment), then the surgeon should be willing to discontinue the trial of intervention—given the concurrence of the surrogate decision-maker and presuming the absence of previous binding instructions. Following the approach outlined in Chapter 2 for informed consent by such decision makers, the surgeon should emphasize that aggressive management was initiated to determine if the patient could benefit and that, unfortunately, it appears that benefit is less likely and harm more likely. Fully informing the surrogate decision maker will help that individual to understand that, though there was justification for initiating the trial, the traditional assumption in favor of aggressive response is now outweighed by the lack of benefit and, in fact, the potential for harming the patient with continued aggressive management is great.

Emergency Patients for Whom Survival with Severe Disability Is a High Probability. Virtually every surgical intervention produces some physical disability. The disability may be as minor as an unsightly scar or as major as a chronic infection, a malunion of a fracture, or a paralysis. All physical disability brings with it risk of mental disability. Surgeons, therefore, confront an important ethical challenge as they attempt to prepare such patients and their families for the disabilities that may result in the short term, intermediate term, and long term following a surgical intervention. As with all treatments involving chronic conditions, coming to terms with long-term disabilities requires a process of reorientation and readaptation. In the face of time constraints, surgeons can usually only imperfectly engage this process so as to prepare the patient and the patient's family for the consequences of a surgical intervention. Surgeons also face a difficulty from these same time constraints on the acquisition of sufficient data to communicate accurate and useful information to the patient or the patient's surrogate, so that decisions can be made. Surgeons as far as possible must come to a judgment regarding whether the treatments that they will offer will be worth the costs and suffering to the patient, given the likely quality of the outcome, all within the constraints of emergency health care.

This difficulty is compounded by the circumstance that, in order to predict well, one must often undertake the trial of intervention and observe the patient for a longer period of time than the patients considered in the previous section, in order to gauge the character of response to the trauma that brought the patient to the emergency room, as well as the trauma that will likely be engendered by the surgeon's intervention on behalf of restoring health. The result is an increased softness of predictions. Though experienced surgeons may not usually experience a press of time in the sense of a need to act at once, still the context for emergency surgical decision making imposes opportunity constraints on the acquisition and assessment of clinical and laboratory data. Often it is simply not possible to judge with sufficient confidence the likelihood of the patient recovering from the presenting trauma, as well as the likelihood of the surgeon's intervention improving long-term prospects for the patient. The burden of proof needed to terminate the traditional obligation to intervene to maintain life and to restore health and thus justify stopping a trial of intervention, can frequently not be met because of the softness of the data in an emergency context. Clinical ethical judgments as to whether an intervention will only marginally extend life, achieve only a poor quality of outcome, or have only a very low likelihood of success can often not be made when one is first confronted with the judgment whether to treat or not to treat. Because of this softness, there are good grounds to qualify all but the most well-founded judgments of futility or of the marginal usefulness of surgical interventions with respect to emergency patients.

Emergency Patients with a Low Probability of Survival but with Good Quality of Life among Survivors. A fourth group of patients that challenges the traditional assumption in favor of aggressive response to emergency surgical patients is defined by those with a low probability of survival but good quality of life among survivors. At stake here is the role of costs in determining the appropriateness of therapeutic interventions. Unfortunately, little policy has developed to guide decision making in such circumstances.

Informed Consent from Patients in Emergencies

The practice of gaining informed consent from patients prior to surgical or medical intervention rests on a complex cluster of moral concerns, as explained in Chapter 2. If the patient agrees to be treated, the surgeon acts with the patient's authorization, and the surgeon has a right to be doing what the surgeon has engaged in. In an emergency context, for surgeons to establish that they are acting with the leave of a patient, it may be enough if the patient recognizes in a general manner what the surgeon intends to do and then agrees to the undertaking. It is another and more complicated matter to argue that a patient has the right to enough information to gauge fully whether a proposed surgical intervention will advance the patient's interests. A great deal of information and reflection may be needed for a patient to make such a judgment with completeness and full maturity. Also, a significant amount of interaction may be needed to satisfy the autonomy interests of many patients. Unfortunately, for emergency surgical patients, an over-elaborate demand for information in the informed consent process may unduly burden the therapeutic goals that surgeons recognize must be pursued with dispatch. The reasonable person standard (see Chapter 2), we believe, should be adapted to the emergency situation. The surgeon should provide only that information necessary for a reasonable person simply to accept the offered intervention, to refuse it, or to seek an alternative. All the information that a non-emergency patient might want is not necessarily provided, but more information is advanced than many surgeons might sometimes be inclined to offer.

It is usually feasible in emergency circumstances only to assess rapidly whether a patient is competent. To be competent simply to choose or refuse emergency surgical intervention, a patient need not be competent in all areas. It is enough if the patient in ordinary terms understands intellectually what is at stake in the choice being made, is able to appreciate the context of the choice intellectually and affectively, and comprehends quickly the causal connections between the choice or refusal of particular interventions and likely outcomes.[8] The patient's understanding need not match that of the surgeon or of the non-emergency patient. Often, the surgeon will quickly act to determine competence, ascertain whether the patient is of age or other legal status to be able to consent, and then provide sufficient information to make an informed decision. If the patient does not appear competent and immediate intervention is needed to save life, limb, or serious health interests, the surgeon is usually obliged to proceed without consent, as explained above.

The practice of surgeons intervening to save life, limb, or serious health interest when there is no good evidence that a patient is competently refusing such intervention or when there is no advance directive in place expressing a prior applicable competent refusal can be understood in terms of the costs of false-positive determinations of competence. If one fails to provide emergency life-saving treatment because of a false-positive determination of competence, the patient will die. The patient will die because of a seeming refusal, which is in fact a false refusal, for authoritative refusals presuppose competence on the part of the patient. The greater the cost to the patient from a false-positive determination of competence, the greater the concern should be to ascertain whether the patient is truly competent.

The costs associated with false-positive determinations of competence account for a seeming disparity. If a patient appears competent and agrees to lifesaving treatment in an emergency, that seeming competence is not usually questioned. The costs of a false-positive determination will generally not be great. The patient will recover if the treatment is successful. If the treatment chosen by the patient or patient's surrogate is a standard and surgically appropriate one, it can in general be presumed to be the kind of treatment a competent person will have accepted. However, if a patient refuses a standard lifesaving treatment in emergency contexts because the costs of a false-positive are high, the patient's competence is immediately brought into question. When time and opportunity permit, a psychiatric consultation should be sought, if this is likely to enhance the quality of the determination of competence. The greater the health costs to patients in an emergency circumstance of refusing particular standard interventions, the greater the burden patients have to establish their competence or to have left effective and available advance directives to clarify the matter.[9] The moral concern to respect patients and to protect their best interests in emergency circumstances brings into question refusals of lifesaving treatment that are not clearly and convincingly competent refusals when the costs of refusal are high.

Informed Consent: The Long Version. When there is time, which is often the case in surgical emergencies, surgeons should inform patients or their surrogates more completely regarding the need for a surgical intervention, the possible alternatives, and the significance of the available alternatives. In the process of informed consent the focus should fall on the short-term, intermediate, and long-term consequences of both refusing any of the alternatives, as well as accepting any of the surgical interventions. Surgeons should therefore understand that they have a responsibility to begin planning for the physical and mental rehabilitation that may be needed to adapt to the consequences of the trauma that brought the patient to the surgeon, as well as the surgeon's own interventions. When involved in such care, the surgeon should include family members, who are not strictly necessary to acquire valid consent, insofar as this meets with the patient's approval.

The view that decision-making authority regarding patients is possessed by the family as a social unit is not universally well received, though many states now explicitly provide a chain of surrogate decision-makers that reflects traditional family structures. When there are concerns whether the patient wishes the family to be engaged in decision making with the patient, the surgeon should explore with the patient when possible the extent to which the patient wishes the family involved.

Treatment Without Consent. Most applicable medical law requires surgeons to provide a standard of care that would be rendered by a similar prudent practitioner offering a service under similar emergency circumstances. Emergency care is usually recognized as a special circumstance. If the surgeon waits to intubate a patient in order to locate a surrogate decision maker or establish a patient's previous wishes when the patient is no longer breathing, the patient is likely to suffer severe central nervous system damage, if not death, from such delays. As a consequence, given urgent surgical conditions, a surgeon may be required to perform interventional procedures in the absence of direct consent from either the patient or a surrogate. These interventions may include the establishment of an airway, be it through oral tracheal intubation, surgical tracheotomy, or urgent crycothyroidotomy. On rare occasions a surgeon may be required to perform a thoracostomy or a tube thoracostomy in the emergency center even on patients who during their last gasp appear to be saying "leave me alone." Such seeming "refusals" may be discounted in true emergency contexts when it appears that the patient's competence has been undermined by trauma, hypotension, or the influence of mind-altering medications or drugs. Again, ethics, law, and public policy do not contemplate that a physician should fail to reestablish respiration and heartbeat because the patient is unable to give consent, because a thorough search for an advance directive has not been completed, or because a diligent attempt to find a surrogate to acquire authorization has not been fruitful. When delay is likely to lead to loss of life, limb, or serious health interests, the standing moral practice is to intervene.

The Quick Consent. In truly emergent circumstances, surgeons should act to intervene to save life, limb, and serious health interests and will generally make do with any consent that has the appearance of competence. For example, during moments of evaluation and resuscitation a surgeon may be heard to say, "Mr. Smith, I am going to need to put a catheter into your bladder and a tube into your chest, OK?" The perfunctory grunt or a feeble "OK" is taken to mean the surgeon has "quick permission." On other occasions the surgeon may say to the hypotensive patient, "You are going to need an operation, put your mark on this paper," or rush to the family and say, "We are on our way to the operating room; can you give us permission to operate? Please sign quickly." The clinical ethical goal is to show as much respect for patients as is possible under rushed and difficult circumstances. Insofar as is possible, authorization is sought from the patient. As time allows, more is said regarding the procedure so as better to engage the patient's and the patient's surrogate decision maker's understanding of and agreement regarding what should take place.

Surrogate Consent. Time permitting, when a patient is not competent to consent, and when there is a valid surrogate decision maker available, the consent of that valid surrogate should be obtained before an emergency intervention is undertaken. Generally, surrogate decision makers who do not serve under proxy appointments with special instructions can only choose among those therapeutic options that would fall within the range of choices embraced by reasonable and prudent persons. Surrogate decision makers thus serve to protect the best interests of the patient in choosing among reasonable options as the patient would have chosen. In so choosing, they not only protect the patient's view of best interests, but serve as an extension of the patient's autonomy. Surrogates are often poor authorities regarding a patient's best interests, though they may be in authority to make certain choices.[10-12] Without special authorization, they do not have the moral standing to delay or deny an intervention needed immediately to save life or limb. For example, the religious conviction of the surrogate may be different from the person over whom he serves as a proxy and cannot be imposed on the patient. A Jehovah's Witness may not deny an emergency blood transfusion to a person who has not validly asked for such a withholding of a lifesaving treatment. So, too, when the surgeon judges that a minor child must immediately have blood to save life, Jehovah's Witness parents legally may not deny blood transfusions to their children who are immature minors. When the parents or the surrogates refuse permission, a process for seeking the advice of the court and an alternative surrogate decision maker such as an ad litem attorney is usually provided by most hospital by-laws and required by law. Also, should a parent (especially a mother) of a minor require blood products or other interventions in order to prevent death, and the death of the patient would result in an orphan, some hospital policies and state law have allowed for the imposition of a surrogate decision maker to protect the minor's interest.

In some situations, when the family or surrogate decision maker reaches a conclusion totally different from the previous wishes of the patient or the surgeon's considered judgment of the patient's best interests, and if the patient is incompetent, the surgeon's responsibility is to protect the patient's authoritative past wishes or the patient's best interests and to deal kindly with the surrogate decision maker and the family. When conflicts arise, various methods of conflict resolution should be considered, including consultations from multiple physicians, attorneys, hospital administrators as well as the Ethics Committee of a hospital. When patients cannot choose for themselves and a surrogate decision maker has become involved in the case, the surgeon is bound by hospital policy and state and federal laws. In general, however, the surrogate decision maker has only the moral right to choose among those interventions that would be accepted by reasonable and prudent persons. Without past authorization of the patient, a surrogate decision maker does not have the moral right to demand intervention that would be considered harmful by the surgeon.

In the absence of a family member, surrogate consent may be given by the courts. Different jurisdictions have different definitions concerning when and how a judge or an ad litem attorney may participate in decision making for permission to perform emergency surgery. Under rare circumstances, some hospitals have a policy stipulating that emergency surgery can be performed if three independent physicians (the "three doctor rule") write a note in the chart that a family member cannot be found, that the patient is not competent, and that emergency surgery is required. All these various policies, when appropriate, reflect a moral concern to protect the best interests of the patient, to provide some protective process when possible, and to give at least a symbolic acknowledgment of the significance of patient autonomy.

The Family, Moral Authority, and Confidentiality in the Context of Treating the Emergency Patient. Communication with family and friends of the patient is an important part of the art of medicine. The surgeon must remember, however, that under some emergency circumstances the patient may not wish for information to be communicated to even the closest of family members or friends (see Chapter 3). Certain diseases and/or conditions representing communicable diseases must be reported by law. From a public health standpoint, family and other associates of the patient may need some information because of a legal obligation to protect third parties. Under some circumstances, such as a drug overdose or when an injury has occurred at an unfavorable location or time, an adult fully alert patient may have good reason specifically to request that family not receive information concerning the patient's emergency surgical condition, even if they would otherwise be the legally designated surrogate decision makers. Under such circumstances, alternative decision makers should be established. The surgeon should advise the use of a medical proxy to establish a decision maker outside of the family. Under such circumstances the surgeon's duty is to the patient rather than to the family. Under extremely rare conditions, the surgeon may even ask the hospital administration that the patient be admitted under an assumed name and be placed under a protective watch to maintain anonymity. In the absence of such a patient request, family surrogate decision makers have the legal right to understand the complexity of a patient's acute surgical condition, insofar as this is necessary for their serving as proxies.

Advance Directives. Patients can use advance directives to withhold authority even for emergency surgical interventions (see Chapter 4). However, there are practical difficulties in having such directives function in emergency settings. Family members may or may not be aware of such directives. Most emergency medical service personnel who arrive on the scene of an accident do not have access to advance directives. Therefore, emergency resuscitation, including establishment of an airway, and other resuscitation is usually begun at once. By the time a family member notifies the surgeon that an advance directive exists, the patient may already have been resuscitated, be on life support in an intensive care unit, or even be in an operating room. When advance directives have been appropriately executed, it is appropriate to follow the advance directive within the confines of the description of what may and may not be done under specific circumstances. In general, when there is unclear evidence that a patient might have desired a form of treatment or refused a particular treatment, such evidence is generally not binding, if it goes against the clear best interests of the patient needing an emergency intervention.

There has been a significant interest in increasing the ability of patients to have their advance directives honored, even in emergency situations. This has been reflected in the development of laws honoring out-of-hospital, do-not-resuscitate (DNR) orders, as well as special bracelets indicating that patients have completed an advance directive, have a terminal illness, and should not receive emergency medical intervention. In addition, given the increased ability securely to store information electronically, it will become ever more feasible to record electronically the availability of an advance directive, so that it can be accessed to increase the opportunity of patients to have their wishes known in emergency circumstances.

Even with an increased ability to store and access information regarding advance directives, one will still in most cases need to determine whether such directives apply in emergency circumstances. Most people who complete advance directives are not at that time suffering from a terminal or fatal illness. In completing an advance directive, most are expressing their wishes regarding the limitation of treatment when treatment will only prolong the process of dying.[13] Therefore, the onus will fall on the surgeon to determine whether the conditions of an advance directive apply. Insofar as time is of the essence, and insofar as laboratory and other data are difficult to acquire with dispatch, it may be necessary to initiate a trial of intervention to sustain life. As already observed, it may subsequently be justified to withdraw treatment. It should be at least as easy to withdraw treatment as withhold it, once one learns that the conditions of an advance directive have been fulfilled and that further treatment would be in violation of the established and applicable wishes of the patient. If such is not the policy, there will be a temptation to forgo appropriate trials of treatment.

Advance directives have their force only when they are expressed in a DNR order. If the condition of the patient becomes better appreciated after an emergency admission so that an initial judgment that the patient is terminal must be revised, making a living will no longer effective, a DNR order that may previously have appeared to be appropriate should then be rescinded. Many hospitals have a policy that a DNR order must be rewritten every 24 hours with a progress note indicating why the DNR order is still required. Instances have occurred in which a DNR order has been written during a crucial time in a patient's early treatment only subsequently to find that the patient has recovered sufficiently to go to a hospital nursing unit with a significantly improved long-term prognosis. On the nursing unit, the non-provision of resuscitation following a cardiac arrest might then violate the patient's wishes. A persisting DNR order would lead to the patient's not being resuscitated, because it would falsely indicate that the treatment was inappropriate or patient's consent had been withheld. DNR orders should be written for specific times for specific patient conditions and then reconsidered. This is especially the case with respect to evaluation within the context of emergency intervention. Once initial judgments can be reassessed and data appear that may not have been apparent during the emergency admission, the order must be revised at once. After the initial period of emergency intervention, the surgeon should develop a new rapport with the family and patient. The therapeutic contract for subsequent care and management should be developed anew.

Clinical Topics in Maintaining the Standard of Emergency Surgical Care

The ethical issues that bear on the relationship between the surgeon and the emergency patient cannot be fully understood until they are placed within concerns that go beyond this dyad and include the commitment of surgery to maintaining an appropriate standard of care for emergency patients in general. The sections that follow recast concerns regarding decision making, consent, and attention to patients and patient surrogates in terms of the appropriate character of the surgical care that should be offered to emergency patients. Understanding the nature of the appropriate standard of care has a bearing on the significance of futile treatment, inappropriate treatment, marginal treatment, and extraordinary treatment. Understanding the nature of the appropriate standard of care is foundational to the responses that surgeons ought to give to those who request treatment that appears inappropriate. Indeed, nearly all of the ethical issues that arise in the provision of surgical care to emergency patients are framed by conflicts of standards of care, standards fashioned by surgeons versus standards fashioned by other specialties, as well as constraints imposed by managed care organizations.

Responding to Inappropriate Demand for or Refusal of Surgery by the Patient or Patient's Surrogate Decision-Maker

Patients, through themselves and through their surrogates, have the right to withhold authorization for lifesaving treatment, even in emergency circumstances. They can thus deprive surgeons of the authority to provide appropriate care (see Chapter 2). When the treatment refused has an expectation of reversing a condition threatening life, limb, or serious health interests, the surgeon has a responsibility to continue attempting to gain consent in the face of a competent refusal. Yet patients do not have a right to demand inappropriate care, even in emergency circumstances. Surgeons are not ethically obligated to provide treatment that they reliably judge will cause more harm than benefit or that will violate appropriate standards of care. For example, if a patient who is in extremis and obviously terminal requests a surgical intervention that would cause more harm than benefit, the surgeon should carefully explain why the intervention is inappropriate. Simple, honest, and compassionate responses in such cases reflect the art of surgery more than its craft. If the surgeon judges that the surgery requested is unnecessary, that the surgery will not reverse a condition, that the surgery may make the patient worse, or that the surgeon is unprepared to perform the surgery, the surgeon should recommend against and should refuse to perform the surgery. Just because the surgeon is on call does not mean that a surgeon has an ethical obligation to perform a procedure that is unwarranted or is beyond that surgeon's capability. Surgeons who refuse to provide treatment because it would be inappropriate should record their judgments and the grounds for their judgments in the progress notes. Patients and their surrogates should be put on notice that they must seek some other surgeon, if available, to provide the care they wish. Should the patient refuse to accept the recommendations of the surgeon, the physician and patient have the option of seeking another caregiver, unless it is a treatment that clearly violates the established standard of care (i.e., involves a modality of treatment that has not been medically proven). Surgeons are ethically obligated not to provide harmful care, even if there is no other physician available.

When the surgeon is the only caregiver available and the patient or patient surrogate demands treatment the surgeon deems inappropriate, involvement of the administration of the hospital or other legal entities may be necessary. In some instances a psychiatric consult may be sought to determine whether or not the patient is competently requesting inappropriate treatment. If the surgeon cannot persuade the patient to accept appropriate care, the patient does not have the moral authority to force the surgeon to accept the wishes of the patient, if in the best judgment of the surgeon the request of the patient or the surrogate decision maker would be harmful. The surgeon should carefully and kindly review the grounds for this judgment. When in doubt, traditional assumptions should guide the surgeon: procedural details should not delay treatment needed immediately to save life, limb, or serious health interests in the absence of a clear and competent refusal.

Institutions also have an ethical obligation to avoid providing inappropriate care, as well as to assist surgeons in avoiding the provision of such care. This institutional ethical obligation can often be met by the creation of review processes, bioethics consultation procedures, as well as the establishment of institutional futility policies.[14] As with surgeons, institutions have an ethical obligation to develop policies proactively, so as to create procedures as well as clear understandings of how surgeons will be assisted in making difficult decisions on behalf of maintaining appropriate standards of emergency surgical care. Because emergency decisions require speedy response, institutional policies should be designed to take into account the special decision-making burden that emergency decisions place on surgeons.

The Relationship Between the Surgeon and Emergency Physicians

Virtually all surgical associations and surgical practice guidelines mandate that surgical conditions (especially in emergency situations) are in the domain of a surgeon. The emergency physician in many instances is a key member of the team (see Chapters 15 and 16), but the emergency physician's primary duty is to identify an emergency surgical problem and promptly summon the appropriate surgical specialists to provide the cognitive and technical care of the patient. The standards of surgical care for an emergency surgical condition are established by surgeons, not emergency physicians or any other disciplines of medicine. For a life-threatening emergency surgical condition, from the moment that the surgeon is contacted, the surgeon is the patient's physician. The emergency physician becomes the consultant. In all instances the patient's primary physician (in this instance the surgeon) is responsible for orders, decisions, and therapeutic interventions. It is inappropriate for other physicians to superimpose their opinions or therapeutic interventions on the patient unless so requested or allowed to do so by the primary physician. By its very nature, emergency medicine does not dedicate sufficient time during residency training or practice to develop surgical judgment or surgical technique. The emergency medicine curriculum is designed to develop skills to recognize the need for a surgical intervention, not to perform the cognitive or technical tasks required for surgical decision making. Should the emergency physician attempt to perform surgical procedures or surgical decision making, thereby delaying a request for a surgeon in an emergency surgical situation, the surgeon has the duty to pursue through the hospital quality assurance mechanism a review of such interference as a violation of practice guidelines.

Dealing with Managed Care Organizations

Managed care organizations (MCOs) under different names and structures are increasing their penetration into the medical marketplace (see Chapters 17, 18, and 19). They are dramatically altering practice patterns among all physicians, even practice involving emergency surgical patients. The emergency surgical patient presenting to a regional emergency care facility such as a trauma, burn, heart, resuscitation, or critical care center presents special problems by creating a potential conflict between the MCO and the surgeon treating an emergency surgical condition. Economic and ethical issues immediately arise. The problem is most acute when a patient with a complex emergency surgical condition requiring an extensive and expensive workup and treatment presents to a facility that is not one of the prearranged facilities of the managed care organization. Issues of notification, authorization, clearance, and expenditures are immediately imposed on an arena where the surgeon is concerned with developing as complete a database as possible while urgently seeking to provide critical care and/or surgical intervention to the patient. MCOs for their part are also focused on maintaining an acceptable level of costs for their subscribers by avoiding marginally useful diagnostic and therapeutic interventions, including marginally useful hospitalizations. MCOs therefore attempt to avoid hospitalizations of their patients unless medically necessary. They are also focused on minimizing hospital costs through practice guidelines, prepaid contracts, and the like. They wish to avoid having their patients hospitalized in institutions where they cannot easily exert control over costs.

The habits of surgeons in approaching emergency surgical conditions and those directing an MCO are often at awesome counter-purposes. Prime examples are the inquiries generated by MCO clerks regarding emergency surgical patients admitted in life-threatening emergencies to trauma centers or hospitals affiliated via the emergency medical services (EMS) systems of a city. Such patients are frequently unstable in the intensive care unit and require multiple operations that are often beyond the scope or ability of the hospital affiliated with the managed care organization. Despite this, numerous inquiries are frequently made under the guise of attempting to save money by transferring the patient, if possible, to the hospital affiliated with the patient's plan. These inquiries are generated even in emergencies because of the standing focus on controlling costs. Their intent is often inconsistent with the surgeon's moral responsibility to the patient.

Even when the treating surgeon gets through to the medical director of the MCO to indicate the appropriateness of the care being provided and the inappropriateness of a hospital transfer, there may be innumerable, interminable, and time-consuming questions required to justify the continued hospitalization in the tertiary care facility of the hospital to which the patient was admitted on an emergency basis. The surgeon must always defend the patient's best interests. If an institution fails to support the surgeon in this, the surgeon has an ethical obligation to inform the patient or patient's surrogate of the risks involved in any transfer. The surgeon must weigh the ethical obligation of caring for the patient with the prior financial arrangements made by the patient through membership in a particular MCO. Such an assessment should focus on the patient's continued critical condition, planned reoperations, and the capability of the physicians at the managed care planned hospital to which the patient may be transferred to provide adequate care. The physician should honestly disclose to the patient or the patient's surrogate risks to health and finances involved in choices regarding the locus of treatment. Furthermore, once a patient is transferred from the surgeon at the tertiary care facility, that patient is most often transferred not to another surgeon, but to a "gatekeeper" who then decides to which specialist the patient should be referred. These decisions are often driven as much by financial concerns as by concerns regarding the quality of care. Until the patient or the patient's surrogate agrees to a transfer, the surgeon should attempt to maintain the standard of care and inform relevant persons regarding risks.

Morally Inappropriate Treatment

Surgeons may find themselves asked to provide or withdraw treatment in manners they find morally objectionable. Patients have a robust right to refuse life-saving treatment. A surgeon in some circumstances may find it morally impossible to be involved in the care of a patient when the surgeon considers the treatment requested to be immoral. Surgeons possess as much of a moral right to their own moral and religious integrity as do patients. Unlike patients, surgeons have the obligation to be clear in advance about their moral commitments regarding the provision or non-provision of treatment. They should understand their own moral views prior to being confronted by a patient with a particular problem. As physician-assisted suicide and euthanasia become legally accepted in the United States, many surgeons will recognize that they are morally and religiously obliged neither to provide such treatment nor even to refer for treatment. The latter may involve significant legal hazards. Surgeons must be clear about their moral and religious commitments, as well as the price of moral and religious integrity. Institutions with special moral and religious commitments will face similar hazards.

Maintaining the Standard of Care in Interactions with Police, Adult, and Child Protective Services and Other Governmental Agencies

The surgeon encountering patients with emergency surgical conditions interacts with numerous governmental and quasi-governmental agencies, including the city, county, and state police; drug enforcement agencies; alcohol, tobacco, and firearms agencies; child and adult protective services; health departments; disease registries, and so on. The federal, state, and local laws, as well as quasi-laws under the guise of federal, state, and local regulations include multiple new laws and regulations. MCOs, including health maintenance organizations (HMO), preferred provider organizations (PPO), and other entities, have their own set of regulations and paperwork. The entirety of these regulatory oversights consume up to one third of a surgeon's time and effort. In all of this, health care and especially surgery are the surgeon's primary responsibility. The enforcement of laws and regulations is primarily the responsibility of government and law enforcement and the quasi-governmental agencies. The moral rule of thumb to both is generally to "each his own," insofar as that is possible. The surgeon has a duty to comprehend and know about applicable laws, regulations and guidelines. Under emergency situations, these laws, regulations and guidelines may at times interfere with evaluation and treatment. The surgeon's primary responsibility is to the health and welfare of the patient who presents in an emergency surgical condition. When turf issues tend to arise, consultation with hospital administration, chiefs of service and chiefs of staff, and even the legal administration of the hospital and surgical practice, may be necessary. Surgeons may even at times find themselves ethically obligated to ignore the law. In such cases, they should understand the consequences.

Clinical Conclusions

Emergency patients present with problems that require immediate evaluation and intervention to save life, limb, or serious health injury. Decisions must be made under circumstances of constrained time, the perception of such constraint, and an emotional sense of urgency. The data available to guide choices are often soft and require further evaluation. Often, that evaluation will not be available until after a decision must be made. The data regarding the patient's competence are also frequently soft, and a full ascertainment of the patient's ability to choose can only be completed after an intervention is necessary. Within these constraints, surgeons must act to respect patients and protect their best interests. They must do this while attempting to maintain the standards of good emergency surgical care, often in the face of interventions by various third parties. With respect to particular cases, as well as to maintain good health care policy to protect emergency patients, surgeons must remember that theirs is one of the three traditional learned professions. This will require aiding patients, surrogate decision-makers, and the families of patients, not to mention MCOs and other institutions, to come to terms with the painful limits of finitude. Surgeons as doctors and as teachers must instruct patients regarding our human finitude, which limits choices especially in emergency circumstances. Surgeons have much to contribute to our culture's appreciation of how to use possible life-saving interventions in the press and urgency of emergent needs.

References

1. H. Tristram Engelhardt, Jr., *The Foundations of Bioethics*, 2nd ed. New York: Oxford University Press, 1996.
2. Stephen Wear, *Informed Consent: Patient Autonomy and Physician Beneficence within Clinical Medicine*. Dordrecht: Kluwer, 1993.
3. Henrik Wulff, *Rational Diagnosis and Treatment*, 2nd ed. London: Blackwell Scientific, 1981.
4. H. Tristram Engelhardt, Jr., and George Khushf, "Futile Care for the Critically Ill Patient," *Current Opinion in Critical Care* 1 (1995): 329–333.
5. Society of Critical Care Medicine Ethics Committee, "Consensus Statement on the Triage of Critically Ill Patients," *Journal of American Medical Association* 271 (1994): 1200–1203.
6. Michael A. Rie, "Ethical Issues in Intensive Care: Criteria for Treatment Within the Creation of a Health Insurance Morality," in *Critical Choices and Critical Care*, Kevin Wm. Wildes., ed. Dordrecht, The Netherlands: Kluwer Academic Publishers, 1995, pp. 23–56.
7. Nancy M. P. King, *Making Sense of Advance Directives*, rev. ed. Washington, DC: Georgetown University Press, 1996.
8. Thomas Grisso and Paul Appelbaum, "Comparison of Standards for Assessing Patient's Capacity to Make Treatment Decisions," *American Journal of Psychiatry* 152 (1995): 1033–1037.
9. James F. Drane, "Competency to Give an Informed Consent," *Journal of the American Medical Association* 252 (August 17, 1984): 925–27.
10. Marion Danis, Joanne Garrett, Russell Harris, et al., "Stability of Choices about Life-sustaining Treatments," *Annals of Internal Medicine* 120 (1994): 567–573.
11. Linda Emanuel, Ezekiel Emanuel, John Stoeckle, et al., "Advance Directives: Stability of Patients' Treatment Choices," *Archives of Internal Medicine* 154 (1994): 90–96.
12. Joel Tsevat, E. Francis Cook, Michael L. Green, et al., "Health Values of the Seriously Ill," *Annals of Internal Medicine* 122 (1995): 514–520.
13. Anita W. Broadwell, Eugene V. Boisaubin, J. Kay Dunn, and H. Tristram Engelhardt, Jr., "Advance Directives on Hospital Admission," *Southern Medical Journal* 86 (1993): 165–168.
14. Baruch A. Brody and Amir Halevy, "A Multi-institution Collaborative Policy on Medical Futility," *Journal of American Medical Association* 276 (1996): 571–574.

6

Acute, High-Risk Patients:
The Case of Transplantation

ROBERT M. ARNOLD
BYERS W. SHAW
RUTH PURTILO

Acute, high-risk surgery involves operations on patients who often face a significant risk of morbidity and mortality without surgery, but for whom surgery itself involves significant risk of morbidity and mortality. Indeed, nonsurgical management may clearly involve higher risk than surgical management, making surgical management seem an obvious choice. Thus, at first glance, the informed consent process for surgery for these patients seems straightforward. Information should be provided to the patient, as described in Chapter 2, and a recommendation for surgery made.

On closer examination, matters are not quite so straightforward. High-risk surgery requires patients to balance a better long-term survival against a significant short-term risk of mortality and morbidity. Informing patients of the various operative and nonoperative statistics is thus critically important. What and how much information to give will be discussed in this chapter. Institutional and economic changes in the way surgery is practiced raise new issues for the consent process.

Organ transplantation involves an important and unique subpopulation of acute, high-risk surgical patients. Ethical issues in transplantation are not addressed at length elsewhere in this volume. As the reader knows, for heart and liver transplantation, the alternative to transplantation is almost certain death, yet surgery itself is often high risk. We therefore address challenges to the informed consent process for transplantation. We also consider a number of clinical topics that are especially pertinent to organ transplantation, especially those that pertain to allocation of scarce resources.

Ethical Analysis and the Management of Scarcity

Informed Consent

As discussed in Chapter 2, informed consent is the primary means of promoting a patient's autonomy in the surgeon-patient relationship. Before the 1960s, the traditional ethic guiding physician behavior was beneficence. In other words, the surgeon did what he or she thought was best for the patient. The patient's role was largely passive and consisted of assenting to or refusing therapy. Informed consent is based on the principle that the patient's view of his or her interests, rather than the surgeon's, should guide clinical decision making. According to this theory, although the surgeon and the patient may negotiate decision making jointly, the patient is the final arbitrator of what should be done to his or her body.[1]

In order to promote the patient's ability to participate in decision making, the surgeon must ensure that the patient understands the risks and benefits of the proposed therapy, as well as the most common alternative therapies. One controversial issue is how much information the surgeon must provide a patient. Legally, the most common standard, the reasonable person standard, states that surgeons must provide information that a reasonable person would need to know in deciding whether to undergo the proposed treatment.[2] Ethically, the surgeon should also provide any other information that he or she believes a particular patient might need to make an informed decision (see Chapter 2). Two issues regarding consent are especially pertinent to acute, high-risk patients; disclosure of surgeon- or institution-specific operative risks; and for transplantation, the use of "marginal donors."

Disclosure of Operative Statistics. The reasonable person standard obliges physicians to tell patients about a therapy's likely complications. In particular, if a treatment is more likely to result in injury, disease, or a patient's death than an alternative, the patient should be informed of these facts. Information pertinent to such disclosure exists in computerized databases that collect data on surgeon-specific mortality rates for procedures. In 1988, the Health Care Financing Administration (HCFA) released data regarding hospital mortality rates for Medicare patients. Subsequently, both New York State and Pennsylvania released statistics regarding hospital- and physician-specific data for open heart surgery. Recently, federal data regarding hospital-specific mortality for transplantation has been published.[3-5] This information and subsequent reports in the medical literature show large differences in hospital-specific mortality. For example, 2-year survival for liver transplantation ranges from 60% to over 85%, with larger programs having better survival rates.[6] Data on cardiopulmonary bypasses also show wide institution-specific differences. Institutional differences are probably as important as surgeon-specific differences because a patient's outcome is greatly influenced by the care and attention of the surgery team. Provider- and institution-specific data will become more pervasive with the growth of outcomes-based research. The question thus arises, "Should surgeons tell high-risk patients about either the surgeon's personal or the hospital's morbidity and mortality data?"

At first glance, the answer seems to be "yes." What reasonable person, facing high-risk surgery, would not want to know if his or her surgeon's outcomes were better or worse than another doctor he or she might see? Informed consent seems to require that a surgeon discuss his or her mortality statistics and explain to the patient how they differ from those of other surgeons, especially when the difference is substantial. Indeed, one state supreme court has taken just this view, a case discussed in Chapter 2.

Some surgeons object to this argument. In their opinion, not only should these statistics not be required as part of informed consent, they should not be released to the public. They fear that the release of provider-specific data to the public will be misinterpreted by patients, will unfairly treat or even libel surgeons, and may lead to poorer patient care.[3]

Let us examine the claim that patients cannot interpret the data. Informed consent assumes that given sufficient time, patients will be able to understand the risks and benefits of surgery and its alternatives. Effective informed consent also assumes that it is the surgeon's obligation to explain complex information in a way that the patient can understand and appreciate.[7] For example, with sufficient education a patient contemplating a renal transplant can understand the risks and benefits of a transplant and the subsequent immunosuppressants, as well as the risks and benefits of dialysis. It is unlikely that the ordinary patient who sufficiently comprehends this information will not be able to understand comparative statistics rating various surgical programs. In the context of effective consent the worry about patients misinterpreting comparative data seems unfounded.

A different objection concerning the release of comparative statistics is, however, more tenable: the data are misleading or inaccurate and thus should be withheld from patients to avoid confusing them.[8,9] There are several reasons one might be concerned about the accuracy of available statistics. The most common concern is that the data are not sufficiently risk-adjusted. Thus, surgeons or institutions that treat acute, high-risk patients may have poorer ratings, leading patients to assume, incorrectly, that these surgeons are worse than those with higher ratings. If forced to disclose these statistics to patients, surgeons might respond out of self-interest and refuse to operate on higher-risk patients. A recent survey found that less than 10% of Pennsylvania cardiologists and cardiac surgeons who responded discussed data regarding surgeon- or hospital-specific risk-adjusted differences in mortality for coronary artery bypass graft (CABG) with more than 10% of their patients. Complaining of inadequate risk adjustment and unreliable data, 63% of surgeons surveyed said that release of this data made them less willing to operate on severely ill patients.[9]

This objection emphasizes that the organization, typically the government or a third-party payer, releasing the provider-specific information has an ethical obligation to ensure that any data released are accurate and as free from potential bias as possible, are presented in ways that don't mislead (e.g., risk-adjusted versus "raw" data), and have a clear statistical relationship to providers' future performances. If different statistical models result in differences in surgeons' performance, the differences should be noted, and assumptions underlying the particular models used should be explained in a manner understandable by the intended user of the information.

However, we believe that refusing to provide any surgeon-specific outcomes data is too extreme. First, no model can perfectly adjust for the multitude of patient, surgeon, or institutional variables that influence morbidity and mortality. Thus, the data will never entirely reflect reality. However, the information that patients currently use to choose providers also does not perfectly reflect surgeons' quality. One would need to show that the haphazard qualitative data that patients are now using to select surgeons is more equitable than any system that attempts to measure the quality of care, a very difficult, if not impossible, task. Second, a variety of models are available for measuring surgeon- and institution-specific quality of care. These alternative models have different methodological biases. A surgeon can present the model he or she believes most accurately represents his or her skill and explain why he or she has chosen this presentation. Alternatively, the surgeon can discuss why he or she believes that the model does not adequately reflect her or his skill.

Finally, what should we do if, as a result of the ethical requirement that surgeons tell patients about their surgical statistics, surgeons refuse to operate on sicker patients? There is a long moral tradition in medicine that requires physicians to put their patients' interests ahead of their own self-interests. This is called a fiduciary relationship and is based on the fact that patients are in a vulnerable position, both because of their sickness and because of their lack of knowledge about medicine. The codes of ethics of both the American Medical Association (AMA) and the American College of Surgeons (ACS) stress the centrality of the fiduciary relationship. Thus, an ethical surgeon would not make a decision about whether to operate on a patient based on the effect of that decision on his or her statistical rating.

Limits on Disclosure. Some argue that requiring surgeons to provide statistical information to patients about success rates opens up a Pandora's box, in which surgeons must tell patients an endless number of surgeon- or institution-specific details. How does one decide what information a patient may want to know? Does a surgeon need to tell the patient how he or she did in medical school or on surgery rotations? What about Board scores? Are these relevant and necessarily reportable? Less tangible factors, such as fatigue or personal distractions, may also influence a surgeon's performance. Is a surgeon obligated to provide this information to a patient? These questions should be addressed in terms of the relationship between the information in question and the outcomes variables about which a reasonable patient facing high-risk surgery can be expected to be concerned. How a surgeon did in his or her third-year surgical clerkship is at best only tangentially related to his or her skill as a surgeon. This is not information that a surgeon is required to tell a patient. On the other hand, a reasonable patient would probably want to know his or her surgeon's experience and expertise in performing the required surgery. The stronger the correlation of the information to the surgery's success, the stronger the obligation for the surgeon to inform the patient of its existence. The justification for this approach is that in acute, high-risk surgery, effective informed consent requires that the patient have sufficient information to make a decision that maximizes his or her values, which are seriously at stake because of the very nature of high-risk surgery. Which surgeon to choose is just as important a decision as whether to have the surgery. These assessments may be appropriately influenced by differences in outcomes.

Informed Consent and Changes in the Organization of Surgery. Changes in the way health care is dispensed and provided may have a profound impact on informed consent. Increasingly, patients are finding their choice of providers being dictated, at least to some degree, by their insurers. For example, many insurers contract with one or two surgical teams to perform expensive high-risk surgery, such as CABGs or liver transplantations. To function more efficiently, surgeons in such settings function as interchangeable units. For instance, the surgeon who interviews a patient preoperatively in the office for lung reduction surgery may not be the same surgeon who performs the operation a week later. These changes in the organization of surgery have several implications. First, under this system of payment, responsibility for providing informed consent shifts away from individual surgeons and onto the team of surgeons. The outcomes statistics most relevant to the patient are the team's statistics, not an individual surgeon's performance figures. Second, in this environment the critical question has changed from which surgeon to choose to which institutional provider to choose. A reasonable person choosing an insurance company might want to know how an insurance company decides to contract with some rather than other surgeons where the patient lives and works. According to the requirements of informed consent as explained in Chapter 2, the insurance company or managed care organization (MCO) should be required to provide potential clients with information about the criteria it uses to select providers. This requirement includes information about the weight given to outcome statistics versus their price differential. Many insurance companies would object to providing this information, arguing that the information is proprietary data needed to maintain a competitive advantage over other MCOs. Whether MCOs should be subject to the principles of health care ethics rather than business is of growing importance (see Chapter 19).

Informed Consent Issues in Transplantation: Marginal Donors. Medical unsuitability is the most common reason for rejecting a family's offer of a liver for transplantation. In Europe, for example, of 1,240 potential donors, 511 livers were not used. In 374 of these cases, the reason for rejecting the organ was because of medical unsuitability.[10] Organ procurement organizations often unilaterally reject possible donors because of age or specific medical conditions.

Many of these "medical contraindications" are based on expert opinion, rather than objective data documenting that individuals who receive these organs have greater morbidity or mortality. The growing shortage of organ donors has led centers to reevaluate these guidelines. For example, the age restrictions for renal and liver donors have been modified from less than 55 years of age to up to 75 or even 80 years of age. Other centers are taking donors who have either diseases or organ abnormalities that, in the past, have precluded donation.[11,12]

What should potential recipients be told about such "marginal candidates"? Currently, recipients are given only relatively general information about the donor such as age, race, and sometimes the cause of death. There is little reason to give other personal or social information, because there are no medical data suggesting that these characteristics influence the patient's outcome. A reasonable person thus has no justification for obtaining more detailed information about the donor.

Would a reasonable person want to know that his or her organ comes from a "marginal donor?" At first glance, the answer is obviously "yes." The "average" risk that an organ won't function should already have been described to the patient and accepted prior to his or her being placed on the waiting list. Assume that a "marginal donor" organ has a significantly higher risk of failure post transplant. If a surgeon intends to subject the patient knowingly to a risk that is substantially greater than average, then there is an undeniable obligation to inform the patient or the patient's surrogate.

Some might object to this claim, arguing that the increased risk does not matter to an acutely ill patient who will die without a transplant. Why should surgeons have to give such a patient information that will not change his or her decision?

This argument misinterprets the ethical requirements of informed consent. Ethically, informed consent requires that the patient understand both what is going to be done and that he or she has the final decision to authorize whether or not it should be done (see Chapter 2). The fact that the patient is highly likely to consent to the procedure regardless of the information is irrelevant to the issue of granting authority to the surgeon to perform an operation or procedure. The information may be valuable in preparing the patient regarding what his or her future is likely to involve. Data indicate that when a patient is told about his or her surgery and the likely postoperative course, he or she recovers more quickly.[13] The information may lead one to take preparatory steps before the operation. Knowing that the surgery is highly risky, a patient may be more likely to get his or her personal affairs in order (see Chapter 10). Even if the information does not change the patient's behavior at all, some argue that the theory of informed consent requires that the patient be told because of his or her right to know what is going to be done to his or her body.

It is also not obvious whether this information might change some patients' decisions regarding transplantation. While it is unlikely to change the decision of a critically ill patient waiting for a liver transplant, it may affect the decision-making process for less critically ill patients or those awaiting non-irreplaceable organs. For example, a patient who is doing well with dialysis may decide to forgo a higher-risk renal transplant to wait for a "good donor."

A more powerful objection to requiring that surgeons tell patients about "marginal donors" is that the data often do not support their designation as "marginal." Remember that the designation of a donor as marginal is not based on outcomes studies. The criteria for acceptable donors are based on experts' beliefs about how well an organ will do if transplanted. These beliefs were often formulated over a decade ago, when preservation and intraoperative and postoperative techniques were in their infancy.

Recent studies have shown similar one-year outcomes for marginal and normal heart, liver, and kidney transplants.[14,15] If these numbers are replicated by other studies, then one could conclude that marginal donors produce outcomes similar to those of traditional donors. The obligation to provide more information to patients about marginal donors hinges on the assumption that these organs place the patient at a significantly higher risk than that to which they had previously consented. If this turns out not to be the case, the obligation to provide patients with more information about marginal donors disappears. Indeed, the phrase would then justifiably no longer be used.

For many types of marginal donors, insufficient data exist about the short- and long-term outcomes. What should be done in instances in which there is professional opinion but no empirical data about marginal donors' effectiveness? Most people would want to know that, despite the lack of empirical information, there is a professional consensus that these organs have a significantly higher expected rate of failure than "non-marginal"organs. It is also appropriate to tell patients about the limits of medical knowledge. Informed consent requires helping the patient understand the situation so that he or she can make an educated decision (see Chapter 2). Sometimes, to understand a situation, the patient needs to understand what is not known as much as what is known. For example, to make an informed decision regarding whether to have a partial lobectomy for emphysema, the patient would need to understand that the medical community is uncertain whether the surgery works. The patient also needs to understand the reason, in spite of this uncertainty, that the surgeon believes that it is reasonable to undergo the procedure.[16] Similarly, in these cases of uncertainty, a surgeon should inform the patient of the surgeon's concerns regarding the organ's quality and how this might affect the patient's postoperative course. The surgeon can also talk with the patient about why the surgeon believes that proceeding with the surgery is, despite these increased risks, in the patient's interest.

These requirements for informed consent parallel surgeons' ethical obligations in high-risk surgery. However, there are pragmatic issues in transplantation that may limit the requirements for informed consent in this particular setting. One of the unique features of transplantation is its dependence on a nonrenewable resource—the organs. Requiring extensive informed consent about specific organs' "marginal quality" may exacerbate the shortage. Organs have a very specific, relatively short, shelf-life. Thus, after procuring the organ from a donor, there is a relatively short window of opportunity to get the organ to the potential recipient and perform the surgery. Imagine that the first possible recipient, after learning about the donor-specific qualities, refuses surgery. One would then go to the next potential recipient and begin the same process again. It is possible that requiring this process repetitively may increase "wastage" of organs, thus exacerbating the shortage of organs. In these cases, there may be a conflict between the surgeon's obligation to ensure adequately informed consent and the attempt to optimize the benefit one can obtain from scarce organ resources.

Whether this conflict would justify a modification of the informed consent process is likely to be controversial. The answer will depend on answers to questions such as, can harm be avoided and full information be provided? Surgeons might be able to talk to patients prior to the specific situation about whether they would be willing to accept marginal donors. What is the magnitude of the harm of providing full information? How many patients will refuse marginal donors and thus, how many organs will be wasted if surgeons are required to provide more information? It is unlikely that many liver or heart transplant recipients, for example, will refuse even marginal donors. Still, this theoretical conflict between individual autonomy and the social harm caused by the shortage of organs marks transplantation surgery and will arise again.

Clinical Topics in Organ Transplantation

The process by which a patient with end-stage organ failure obtains an organ consists of a variety of steps, each of which raises ethical issues. Here we consider institutional policy, ability to pay, age-related criteria, exclusion based on alcoholism, the changing financial environment and decisions to list a patient, and national allocation criteria.

Institutional Policy

A central principle in most ethical theories, emanating from considerations of justice, is that similar cases should be treated in a similar fashion. To avoid violating this egalitarian principle, it is essential for the transplant team to develop and adhere to written policies regarding the criteria the team will use for accepting patients on their waiting list. Because organs are a societal resource, it is essential that the public have a central role in developing these policies.[17-20]

Ability to Pay

Once a patient is referred to a transplant center, his or her suitability for transplantation must be determined. One nonmedical factor used at most centers to determine if a patient should be listed is his or her ability to pay for the transplantation. Although this is not an issue for kidney transplantation, because of the federal end-stage renal disease program, it is an important consideration in heart, liver, and other organ transplants. Two major arguments are given in the literature for eliminating the patient's ability to pay as a criterion for being placed on the transplant list. First, some argue that it is unfair to treat extrarenal transplantation differently from other costly medical interventions with similar benefits. If society funds bone marrow transplantation for leukemia, a similarly costly and risky procedure, then it also ought to fund other transplantation. It is unfair to single out specific types of transplantation in an attempt to save money. (What ethical justification is there to fund renal but not liver transplantation?) This argument would preclude the development of state policies that would fund some expensive, high risk interventions but not transplantation. This argument, however, would not preclude a society from deciding not to fund any high-cost interventions for those who cannot afford insurance.

Second, it is argued that it is "unfair and even exploitative for society to ask people, rich and poor alike, to donate organs if access to donated organs will be determined by ability to pay rather than medical factors . . ."[21] Allowing commercialization of organ distribution but not procurement seems to harm the poor twice—they can neither reap the benefits of selling their organs nor receive the benefit of obtaining one. These two arguments have convinced most commentators that one's financial status should not be a criterion in determining whether or not one is eligible to receive an organ transplant.

Age-Related Criteria

The upper age limit for renal transplantation varies considerably across centers.[4] Most programs have not publicly justified the inclusion or exclusion of age-related criteria to determine eligibility for transplantation. This is unfortunate, because there are a variety of reasons, some more justifiable than others, for excluding elderly patients from receiving transplants. One argument is that elderly patients are less likely to do well after renal transplantation. Giving priority to patients with a greater possibility of benefit from medical treatment is widely accepted among both ethicists and policy makers. Whether the elderly actually do less well after transplantation, however, is controversial (at least for patients under 75 years of age). Moreover, how great the differences in benefit would have to be to be ethically significant is an issue about which reasonable people disagree.

How to define benefit is also controversial and complicates the claim that elderly do "less well" after major surgery. Is the surgery defined as a success solely if the patient lives a certain period of time? According to this criterion, the elderly may do as well as younger patients. Or does benefit assume that the patient has a certain quality of life?[1] The latter claim is adopted by those who argue that the elderly should have a lower priority for transplantation because their co-morbidities result in a lower quality of life.

There are two problems with this approach. First, when discerning the contraindications to a medical treatment, one should define the exclusion criteria precisely, so as not to exclude those who may benefit. The variables one really cares about, the patient's co-morbidities and functional status, are imperfectly correlated with age. Excluding a patient based on his or her age will exclude some elderly individuals with no co-morbidities who will do well after surgery. Given that important variables can be measured directly there is no need to use age as a surrogate variable. Second, and more serious, is the difficulty of determining what is meant by quality of life and deciding that the elderly have a lower quality of life than younger individuals. Quality of life is a very subjective concept, depending on an individual's values and life goals. There is no legitimate reason to insist that an elderly patient is less satisfied with his or her life than younger patients.

A different argument suggests placing an upper limit on an organ recipient's age, based on what constitutes a just allocation of societal resources. According to some, fairness—rather than probability of success—argues for giving priority to younger patients. This claim is controversial and is part of a larger argument about how resources should be distributed in a just health care system. It would be improper, we believe, for individual surgeons to make his or her decision to place a patient on the transplant list on the basis of this controversial line of reasoning.

Exclusion Based on Alcoholism

Alcoholism is another criterion used to exclude patients from transplantation, or to lower a patient's priority for liver transplantation. Because of the severe shortage of livers, either excluding or assigning a lower priority to patients with alcoholism may functionally serve the same purpose: these patients may be prevented from obtaining the necessary surgery in time. Four arguments justify excluding, or assigning lower priority to, patients suffering from alcoholism.[15,17,22,23]

The first argument asserts that patients with alcoholism should be assigned lower priority for liver transplantation for strictly medical reasons. Thus, some would give patients with alcoholism lower priority because it was believed that those patients would have a lower probability of benefit. However, a number of studies have shown that transplanted patients with chronic liver disease induced by alcoholism have survival rates similar to patients who require liver transplants for other reasons.[24] Moreover, recidivism rates, particularly in individuals who have stopped drinking for a period of time pre-transplant and/or are involved in rehabilitation, are low enough to make predictions of future abuse a weak indicator of transplant outcomes. Thus, there is insufficient medical justification for excluding patients with previous alcoholism who have begun abstaining in anticipation of transplantation. The statistics for patients who continue to drink actively are more controversial.

The second argument for excluding patients with alcoholism from transplantation is a belief that these individuals have caused the harm that they are suffering. Given the shortage of organs, some believe that it is ethically justifiable to distinguish between those who develop the disease "through no fault of their own" and those whose disease is a consequence of their own behavior. According to this view, patients can and should be held responsible for seeking and obtaining treatment for alcoholism. If a patient fails to receive treatment for his or her addiction and develops cirrhosis, he or she is partially to blame for his or her condition and thus should receive lower priority for organ transplantation.

This argument is controversial. The bulk of the literature argues that there is no ethical justification for discriminating against patients whose cirrhosis is induced by alcohol. Critics point out that consistency would require that transplants be denied to any patients who engaged in activities precipitating the need for organ replacement. Thus, patients who smoke and need a heart transplant due to ischemic cardiomyopathy, as well as those with end-stage renal disease related to non-compliance with hypertensive medications, would also have to be excluded from transplantation. But they are not and so patients with alcoholism should not be arbitrarily denied access to liver transplantation.

Attempts to determine patients' responsibility for medical conditions on the basis of lifestyles or activities introduce three problems. First, it is almost impossible to determine the degree to which a person's illness is due to voluntary behaviors versus genetic factors or environmental conditions. For example, research indicates that some individuals have a greater predisposition to alcoholism. Studies show, for example, that the effect of alcohol on one's liver is genetically determined. Women are more likely to suffer cirrhosis than men after correcting for the amount of alcohol imbibed. Thus, this policy would treat women more harshly for engaging in the same behavior as men. Second, the argument for patients' responsibility assumes that patients are aware of, and have access to, programs to alter their behavior. One should not hold individuals responsible for consequences they did not (and should not have) foreseen. Finally, these policies may result in an invasion of privacy. To gather the information needed to determine individual responsibility for disease will be very difficult and require intrusions into an individual's personal life. Given these problems, critics argue that assigning lower priority to patients with alcoholism is unfair.

A third argument for giving patients with alcoholism lower priority is that "those whose condition is a result of their morally blameworthy behavior ought be excluded from transplant candidacy because they don't deserve transplant."[22,25] This view places less emphasis on the reason for the liver failure and more on the potential candidate's moral behavior. By engaging in morally reprehensible behavior, patients with alcoholism deserve to be placed lower on the transplant list. This argument is also used as justification for withholding valve replacements from patients who abuse intravenous drugs. Arguing that liver failure due to alcohol abuse is "ethically worse" than that due to one's genetic structure assumes that there is an ethical prohibition against alcohol consumption. This view requires that we have access to the morally correct view—that is, a privileged conception of what constitutes morally reprehensible behavior. There is a general consensus that in a liberal society there "is absolutely no agreement—and there is likely to be none—about (what) constitutes moral virtue and vice and what rewards and penalties they deserve."[23]

A final argument for giving a lower priority to patients with alcoholism relies on their disadvantaged social status. According to this view, allocation of scarce resources should maximize social benefit. This argument is reflected by physicians and surgeons who complain that resources spent on noncompliant, socially disadvantaged patients would be better spent on others. The statement includes a strong judgment that an individual's value is synonymous with his or her social worth to others.

Three problems associated with determining an individual's social worth deter most analysts from supporting this position. First, some critics argue against prioritizing prospective transplant recipients using social worth criteria because such determinations overlook the moral equality of all patients. Second, how would one rank or compare an individual's contributions? Which are more important—aesthetic, political, or health-related contributions? Does a single CEO have a more social worth than an artist or a secretary who is the sole support of her extended family? Third, predicting an individual's life after transplantation and hence future social worth is even more difficult.

The Changing Financial Environment and Decisions to List a Patient

MCOs are now paying a flat fee for liver transplantation, determined by competitive bidding among a number of different centers. The ethical question is whether the estimated cost of a patient's transplant can be taken into account when deciding to list the patient. By listing healthier patients, a program can decrease the cost of transplantation, as well as increasing the probability of good morbidity and mortality statistics. If one surgery program engages in this process, called "cherry-picking," and another program does not, the latter program will have a higher cost per transplantation. If the cost exceeds what the MCO or insurance company is willing to pay, the latter program will become financially unattractive. To survive, the second program may also exclude higher risk, expensive patients from the waiting list. The result will be that patients who may be in the most dire need of transplantation would not be listed.

Most people agree that the cost of a patient's transplant is not an ethically relevant reason for excluding a patient (although sicker patients' high mortality may be a relevant reason). In today's fiscal environment, a program holding this position may not survive economically. This problem is the result of a system that prioritizes economic gains over other considerations. To correct cherry-picking, surgeons need to convince MCOs and payers to include nonfinancial factors in their decisions. Whether physicians will succeed in this complicated political process is unclear (see Chapters 17, 18, and 19).

National Allocation Criteria

Before 1987 there were no national policies regarding how patients on each hospital's waiting lists should be prioritized. Each organ procurement organization (OPO) devised its own process for determining how to allocate the organs procured. Often these criteria were not published and decisions were made informally by a few individuals (either surgeons or individuals in the OPO). A national task force criticized this policy in 1986, arguing that it resulted in unjustifiable inequities in distribution and that it did not rely on fair or publicly known procedures. A national organ procurement and transplantation network was subsequently mandated by federal legislation and is currently run by the United Network for Organ Sharing (UNOS). UNOS members include every transplant program, organ procurement organization, and tissue-typing laboratory in the United States. Policies governing the transplant community are developed by the UNOS membership through a series of regional meetings, deliberations at the national committee level, and final approval by an elected board of directors, equally representing physicians and non-physicians. The majority of non-physicians on the board have close professional or personal connections to organ transplantation, such as working for an OPO or having received a transplant. As a condition of receiving Medicare funds, hospitals and OPOs must be members of UNOS' national network, although compliance with UNOS' policies is currently voluntary.

In May 1987, UNOS established criteria for distributing organs. The latest statement of principles and objectives for equitable organ allocation was passed by UNOS in 1994.[25] This policy tries to "strike a balance" among the following ethical considerations: enhancing the overall availability of organs; allocating organs based on medical criteria (which itself requires a balancing between a patient's need for a transplant and the likelihood that the transplant will benefit the patient); equalizing patients' waiting times; and respecting patient autonomy.

Local Allocation. Currently, "organs are first made available for patients in the donor's local area . . . If no patient is available locally, organs are offered for patients within the donor's geographic area . . . and then nationwide."[26] The location of OPOs and preexisting city and state boundaries are used to define these "local areas." Unfortunately, these arbitrary definitions result in large variations—one to nine million—in the number of people located in a single "local area." Potential recipients are also not equally distributed throughout these "local areas," nor are transplant centers. The result is considerable disparity in waiting time relative to the location of one's chosen transplant center. For example, waiting time for kidneys ranges from 72 days (about 2.5 months) in one local area to 1,078 days (nearly 3 years) in another. These variations seem unfair.

Much could be done to decrease local inequities in waiting times. For example, given the improved ability to decrease cold ischemia time and transport organs, it might be possible to allocate organs over larger geographic areas. Moreover, UNOS could pay more attention to equity when defining what constitutes a local area. Currently, the local and regional areas are based on OPO service areas. These boundaries are established by the federal government and are not based on consistent geographic or population-based criteria. By taking into account the average number of organs procured per year, the distribution of transplant centers, and the geographic distribution of patients waiting for a transplant, it would be possible to redefine local areas, to decrease inter-regional inequities.

Institutional and economic pressures work against revising local boundaries to decrease inequities. Such revisions are likely to increase the number of organs going to busier transplant centers with longer waiting lists. Because the number of organs procured is relatively flat, this change would tend to decrease the number of organs that go to less active centers with shorter waiting lists. This decrease in transplantable organs will result in fewer transplants, and less revenue or prestige for a medical center trying to promote its transplant program. Such programs may therefore object to these changes, saying they favor larger, older transplant centers that have longer waiting lists. UNOS' governing body consists largely of OPO staff and representatives of all transplant programs, so its policies are likely to reflect the views of the numerous small and mid-sized programs rather than the largest centers.

These debates illustrate how transplant surgeons' own self-interest may come into conflict with developing just allocation systems. Organ transplantation, in addition to being a life-saving procedure, is also big business. Transplant centers bring their institutions prestige and money. The rules for determining organ distribution are made by those who have economic and personal interests in maximizing the number of organs that go to their center. One of us has characterized this situation as having the foxes guarding the chicken coop.[6]

Why, one might ask, should transplant surgeons be involved in determining the distribution rules in the first place? Organs are societal resources, rather than a commodity owned by transplant surgeons.[20] Moreover, the formulation of a rationing policy is not a medical question, but a philosophical one. The philosophical issues concern determining how to best balance important societal values. Thus, we believe that such decisions are better made by committees that are more representative of the entire community. Surgeons, under this model, could serve as an intellectual resource, but not as the primary decision makers. We believe that UNOS should seriously reevaluate who makes the rules regarding distribution and the credibility of this process.

The Case of Re-Transplantation—Justice and Efficacy.[27] Whether patients who need a re-transplant should get the same priority as those awaiting their first transplant is another ethical question that UNOS attempts to answer. Some transplant surgeons argue that patients who need a re-transplant should go to the top of the list. Surgeons believe that because they put in the organ that is now failing, they have an obligation to replace it with a new one.

Psychologically, it is understandable that surgeons find it difficult to watch a patient whom they have cared for die of organ failure. However, this does not justify giving patients needing re-transplants priority over patients who have never had a transplant. Three reasons argue against prioritizing re-transplants. First, the transplant surgeons often have relationships with patients prior to receiving a transplant. It is unclear why the fiduciary relationship with a patient whose first transplant "failed" is more important than the one developed with a patient who has never gotten a transplant or why a transplant surgeon's relationship with his or her patient is more important than the relationship other surgeons have with their patients with end-stage organ failure. Second, transplant surgeons are under no special obligation to fix the "wrong" of organ rejection. The patient undergoes transplantation in the anticipation that the new organ may save his or her life, but the procedure does not come with a guarantee. If the patient had not had a liver transplant in the first place, he or she would have already died. Third, even if a surgeon has a special relationship to the patient needing a re-transplant, this does not justify placing the patient higher on the transplant list. The surgeon's obligation is to do everything that he or she can, using the patient's resources, to promote the patient's well-being. This limits the scope of the surgeon's power. He or she cannot lie or steal, for example, to obtain resources to which the patient does not have a just claim. The question in this case is whether the patient who needs a re-transplant has a special claim overriding the claim of a new transplant candidate. The fact that the surgeon prefers performing a retransplant on a patient with whom that surgeon has developed a special relationship does not add ethically relevant weight to the situation. As previously explained, organs are a societal resource subject to principles of just distribution. In and of itself a transplant surgeon's relationships with a patient are not sufficient to give the patient priority for a transplantation.

An alternative position holds that a re-transplant candidate should have lower priority because he or she already had his or her chance at transplantation. This view is supported by our common-sense dictum that one should not get a second piece of pie before everyone gets one piece. However, this argument assumes that the only good requiring fair distribution is organs. A broader view of the health care resources pie takes into account previous access or use of health care resources. Imagine two candidates, one of whom has received a transplant. The transplanted individual had to struggle to overcome poverty and has had inadequate access to health care. Aside from her liver failure she is healthy and rarely hospitalized. The patient who is awaiting his first transplant, on the other hand, has multiple co-morbid conditions requiring hospitalizations, has excellent health insurance, and received superior medical care. Distributing the organ based on who has had less of the health care pie is less clear-cut in this case.

For this reason, the AMA and UNOS do not distinguish between transplant and re-transplant candidates. These organizations believe that allocation should be based primarily on the patient's medical needs and that "past use of resources is irrelevant to present need."[17]

One can agree that past use of resources is irrelevant to a just allocation system and still argue that re-transplant candidates should receive lower priority than primary transplant candidates. The UNOS system does take into account an individual's probability of successful transplantation. For example, both hearts and livers are preferentially distributed to individuals whose ABO types match the available organs because these patients, on average, are 20% more likely to survive.

The medical question is whether re-transplant candidates have similar survival rates when compared with candidates who are receiving their first transplant. There is general agreement, for example, that individuals who reject their first heart transplants within the first 30 days have a much higher mortality after a second transplant than do primary transplant candidates. It is inconsistent to factor efficacy into the allocation system in one case but not the other.

The survival advantage for primary liver and heart transplant candidates over re-transplant candidates is roughly 20%. For this difference to be ethically relevant, however, one needs to ascertain whether primary and re-transplant patients are equally ill. To turn re-transplant candidates away because they are sicker and therefore have a lower chance of survival seems to violate the surgeon's duty to help the most urgently ill patient. In these situations the UNOS policy would need to balance the conflict between efficacy and need.

Data comparing primary and re-transplant candidates with similar levels of acuity are controversial. Statistics vary, depending on the severity of illness scale used. We therefore recommend that UNOS convene a group of experts to periodically examine the survival data. If groups of re-transplant candidates have significantly lower survival rates than similarly situated primary transplant candidates, we believe the former should receive lower priority for transplantation. If the differences in outcome are due to differences in acuity of illness, UNOS should specifically address how it will balance the competing values of efficacy and need.

Clinical Conclusions

We have argued that the surgeon should disclose comparative outcomes-based statistics to high-risk surgical patients, inasmuch as this information would be of vital interest to the reasonable person confronted with the choices involved in acute, high-risk surgery. We have also argued that public disclosure of such information is appropriate, provided that this is done in ways that are not misleading. At the same time, we recognize appropriate limits on the consent process.

We also considered topics of informed consent that relate particularly to transplantation and have argued that where the use of organs from marginal donors affects outcomes, this information should be provided to potential recipients.

Because of its paradigmatic importance in acute, high-risk surgery, we have given particular consideration to transplantation and the ethical issues that it raises for surgeons. Transplantation differs from other aspects of medicine and surgery in one vital aspect: scarcity of organs is a highly visible and a controlling feature of the enterprise. This scarcity of organs forces transplant surgeons to deal more explicitly with ethical quandaries related to justice than do most other surgeons and physicians. We have argued for the necessity of ethically well-groomed institutional policy for determining who is listed for transplantation, and against using ability to pay, age, and a history of alcoholism as criteria for such listing. We also have raised doubts about UNOS' composition and their approach to local allocation of organs. Finally, we discussed the question of how to think about organs for re-transplantation.

References

1. President's Commission for the Study of Ethical Problems in Medicine and Biomedical and Behavioral Research, *Making Health Care Decisions: The Ethical and Legal Implications of Informed Consent in the Patient-Practitioner Relationship.* Washington, DC: US Government Printing Office, 1982.
2. Paul S. Appelbaum, Charles W. Lidz, and Alan Meisel, *Informed Consent: Legal Theory and Clinical Practice.* New York: Oxford University Press, 1987.
3. Darius F. Mirza, Bridget K. Gunson, Renato F. DaSilva, et al., "Policies in Europe on 'Marginal Quality' Donor Livers," *Lancet* 344 (1994): 1480–1483.
4. Mark V. Pauly, "The Public Policy Implications of Using Outcome Statistics," *Brooklyn Law Review* 58 (1992): 35–53.
5. Aaron D. Twerski and Neil B. Cohen, "Comparing Medical Providers: A First Look at the New Era of Medical Statistics," *Brooklyn Law Review* 58 (1992): 5–34.
6. Byers W. Shaw, "Something Juicy," *Liver Transplantation and Surgery* 2 (1996): 245–246.
7. Robert M. Arnold, Lachlan Forrow, and L. Randol Barker, "Medical Ethics and Doctor-Patient Communications," in *The Medical Interview*, Mack Lipkin, Sam M. Putnam and A. Lazarre, eds. New York: Springer, 1995, pp. 345–367.
8. Jesse Green, "Problems in the Use of Outcome Statistics to Compare Health Care Providers," *Brooklyn Law Review* 58 (1992): 55–73.
9. Eric C. Schneider and Arnold M. Epstein, "Influence of Cardiac Surgery Performance Reports on Referral Practices and Access to Care: A Survey of Cardiovascular Specialists," *New England Journal of Medicine* 335 (1996): 251–256.
10. Eythan Mor, Goran B. Klintmalm, Thomas A. Gonwa, et al., "The Use of Marginal Donors for Liver Transplantation. A Retrospective Study of 365 Liver Donors," *Transplantation* 53(1992): 383–386.
11. Eleanor L. Ramos, Betram L. Kasiske, Steven R. Alexander, et al., "The Evaluation of Candidates for Renal Transplantation: The Current Practice of U.S. Transplant Centers," *Transplantation* 57 (1994): 490–497.
12. Terri Randall, "Criteria for Evaluating Potential Transplant Recipients Vary Among Centers, Physicians," *Journal of the American Medical Association* 269(1993): 3091–3094.
13. Lawrence D. Egbert, George E. Battit, Claude E. Welch, et al., "Reduction of Postoperative Pain by Encouragement and Instruction of Patients," *New England Journal of Medicine* 270 (1974): 825–827.
14. J. Wesley Alexander and William K. Vaughn, "The Use of 'Marginal' Donors for Organ Transplantation: The Influence of Donor Age on Outcome," *Transplantation* 51 (1991): 135–141.
15. Alvin H. Moss and Mark Siegler, "Should Alcoholics Compete Equally for Liver Transplantation?," *Journal of the American Medical Association* 265 (1991): 1295–1298.

16. Jay Katz, *The Silent World of Doctor and Patient*. New York, NY: The Free Press, 1984.
17. American Medical Association, Council on Ethical and Judicial Affairs, "Ethical Considerations in The Allocation of Organs and Other Scarce Medical Resources among Patients," *Archives of Internal Medicine* 155 (1995): 1083–1087.
18. Dan W. Brock, "Ethical Issues in Recipient Selection for Organ Transplantation," in Organ Substitution Technology: Ethical, Legal and Public Policy Issues, Deborah Mathieu, ed. Boulder CO: Westview Press, 1988, pp. 86–99.
19. James F. Childress, "Ethical Criteria for Procuring and Distributing Organs for Transplantation," *Journal of Health Politics, Policy and Law* 14 (1989): 87–113.
20. Ruth B. Purtilo, "What Kind of Good is a Donor Liver Anyway and Why Should We Care," *Liver Transplantation and Surgery* 1 (1995): 75–79.
21. Note, "Provider-Specific Quality-of-Care Data, and A Proposal for Limited Mandatory Disclosure," *Brooklyn Law Review* 58 (1992): 85–143.
22. Mark P. Aulisio and Robert M. Arnold, "Exclusionary Criteria and Suicidal Behavior: A Comment on 'Should a Patient Who Attempted Suicide Receive a Liver Transplant?', by Forster, Bartholome, and Delcore," *Journal of Clinical Ethics* 3 (1996): 277–283.
23. Carl Cohen, Martin Benjamin, and the Social Impact Committee of the Transplant and Health Policy Center, Ann Arbor, Michigan "Alcoholics and Liver Transplantation. The Ethics and Social Impact Committee of the Transplantation and Health Policy Center," *Journal of the American Medical Association*, 265 (1991):1299–1301.
24. Owen S. Surman and Ruth B. Purtilo, "Reevaluation of Organ Transplantation Criteria: Allocation of Scarce Resources to Borderline Candidates," *Psychosomatics* 33 (1992): 202–212.
25. Arthur L. Caplan, "Hepatic Transplantation Ethics of Casting the First Stone: Personal Responsibility, Rationing, and Transplants," *Alcoholism Clinical and Experimental Research* 18 (1994): 219–221.
26. UNOS, "Statement of Principles and Objectives of Equitable Organ Allocation," *UNOS Update* (1994): 20–38.
27. Peter A. Ubel, Robert M. Arnold, and Arthur L. Caplan, "Rationing Failure: The Ethical Lessons of the Retransplantation of Scarce Vital Organs," *Journal of the American Medical Association* 270 (1993): 2469–2474.

7

Acute yet Non-Emergent Patients

JEREMY SUGARMAN
ROBERT HARLAND

Treating acute yet non-emergent patients poses a unique set of challenges to the surgeon. These patients typically have only recently learned of their disease, sometimes without feeling ill. For example, occult blood detected in stool obtained as part of a routine physical examination may lead to colonoscopy that in turn leads to the detection of polyps that are precancerous. Such a patient is suddenly given diagnostic information and may not yet have had time to apprehend the ramifications of the diagnosis. The patient may respond in a variety of ways to this situation, from denial to indifference to a rapid, not-so-well thought-through request for surgical management even though there is usually adequate time for patients to form well-considered personal preferences regarding appropriate management. Because management decisions are likely to have profound implications for patients, creating a situation in which such preferences can be formed is most desirable.

The manner that surgeons use to heighten the possibility that patients participate meaningfully in medical decision making requires clinical acumen. For instance, surgeons may need to educate patients about their clinical condition. For patients who have not manifested clinical symptoms, education should include information about why further diagnostic tests are needed and the implications of decision making in this regard. In contrast, patients who have symptoms, such as claudication from peripheral vascular disease, might request immediate surgical correction even though they continue to smoke quite heavily. In this case, education should focus on the pathophysiological mechanism of the disease. Thus, patients with acute yet non-emergent conditions may require education during the decision-making process, but the focus of these efforts needs to be nuanced according to the patient's clinical condition.

Acute yet non-emergent patients, unlike many emergent patients, are often able to meaningfully participate in decision making about a range of viable treatment options, thereby making clinical management in some ways more complicated than in the setting of emergent illness. Treating such patients appropriately requires flexibility and creativity on the part of the surgeon. For example, a trial of nonsurgical management might be employed to allow a patient time to adjust to, get information about, and think through a diagnosis and its treatment options. This possibility of having time to develop a better understanding of a particular clinical situation can and should be incorporated into the informed consent process.

The wide spectrum of risk of medical conditions and the therapeutic options that fall into this clinical category of acute yet non-emergent conditions makes it challenging to outline a set of clear rules with which to guide the treatment of all such patients. Surgeons must nevertheless give these patients adequate information about viable therapeutic alternatives, including surgical and nonsurgical treatment options along with their associated morbidities. It is only in this way that patients will receive medical care that is consistent with their personal preferences for treatment. Nevertheless, the surgeon's approach to acute yet non-emergent patients should be guided by the risks related to patients' medical conditions.

Ethical Analysis

Risk Due to Patients' Medical Conditions

Patients have different clinical interests depending on the level of risk posed by their medical condition as well as the risks and benefits associated with surgical and nonsurgical therapeutic alternatives. The spectrum of medical conditions that we consider in this chapter is displayed in the accompanying table. In this table, we outline the risk of medical conditions (low, medium, high, and uncertain), give a prototype clinical condition for each risk category, and describe possible nonsurgical treatment options along with their associated potential morbidities. Based on current surgical practice, in each prototypical case we assume that for most patients a surgical intervention ultimately would decrease morbidity, and sometimes mortality, from the underlying disorder. While it is obviously possible to describe cases in which a surgical approach would be

Prototype Cases of Acute yet Non-Emergent Patients Facing Different Degrees of Risk

RISK	DISEASE	NONSURGICAL TREATMENT OPTIONS	POSSIBLE MORBIDITY AND MORTALITY OF NONSURGICAL TREATMENT
Low	Non-incarcerated inguinal hernia	Observation; modification of activities	Incarceration
Medium	Peripheral vascular disease with rest pain	Medical therapies; stop smoking	Pain; loss of limb
High	Large abdominal aortic aneurysm	Observation	Rupture; extension with renal impairment; death
Uncertain	Biopsy of breast mass or lymph node	Observation	Progression of possible malignancy

contraindicated, we present these examples in an effort to suggest what a reasonable clinical approach would be in most situations. For instance, when considering high-risk conditions such as large abdominal aortic aneurysms, we are interested in a prudent clinical approach to most patients with this condition, not how this approach would be modified if a particular patient had a coexisting risk factor for operative therapy, such as a recent myocardial infarction or severe chronic obstructive pulmonary disease, for which nonsurgical options might be indicated.

Mixing in Personal Values

The ethical challenges associated with treating patients with acute yet non-emergent underlying conditions emanate not only from the variety of medical conditions in this category, but also from other factors, especially patients' preferences for treatment. Because, as Chapter 2 makes clear, patients who have adequate decision-making capacity have an ethical and legal right to refuse any medical intervention, many of the ethical challenges posed to the surgeon relate to ensuring that patients receive optimal clinical care while simultaneously respecting their *well-considered* personal preferences. The emphasis here is on well-considered personal preferences, not first responses or quick judgments. Therefore, surgeons need to respond appropriately to a quick refusal or acceptance of surgical management by patients and their surrogates. Frequently this response requires compassionate and careful questioning about these seemingly reflexive decisions. Such a tack is commensurate with the process of obtaining meaningful informed consent for therapy.

Informed Consent

Comprehensive discussions of the informed consent process are found in Chapter 2 and elsewhere[1] and therefore will not be repeated in detail here. Based on these discussions, we assume that adult patients with adequate decision-making capacity have the ethical and legal right to provide informed consent for medical and surgical interventions. Informed consent is a process in which adequate information is disclosed by surgeons in a manner in which patients can understand it. Following this disclosure, patients can then voluntarily authorize their agreement to participate, usually by signing a consent form. It is incumbent upon the surgeon to attend to each aspect of the informed consent process. Adequate decision-making capacity implies that patients are able to take in new information and use it to make a reasoned decision that is consistent with their personal values. In the setting of many surgical illnesses, fear, pain, and intercurrent medical illness must be considered when assessing decision-making capacity. If the patient has adequate decision-making capacity, the informed consent process may continue with a disclosure that includes a careful description of a proposed surgical intervention and its alternatives. It is essential that the procedure itself, as well as the medical and nonmedical implications of the procedure, be described in a way that is understandable to patients. Moreover, an adequate disclosure incorporates a discussion about both the short-term and long-term benefits and risks of surgical versus nonsurgical management. These benefits and risks encompass not only medical factors, but also nonmedical factors, such as the effect different alternatives may have on the patient's self-image and quality of life. Patients must then be able to make a voluntary decision about whether to undergo the proposed procedure. Finally, if patients decide to have the procedure, they authorize their agreement either orally or by signing a consent form. While consent forms need not recount all the details of a lengthy and informative discussion with patients, key points about planned procedures and their risks as well as a statement that consent is voluntary should be included on properly crafted forms.

In treating patients with acute yet non-emergent conditions it is virtually always possible to disclose to the patient the range of viable surgical and non-surgical treatment alternatives. Using the prototype cases listed in the table as examples of conditions posing different levels of risk, we suggest the type of information that should be included in the disclosure process.

Low-Risk Conditions. For low-risk conditions, many patients seek medical or surgical evaluation because they have been experiencing symptoms. In our prototype case, a non-incarcerating inguinal hernia, symptoms might include discomfort from an inguinal bulge or from gastrointestinal symptoms. Here it is likely that discussing surgical treatment aimed at correction, so that the hernia does not enlarge or subsequently incarcerate, will not be unexpected by patients. In such cases, an adequate disclosure regarding surgical correction includes the type of surgical approach being recommended, how it will be performed, whether this will be done as an inpatient or as an outpatient, the type of anesthesia to be used, the expected length of recovery, and the short-term risks associated with surgery (e.g., bleeding, pain, and infection), as well as the long-term risks (e.g., failure of the procedure to correct the defect permanently). In addition to describing the proposed operative correction, surgeons should discuss the possibility of nonsurgical management, such as observation with modification of activities to limit heavy exertion. The extent to which such an approach is appropriate for a particular patient depends in large part on his or her lifestyle, activity level, personality, and self-image. For instance, nonsurgical management may be appropriate for a sedentary individual who is not terribly concerned about an inguinal bulge, whereas it may be inappropriate for someone who does extensive physical work or exercise.

Medium-Risk Conditions. The disclosure process for patients with medium-risk disorders is similar with respect to the type of information about surgical and nonsurgical options that needs to be provided to patients, including the short-term risks and discomforts associated with surgical management. However, as in our prototype medium-risk case, peripheral vascular disease with ischemic rest pain, patients must be apprised of the clinical importance of, yet practical difficulties inherent in, nonsurgical therapeutic options, such as stopping smoking. Furthermore, surgeons should make it clear that nonsurgical interventions are only likely to halt progression of disease and that these nonsurgical treatments are often an important adjunct to surgical therapy. By disclosing this sort of information, surgeons can enhance the possibility that patients make valid informed decisions about their care and management. This is especially important, because it is patients themselves who are best positioned to make judgments about the influence of different approaches on their own quality of life.

High-Risk, Non-Emergent Conditions. When patients present with high-risk non-emergent conditions, it is again necessary for surgeons to describe the surgical and nonsurgical treatment options. In our prototype high-risk condition, a large abdominal aortic aneurysm, from a clinical perspective the risk/benefit calculus for surgical versus nonsurgical intervention very obviously shifts greatly in the direction of surgical treatment. Surgeons need to make the disclosure process consonant with the risks associated with the clinical situation even though some patients may still opt for facing the risk of rupture compared to the certain discomforts of recovery from surgical correction.

Uncertain-Risk Conditions. Finally, some patients face an uncertain risk for acute yet non-emergent conditions. Two prototype cases here are a palpable breast mass or nontender lymph node. As with any disclosure process for a surgical intervention, surgeons should include a description of the proposed procedure and its risks. However, because of the possibility of a malignancy that might progress without a clear diagnosis and appropriate treatment, it is difficult to describe accurately the range of morbidity and mortality related to nonsurgical observation. During the informed consent process it is incumbent upon surgeons to explore the way in which patients are managing the potential diagnosis of malignancy.

Thus, in order for patients to participate meaningfully in their medical care, it is critical for the surgeon to give them an adequate disclosure about therapeutic options. An adequate disclosure also incorporates a discussion about the implications of their decisions on nonmedical aspects such as quality of life and self-image.

Clinical Topics

Responding to Refusal of Surgical Management

Adult patients with adequate decision making capacity have the ethical and legal right to refuse any type of medical intervention, including surgical management.[2] Nevertheless, this does not mean that all statements made by patients should initially be accepted at face value. Medical ethics, including the obligation of physicians to continue to care for patients with whom they have established a professional, fiduciary relationship, requires a more comprehensive response to an assertion of refusal. When patients refuse surgical management it is important for the surgeon to develop a comprehensive understanding of the basis of their refusals, because the reasons behind such refusals may help outline appropriate courses of action.

The surgeon should respond initially to refusals of surgical treatment by ruling out inadequate or ineffective communication. This involves asking the patient to describe his or her general understanding of the working diagnosis and what surgery has to offer, so that the surgeon can be confident that the patient has an adequate fund of knowledge with which to make a decision that is indeed consonant with the patient's personal values. After all, good decision making requires good information about the clinical realities associated with different courses of management.

Once the surgeon is assured that the patient has a grasp of the necessary clinical information, and if the patient is still refusing surgical management, the surgeon should seek to understand the reasoning behind the patient's decision. In asking for this information, it is important for the surgeon to discern how the patient understands the medical and nonmedical aspects of potential surgical and nonsurgical options. If the patient is not forthcoming with a clear description of his or her reason for refusal, the surgeon might want to ask a series of probing questions. For instance, the surgeon might inquire in such a way to determine whether this refusal is based upon an apprehension over anesthetic risk, a fear of surgery itself, or uncertainty regarding having surgery at a particular institution.

Of course, this approach is only appropriate if patients have adequate decision-making capacity. As when patients are required to make any significant clinical decisions, it is essential to assess whether they have adequate decision-making capacity to authorize surgery. While a full description of how to assess decision-making capacity is beyond the scope of this chapter, adequate decision-making capacity implies that patients are able to take in new information, process it, and engage in a rational process using this information[3,4] (see also Chapter 2).

There is also a host of nonmedical factors that might contribute to refusals of surgical treatment, including patients' previous experiences, poor timing of surgical intervention from the perspective of patients, and financial considerations. Because some patients may fear surgery because of personal experience, the surgeon might want to ask patients about their previous experience with surgery and rectify any misperceptions that they may have about surgery. It is also important to use other questions to determine whether patients are refusing surgery because of unrelated personal events. For example, patients may want to postpone surgery until after an upcoming wedding, birthday, or anniversary. Finally, patients may correctly or incorrectly understand the financial implications a surgical intervention will have for them. Sources of financial concern might be related to insurance considerations or loss of time from work. The surgeon should discuss these factors directly with patients and be prepared to make referrals to appropriate personnel (e.g., business office representatives or social workers), who may be able to provide accurate information so that the patient can make an informed decision.

Having developed a more complete understanding of a particular patient's reasoning behind a refusal, the surgeon is then in a better position to engage in a series of steps to ensure that the patient is being treated in an optimal manner. If corrections of fact about proposed surgical and nonsurgical management options do not result in agreement about the proposed treatment course, the surgeon should consider at least three possible approaches: negotiation, persuasion, and a trial of nonsurgical management. Primary care physicians might also help surgeons and patients make sound decisions by helping present information about therapeutic alternatives or in suggesting an alternative approach to patients who refuse surgical therapy.

Negotiation. Negotiation is a reasonable approach to take with patients who might be refusing surgical management because of the proposed surgical approach, the type of anesthesia to be used, the expected number of days of hospitalization, and the timing of the procedure. Engaging patients in this decision-making process when they are vulnerable due to illness may alone prompt some patients to trust their surgeons sufficiently that they will agree to proceed with a surgical intervention.

Persuasion. In some instances, especially when a patient is faced with a high- or uncertain-risk medical condition, it is reasonable for the surgeon to persuade the patient to undergo surgical therapy. Once the surgeon understands the patient's underlying set of values and fears, it may be possible to use this information to persuade the patient to undergo surgical treatment. For instance, if patients have an uncertain-risk condition, such as a breast mass, the surgeon can help patients understand that the proposed surgical treatment is a way of removing the uncertainty associated with what might simply be a benign condition compared to a malignant one (e.g., a cyst versus breast cancer). By resolving uncertainty, a surgical approach can empower a patient to make future decisions. These subsequent decisions require reliable information, not speculation.

While using persuasion is appropriate in such instances, it is critical that attempts at persuasion are not coercive. Coercion may involve telling patients that if they do not follow a surgical course of management they will be abandoned in some way, including not being seen by a particular surgeon or by being made ineligible for future care within the health care system in which they are receiving medical therapy. Likewise, it would be inappropriate for a surgeon to knowingly overestimate the risk of nonsurgical interventions in order to convince the patient to acquiesce to surgery.

Trial of Nonsurgical Management. Finally, patients may need to experience nonsurgical treatment in order to be able to make a good clinical decision. For these patients, a trial of nonsurgical management is a reasonable course to take. Although nonsurgical management might not remove the risk of some preventable morbidities, using these therapies can allow patients to better understand the clinical realities of their diseases so that they might make an informed and experienced decision. Similarly, some patients may not be prepared to make a decision about surgical therapy in a single clinic visit. In cases such as this, patients can be given a nonsurgical therapy, affording them the opportunity to go home and discuss other clinical options with family and friends.

Managing Refusal of Blood Products

Some patients may refuse surgical treatment as a means of refusing treatment with blood products, whereas other patients are willing to undergo surgery provided that they can be assured that blood products will not be used in their care. The refusal of blood products can emanate from several sources. Perhaps the most common instances of refusal of blood products relate to religious beliefs or fear of contagion.[5]

There is an extensive literature describing the beliefs of Jehovah's Witnesses regarding the use of blood products.[6] In treating patients who are Jehovah's Witnesses it is essential that surgeons understand each patient's personal belief system. This is critical because some Jehovah's Witnesses categorically refuse transfusions of blood and blood products but they may accept blood-conserving methods and artificial blood products. Other Jehovah's Witnesses may, rarely, accept blood products, such as albumin. Therefore, surgeons should have a careful discussion about treatment options with patients who are Jehovah's Witnesses. The goal is to reach a clear, mutually acceptable plan about precisely what will and will not be done in response to significant blood loss.

The onset of the AIDS epidemic has also heightened the anxiety of many patients regarding the use of blood products. Although the blood supply is safer now than it has ever been, a substantial number of patients simply fear receiving blood.[7] When discussing impending surgery, it is essential for the surgeon to describe the actual risks inherent to the transfusion of blood and blood products. Patients need to understand that it is impossible to eliminate risk in the use of blood; risk can be minimized, however. For many patients, consultation with a blood bank might be a useful step.

Regardless of whether patients offer a specific statement about refusal of blood products, given current concerns among the general public about the safety of the blood supply, it is essential that surgeons assure patients that available techniques will be used to diminish blood loss during surgery. In situations where the patient clearly refuses the use of blood products, additional technical procedures such as using cell-saving devices and autologous blood donation must be considered and, if they are expected to benefit that particular patient, they should be offered and recommended.

Patients Who Don't Want to Be Involved

When patients overtly refuse interventions, their participation in the medical decision-making process is quite obvious. In addition, a meaningful informed consent process assumes that patients are active participants. Yet there are some patients who do not want to be involved—at all or very much—in the decision-making process. For acute yet non-emergent patients the trade-offs between risks and benefits, short-term and long-term, as well as medical and nonmedical, are subtle and variable. It is therefore often difficult for the physician to definitively recommend one course of management. Thus, to enhance the likelihood of making an ultimately good choice from the patient's perspective, the patient must contribute to, if not play a very active role in, the decision-making process.

Although it might be clinically expedient simply to make choices for patients, the surgeon has an ethical obligation to encourage patients to play a role in medical decision making. In encouraging patients to participate, the surgeon must create an atmosphere in which patients feel comfortable speaking about their hopes and fears. In addition, in some situations, it may be helpful for the surgeon to express his or her need to gain patients' expertise regarding their own values about which the surgeon has no special insight. Such an approach can make it clear to patients why their input is necessary.

Communicating with Family Members and Friends of the Patient

Caring for acute yet non-emergent patients raises some interesting questions about how best to communicate with their family members and friends. Patients' expectations of confidentiality and the hazards associated with violating confidentiality make this a particularly challenging area of clinical practice.[8] Confidentiality has been an important component of medical practice and ethics at least since the time of Hippocrates. The Hippocratic Oath is clear: "What I may see or hear in the course of the treatment in the regard to the life of men, which on no account one must spread abroad, I will keep to myself."[9] Based on this long tradition, most patients expect that their physicians and surgeons will keep medical information confidential. Given widely differing notions of privacy, it is incumbent upon surgeons to understand what matters each patient considers to be privileged. Some patients expect that all discussions about their medical condition involve only two central players: the surgeon and the patient. In contrast, other patients engage large extended families in a conversation about their medical diagnoses and treatment. To circumvent ethical problems created by violating patients' privacy, the surgeon should ask patients early in their professional relationship about whom they would like the surgeon to share what types of medical information. Such a direct approach promises to obviate subsequent problems (see also Chapter 3).

When discussing the possibility of surgery, the surgeon should ask patients who, if anyone, they would like to have included in the decision-making process. Such questioning is needed because it is inappropriate to automatically assume that all patients want their spouses, parents, or children to participate in these discussions.

Before surgery, the surgeon also needs to find out what patients would like their families to be told immediately following the procedure. For example, in relevant clinical situations does a patient want family members or friends notified that a frozen section from a surgical biopsy reveals a malignancy? Or does the patient prefer to discuss these findings with the physician alone before the family is notified? Or does the patient want to discuss these issues with the physician when family members or friends are present? Posing questions such as these is part of practicing preventive ethics. Following our example, if families or friends are *not* given information about the diagnosis of a malignancy while the patient is in the recovery room, they are in no position to request that the true diagnosis be withheld from the patient, thereby relieving the surgeon of a possible ethical bind subsequently. Therefore, instead of adhering to the custom of surgeons talking to patients' families following a procedure, prudence suggests asking patients in advance about their preferences for sharing medical information with family members and friends. As a rule, if the surgeon has not been given explicit permission by a patient to describe the operative course and diagnosis to those in the waiting room, the surgeon should limit the type of information given to those waiting. Limited information might include a simple statement that the procedure is over, that the patient is going to the recovery room, and that a full discussion about the surgery will take place when the patient returns to a regular hospital room. Obviously, by setting these rules out in advance, the surgeon can do much to assuage the anxieties of family members and friends while not divulging confidential medical information and maintaining the patient's authority in the decision-making process.

Responding to Inappropriate Demands for Surgical Management by Patients or Their Surrogates

Although both medical ethics and the law are clear that adult patients who have adequate decision-making capacity can refuse treatment, the surgeon need not acquiesce to inappropriate demands for surgical interventions. The right to refuse medical treatments is based in a long tradition of protecting individual liberty, both in medical and nonmedical situations. The protected liberty interest is generally a negative one. That is, patients have a right to be left alone. These negative rights are very difficult to limit, unless the individual's actions are causing substantial harm to others. The counterpart of a negative liberty interest is a positive interest that connotes the right to have something done for oneself— that is, to consume resources to advance one's interests. These positive claims come with limits; the argument concerns what the limits should be. While we respect a small set of positive liberty interests in medicine, such interests do not typically seem to be as persuasive as negative liberty interests. Based on this distinction among liberty interests, coupled with the absence of clear and accepted clinical indications, surgeons can find justification for not meeting demands for inappropriate therapies.

Despite an ability to theoretically justify not meeting these demands, responding to them in practice can be tricky. Patients may simply not share the same medical paradigm as surgeons. For instance, patients may believe that a particular surgical intervention is capable of ameliorating their suffering although there is no medical evidence to suggest that this is the case. Imagine, for example, a patient who presents with atypical abdominal pain and is convinced that this is attributable to the appendix or gallbladder. The patient may insist on surgical removal of the offending organ, even though from the surgeon's perspective the clinical exam and laboratory data do not support a diagnosis of surgical disease such as appendicitis or cholecystitis. Faced with situations like this, the surgeon ought to explain his or her reluctance to perform a procedure that exposes the patient to a known medical risk when there is no known medical benefit of treatment. The patient would likely best be served by a period of observation and nonsurgical therapy, while further diagnostic testing is performed and the true cause of the discomfort is determined. Gathering additional consultants to confirm the surgeon's assessment about this standard of care might also be helpful.

When May the Surgeon Refuse to Perform Surgery?

Surgeons may be inclined to refuse to operate in a variety of situations. Sometimes these refusals are justified and other times they are not. It is justifiable to refuse to perform surgery when the procedure is clearly not medically indicated, the surgery is non-emergent, and when there are other sources of medical care available and accessible to the patient. Refusing to perform surgery when it is not medically indicated is justifiable under the ethical principles of beneficence and non-maleficence.[10] According to the principle of beneficence, medical interventions must be intended to promote the patient's medical interests. Therefore, if surgery will not provide medical benefit, it is inappropriate to employ it. Similarly, according to the principle of non-maleficence (which captures the medical maxim "Do no harm"), surgeons must act in such a way so as to avoid only harming patients as a result of medical interventions. If surgery is contraindicated, patients would be exposed to unbalanced and unnecessary harm, a violation of the principle of non-maleficence.

Surgeons may also refuse to perform surgery in non-emergent settings. For example, if a patient has a low-risk underlying medical condition such as a non-incarcerated hernia, and the patient desires to have it corrected on a particular day when the surgical schedule is already filled with more critical cases, it would be reasonable for the surgeon to refuse to perform surgery on that particular day. Although it is desirable to meet patients' requests for timing of procedures and office visits, the surgeon need not meet requests when he or she will be fatigued from handling other more emergent cases.

Finally, in rare cases it might be reasonable for the surgeon to refuse to perform indicated surgery for personal reasons. A valid personal reason would be that the needed procedure is one that the surgeon simply prefers not to do. However, refusals for personal reasons are only justified when there are other sources of care available and accessible to patients.

When refusing to operate, the surgeon should facilitate a referral to another competent surgeon who is willing to take the case. Such a referral must also be a reasonable option on nonmedical grounds. Nonmedical considerations of referral include that the patient need not have to travel an excessive distance to get care, that the patient's insurance still covers the referral, and that the referral will be done in a timely and efficient manner.

Unacceptable Reasons for Refusing to Perform Surgery. In other situations, a desire to refuse to treat patients would not be justified. These situations include patients who pose a somewhat increased risk to the surgeon, such as persons with HIV infection or hepatitis B virus infection, patients who are being discriminated against for nonmedical reasons, and situations in which performing surgery simply would not be lucrative for the surgeon.

Much critical attention has been paid to the obligation of the health care providers to treat those who pose a somewhat increased risk to physicians, particularly patients with HIV infection or AIDS. Following a flurry of assertions about whether or not physicians have an obligation to treat patients with HIV infection or AIDS, there is now broad consensus that this obligation exists.[11-14] The history of medicine reveals that medical and surgical practice have virtually always been associated with some risk to physicians; HIV is merely another form of risk.[15] The initial refusals of surgeons to care for patients with HIV infection or AIDS appear to have been primarily based on both uncertain medical risks as well as discrimination. The former concern is no longer relevant because the actual risk, with appropriate levels of infection control, to the physician of infection during surgery is now estimated to be acceptably low.[16] The latter concern is invalid since it is both inappropriate and intolerable to eschew caring for patients simply because of nonmedical factors, such as race, gender, religious beliefs, or sexual orientation. This claim finds theoretical justification in many analyses of the ethical principle of justice.

Finally, based on the degree to which society contributes to the education of every health care practitioner, we believe that every surgeon has some obligation to care for patients even when the surgeon may not be paid directly for doing so. The scope and limits of this obligation are matters of controversy and conscience (see Chapter 17).

Responding to Advance Directives

The Patient Self-Determination Act now requires that all hospitals that receive Medicare and Medicaid funding inform patients about advance directives, tell them how the institution will follow their directives according to hospital policy and state law, inquire whether patients have an advance directive, and make valid directives part of patients' medical records. Accordingly, surgeons should have a working familiarity with both advance directives and their hospital's policy regarding advance directives.[17,18] See Chapter 4 for a detailed account of advance directives.

Given the attention paid to advance directives at the time of admission, it is prudent for surgeons to devise ways of informing their patients about advance directives, so they are not surprised when they are admitted prior to surgery. Many health care institutions now have brochures and information the surgeon might want to consider giving to patients during their outpatient, preoperative workup, so that patients have this information at a time that is not as stressful as that of hospital admission. This is important because sentinel events, such as impending surgery, precipitate some patients to formulate advance directives. This is especially relevant for patients who have acute yet non-emergent conditions beause they frequently have sufficient time to deliberate about advance directives. In addition, surgeons and their staff should become familiar with their institution's policy regarding the Patient Self-Determination Act so that they know what types of discussions about advance directives patients may have had prior to meeting them.

Now that advance directives have become an accepted part of medical care, the surgeon should be prepared to discuss them with patients. Upon patients' admission to the hospital, the surgeon should ask about their advance directives, how patients would like them used during their care, including the types of situations in which patients might want the surgeon to disregard their written advance directives. If applicable, the surgeon should meet with patients and their designated surrogates so that everyone involved is clear about how decisions will be made during and after surgery. In general, if patients have executed an advance directive, unless there are intervening circumstances that could not be predicted (e.g., a patient who does not desire to be on a ventilator but who suffers an easily reversible event such as anaphylaxis), it is the moral responsibility of the surgeon to adhere to valid advance directives. This includes not following inappropriate last-minute family requests to override a patient's advance directive simply because the patient is no longer capable of making a decision.

Clinical Conclusions

The informed consent process must address the distinctive features of decision making with acute yet non-emergent patients. These patients may not be experiencing symptoms and so the surgeon must deal with the abruptness and surprise of disclosing an unexpected diagnosis. At the same time, there may be some urgency to the patient's problem, constraining the time for the informed consent process so that danger to the patient is avoided. The surgeon should adjust the consent process to take these factors into account. In doing so, the surgeon should at first assume that patients with these clinical conditions are capable of participating in the informed consent process and ought to be encouraged to do so. The range of therapeutic options that are typically available to such patients can make the disclosure step of this process quite challenging for the busy surgeon. Nevertheless, its centrality in ensuring patients' meaningful participation in their health care makes it incumbent upon the surgeon to provide understandable information about relevant treatment alternatives, including their medical and nonmedical benefits and risks.

Surgeons have an obligation to evaluate initial statements of refusals of surgery by patients. The initial evaluation includes not only an assessment of decision-making capacity, but also of the patient's experiences, understanding, fears, and reasons for indicating a refusal of surgery. Once any discrepancies between a patient's understanding of the facts of his or her medical illnesses and the proposed surgical intervention are rectified, the surgeon has an obligation to use a variety of techniques to encourage the patient to have surgery. Depending on the case, it may be reasonable to negotiate the timing of surgery or the surgical approach with patients. Or it may be appropriate to try to persuade, but not coerce, patients into undergoing surgery that is clinically indicated. Finally, it may be appropriate to undergo a trial of medical therapy. However, in the end it is the moral and legal right of patients to refuse surgery.

Although patients have a legal and moral right to refuse surgery, the surgeon need not perform clinically inappropriate surgery. Nevertheless, caring for patients who make such requests can sometimes be difficult and these requests must be handled carefully. Faced with a request for an inappropriate intervention, the surgeon should first share with patients his or her paradigm for understanding why surgery would not be appropriate. It may be prudent to gain consultation from other surgeons in an effort to validate the surgeon's assessment for patients.

The refusal of blood products can emanate from several sources, most commonly from religious beliefs or fear of contagion. Regardless of whether patients make an explicit statement about refusing blood products, it is essential that the surgeon assure patients that the blood bank will use appropriate techniques to screen blood and he or she will strive to limit blood loss during surgery to avoid the use of unnecessary transfusions. As in any medical intervention, the surgeon should understand patients' beliefs and directives regarding the use of blood products so that patients are treated in a manner consistent with their personal values and beliefs.

In treating patients with acute yet non-emergent conditions it is difficult to predict accurately an individual patient's expectations regarding medical information. Given the range of these expectations, from a desire to discuss openly all aspects with a large extended family to sharing information with a close friend to keeping all information within the surgeon-patient relationship, it is critical that the surgeon develop an understanding of each patient's expectations about to whom the surgeon should communicate private medical information.

As health care institutions respond to the Patient Self-Determination Act, it is likely that more patients will ask surgeons about advance directives. Surgeons therefore need to become familiar with advance directives and their institution's policies regarding them. Since upcoming surgery may prompt patients to complete or change their advance directives, the surgeon should include a discussion about them in his or her preoperative discussions with patients.

Surgeons should work with their administrative boards and ethics committees to adopt policies that optimize the likelihood that patients are treated in a medically and morally appropriate fashion. If these policies are to be practical and clinically meaningful, the surgeon should be actively engaged in the process of formulating them.

References

1. Ruth R. Faden and Tom L. Beauchamp, *A History and Theory of Informed Consent*. New York: Oxford University Press, 1986.
2. Mary Faith Marshall, "When the Patient Refuses Treatment," in *Introduction to Clinical Ethics*, John C. Fletcher, Charles A. Hite, Paul A. Lombardo, and Mary Faith Marshall, eds. Frederick, Maryland: University Publishing Group Inc., 1995, pp. 97–113.
3. Paul S. Appelbaum and Thomas Grisso, "Assessing Patients' Capacities to Consent to Treatment," *New England Journal of Medicine* 319 (1988): 1635–1638.
4. Allen E. Buchanan and Dan W. Brock, *Deciding for Others: The Ethics of Surrogate Decision Making*. New York: Cambridge University Press, 1990.
5. Judith C. Ahronheim, Jonathan Moreno, and Connie Zuckerman, "Case 1: A religious objection to a blood transfusion," *Ethics in Clinical Practice*. New York: Little, Brown and Company, 1994, pp. 83–90.
6. Jeremy Sugarman, Larry R. Churchill, John Kevin Moore, and Robert A. Waugh, "Medical, Ethical and Legal Issues Regarding Thrombolytic Therapy in the Jehovah's Witness," *The American Journal of Cardiology* 68 (1991): 1525–1529.
7. Jeremy Sugarman, Neil R. Powe, Alan D. Guerci, et al., "Facts and Fears Regarding Blood Transfusions in Decision Making for Thrombolytic Therapy," *American Heart Journal* 126 (1993): 494–499.
8. Mary Faith Marshall, "Respecting Privacy and Confidentiality," in *Introduction to Clinical Ethics*, John C. Fletcher, Charles A. Hite, Paul A. Lombardo, and Mary

Faith Marshall, eds. Frederick, Maryland: University Publishing Group Inc., 1995, pp. 39–49.

9. Hippocrates, "The Oath," in *Ancient Medicine: Selected Papers of Ludwig Edelstein*, Owsei Temkin and C. Lilian Temkin, eds. Baltimore, Maryland: Johns Hopkins Press, 1967, p. 6.

10. Tom L. Beauchamp and James F. Childress, *Principles of Biomedical Ethics*, 4th ed. New York: Oxford University Press, 1994.

11. Council on Ethical and Judicial Affairs, American Medical Association, "Ethical Issues Involved in the Growing AIDS Crisis," *Journal of the American Medical Association* 259 (1988): 1360–1361.

12. Ezekiel J. Emanuel, "Do Physicians Have an Obligation to Treat Patients with AIDS?" *New England Journal of Medicine* 318 (1988): 1686–1690.

13. Abigail Zuger and Steven H. Miles, "Physicians, AIDS, and Occupational Risk: Historic Traditions and Ethical Obligations," *Journal of the American Medical Association* 258 (1987): 1924–1928.

14. Edmund D. Pellegrino, "Altruism, Self-Interest, and Medical Ethics," *Journal of the American Medical Association* 258 (1987): 1939–1940.

15. John D. Arras, "The Fragile Web of Responsibility: AIDS and the Duty to Treat," *Hastings Center Report* 18 (1988): 10–19.

16. Jerome I. Tokars, Mary E. Chamberland, Charles A. Schable, et al., and the American Academy of Orthopaedic Surgeons Serosurvey Study Committee, "A Survey of Occupational Blood Contact and HIV Infection Among Orthopedic Surgeons," *Journal of the American Medical Association* 268 (1992): 489–494.

17. Joint Commission on Accreditation of Healthcare Organizations, *Accreditation Manual for Hospitals*. Oak Brook Terrace, Illinois: JCAHO, 1995.

18. Public Law 101–508, Sec. 4206 and 4751.

8

Elective Patients

ANDREW LUSTIG
PETER SCARDINO

Elective surgery is an option to be considered in response to non-emergent diseases that exhibit a "gray zone" for clinical judgment, wherein the ratio of risks to benefits has not reached a decisive balance in favor of surgical management. Surgery may be judged to be elective for two types of cases. First, surgery may be viewed as elective in response to chronic diseases and slowly progressive conditions that are relatively benign. For example, in responding to benign prostatic hyperplasia (BPH), single-vessel coronary artery disease, emphysema, or cholelithiasis, surgery may be deemed elective because there is no demonstrable risk of physiological catastrophe if nonsurgical management is adopted as the preferred strategy, at least initially. Uncertainty about the respective ratios of risks to benefits between surgical and nonsurgical management is a function of morbidity and quality-of-life outcomes. Surgical management sometimes results in significant morbidity that may adversely affect the patient's short- and long-term quality of life. Likewise, nonsurgical management, which includes diagnosis, medical management, and symptom relief, may also involve significant associated morbidity and increased risk of mortality. Thus, the patient's own values are crucial in assessing alternative outcomes and making "trade-offs" between associated morbidity and mortality. In a second type of case—for example, localized prostatic cancer—clinical judgment is complicated by the need to avoid a rarely seen but very bad outcome. In such cases, although the ratio of risks to benefits remains less than definitive, prudential clinical judgment lends greater support to surgical management, though still not enough to warrant a univocal recommendation, given the risks of morbidity and adverse effects on the patient's quality of life.

The management of elective surgical patients in both types of cases raises a number of important ethical concerns. First, issues arise about the range and specificity of the data to be provided patients as the basis for their decision to accept or forgo surgical management in favor of other therapeutic alternatives, especially the alternative of conservative or nonoperative management. Second, there are distinctive features to the ethical model of informed consent in the elective context when compared with situations involving emergency or imminent risk. In the elective context, greater time is available for strategies of negotiation, persuasion, and compromise between patient and surgeon in the ongoing management of the patient's underlying medical condition and symptomatology. Third, as an extension of the second cluster of concerns, questions arise when available data about relative outcomes from alternative therapeutic responses are incomplete, in conflict, or insufficient to allow the surgeon to recommend a particular alternative with the degree of confidence one ordinarily associates with more conclusive scientific bases for reasonable medical judgment. This third cluster of issues includes both epistemological and ethical aspects. As a matter of medical epistemology, on what basis does a surgeon offer a reasonable professional medical judgment between or among alternatives in the absence of clear and compelling data? As an ethical matter, how should the surgeon exercise his or her fiduciary obligation to the patient when the expected basis for reasonable medical judgment is itself at issue? More pointedly, how does the surgeon, committed by the principle of beneficence to safeguard and promote the patient's best interest, guard against undue self-interest in making recommendations when, in light of available data, no particular therapeutic option may be strictly indicated or contraindicated over any other? (Self-interest may include doing something in fee-for service medicine or doing nothing in a managed care context.) Fourth, several clinical issues arise in elective surgery that, although not unique to the elective context, are equally relevant to a consideration of the ethical obligations of surgeon and patient, here as elsewhere. Although other chapters in this volume address these issues with greater scope, the ethical analysis of elective surgery also entails at least brief consideration of the following topics: (1) ethical concerns when surgeons are faced with what they deem inappropriate demands for, or inappropriate refusals of, elective surgical management; (2) ethical questions concerning the basis for a surgeon's legitimate refusal of elective surgery; (3) religiously based refusals of blood products; and (4) the status of DNR orders for elective surgical patients that have been written in other settings.

Ethical Analysis

The Process of Informed Consent in the Context of Elective Surgery

Unlike situations involving emergency or acute high-risk patients, where clinical decision making occurs under greater time constraints, the process of informed consent involving elective patients and/or their surrogates is usually characterized by the luxury of time for a more relaxed sharing of relevant medical information, a more extended deliberation (or set of deliberations) within which shared decision making may occur, and a wider window within which various alternatives can be assessed and reassessed, as necessary, according to the patient's progressive medical status.

As a result of these differences, clinical decision making that is responsive to circumstances where elective surgery is one option among several will properly entail a "process" rather than a "discrete event" model of informed consent.[1] To this extent, the same general model developed in Chapter 2 will illuminate the clinical partnership that should obtain in the elective context.

The differences between the context of decision making characteristic of elective surgery and certain features of acute or high-risk surgical situations can affect the entire therapeutic encounter. Granted, even in acute or high-risk situations, the process of informed consent is hallmarked by the centrality of the patient's own values as finally determinative of the treatment to be chosen and pursued (see Chapter 7). Nonetheless, in acute or high-risk situations, the surgeon's own beneficence-based judgment, as a scientifically based clinical recommendation to the patient, will very often lead the surgeon to offer a judgment regarding what constitutes, in his or her considered opinion, the "more reasonable" or "most reasonable" course. That is to say, the basis for the "reasonableness" of the surgeon's recommendation for immediate intervention will typically be more obvious in acute or high-risk circumstances, given the specific nature and urgency of the patient's medical need.

Indeed, much of the medical ethics literature on determining competence reflects this conceptual linkage. According to the so-called "sliding scale" of competence, the "favorability" of the patient's decision may depend, ever more stringently, on the ability of the patient to understand clearly the nature of the risks involved in rejecting the physician's considered opinion. In acute or high-risk circumstances, a number of ethicists would defend a conceptual correlation between the gravity of the harm likely to result from refusing a clearly preferable treatment alternative, judged according to professional canons, and more stringent judgments about the cognitive and affective basis of the patient's own process of making a decision, in light of an objectively measurable likely harm.[2,3]

To be sure, even in medically urgent or high-risk situations, such sliding scale judgments of competence determination remain both controversial and subject to cogent criticism.[1] Critics point out the danger of an unjustified medical paternalism trumping the patient's own values in correlating competence with the likelihood and gravity of harm in failing to heed a medical recommendation. Without assessing the merits of that ongoing debate, it is obviously of much less relevance to the process of informed consent (and the determination of competence) that characterize the context of elective surgery. Indeed, because elective surgery is, by definition, not an option considered under conditions of medical urgency or duress, the choice among alternatives is viewed as more obviously, and less controversially, resting on the patient's values for determining what constitutes an appropriate therapeutic course in two important respects: in light of the time available for trials of various alternatives, including the option of nonsurgical management; and because for some conditions (two of which we will discuss shortly), the risks and benefits of any particular choice among therapeutic options are far less immediately obvious than in high-risk or acute circumstances.

Issues in the Management of Elective Surgical Patients

This chapter will discuss the ethical issues raised in the surgical management of elective patients by discussing, in some detail, two medical conditions—benign prostatic hyperplasia (BPH) and clinically localized prostatic cancer—as examples, respectively, of the two types of cases discussed briefly in our introduction. The medical management of both conditions exemplifies the range of considerations appropriate to the population of elective patients, and each condition raises significant questions about the most appropriate way to pursue meaningful shared decision making in the face of uncertain data regarding alternatives. Moreover, both conditions have been the subject of recent studies and literature reviews.[4-10] Current data indicate an extensive range of practice variations, both geographically and temporally. Thus the notion of rational shared decision making, in the face of such uncertain data and variable practice patterns, requires careful attention to the ethical values and the practical dynamics central to the physician-patient clinical partnership.

Clinical Topics

Informed Consent When There Is Time and When the Patient May Do Well by Declining Surgical Management in Favor of Medical Management

In the face of significant variability in practice patterns and great uncertainty regarding the relative benefits of particular alternatives among which the elective patient will choose, informed consent is a process that requires time, clinical sensitivity to the patient's own values as decisive, and willingness by the surgeon to negotiate (and/or renegotiate) an appropriate course of therapy, over an extended period of time, as follow-up visits continue and interim outcomes are monitored. Informed consent, as the linchpin of the process of shared decision making between physician and patient, is crucially important, for reasons both ethical and medical.

Ethically, informed consent is based on the principle of respect for persons. Persons, as moral agents, must be empowered with sufficient information to make clear, well-reasoned judgments regarding treatment options, especially in situations when the option of nonoperative management may well emerge as the most appropriate course. At least since *Canterbury v. Spence*, the principle of informed consent, according to a reasonable person standard, has been recognized as the ethical lodestar of clinical decision making[11] (see Chapter 2). This constraint on unilateral action by physicians is based on the dignity of persons and their right to make decisions regarding medical treatment, especially those that may involve different degrees of invasive therapy.

It is also clear that shared decision making, with close collaboration and negotiation between physician and patient regarding the most appropriate course of treatment, is often decisive for understanding the very meaning of "harm" and "benefit," in relative terms, for these words are seldom neutral terms in clinical judgment. In many instances, especially choices involving elective surgery as one of several available options, reasonable medical judgment supports a range of therapeutic alternatives. Thus, the patient's own normative assessment will prove decisive in determining what constitutes a relatively beneficial course of therapy, all things considered.

Nonsurgical Management as an Alternative to Elective Surgery

If the model of shared decision making is nearly always relevant, save for emergency circumstances when consent can be assumed, it is *a fortiori* relevant to cases where elective surgery is but one option among several, and the data about preferable outcomes in terms of mortality and/or morbidity remain unclear. In such circumstances, the patient's own values will be decisive in relation to several aspects of the decisions about treatment options: (1) with regard to the judgment about the frequency and severity of present symptoms; (2) with regard to the magnitude and probability of likely risks associated with surgical versus nonsurgical options; (3) with regard to judgments about acceptable quality of life after particular interventions, or in the wake of nonsurgical management; and (4) with regard to differential judgments based on highly variable data regarding the effectiveness of surgical versus nonsurgical options, as well as among nonsurgical options, which are now available with the recent introduction of a number of methods less invasive than surgery.[12,13]

In addition, as some studies suggest, enhanced patient participation in clinical decision making may well redound to the benefit or advance of medical practice *per se*, because choices that are more fully collaborative in nature may well reduce unwanted practice variations and improve the reliability of outcome data that truly reflect actual patient preferences.[4,5,14] A number of practitioners have highlighted the general need for careful attention to actual patient preferences in decision making. That requirement deserves particular emphasis—ethically, legally, and medically—when outcomes data remain unclear, when the relative benefits of particular options remain inconclusive, and when unilateral recommendations by physicians that merely reflect their own professional expertise (here the recommendation for surgery by surgeons) appear unwarrantedly paternalistic.[4,5,14,15]

The Stakes of Forgoing Surgical Management

Elective patients offer an interesting set of variations to the theme of informed consent as a process of shared decision making. For a number of conditions, the requirement that clear and comprehensive information regarding the risks and benefits of alternative forms of available treatment is complicated by the incomplete, unclear, or disputed nature of empirical studies of the benefits and risks of surgical intervention in comparison with other, less invasive, forms of medical management. The two illustrative examples that we will analyze—benign prostatic hyperplasia and localized prostate cancer—offer useful examples of several key elements of our usual understandings of informed consent. (1) What constitutes a fair and unbiased assessment of the risks and benefits of alternatives in the face of significant uncertainty in the medical literature regarding the associated risks of mortality and morbidity among such alternatives? (2) How is an assessment of the "reasonableness" of the patient's decision to be made in the face of such persistent uncertainty? (3) Faced with uncertain data regarding alternatives, what practical steps should be taken by the surgeon to ensure that he or she avoids undue bias toward surgery in his or her recommendation to the patient? (4) What practical strategies can best assure that the patient understands the range of factors relevant to trade-offs between mortality and morbidity in light of the patient's own perspective in making judgments regarding quality of life?

The Meaning of Fair and Unbiased Assessment by the Surgeon of Treatment Alternatives When a Slowly Progressive Disease Is Relatively Benign

Benign prostatic hyperplasia (BPH) exemplifies the first type of case we discussed in our introductory remarks. (That type also includes emphysema, osteoarthritis of the hip, and vascular disease.) BPH is a chronic or slowly progressive condition that primarily affects the elderly, with the mean age at which symptoms develop between 60 and 65 years. BPH arises as a proliferation of fibrostomal cells in the periurethral glands; as growth continues, patients may develop clinically troublesome obstruction to voiding. The primary symptoms of BPH are a complex called "prostatism." Prostatism may include any or all of the following features: decreased urinary flow; difficulties in full voiding of the bladder, ranging from mild to severe; interruption(s) in urinary flow; continued dribbling after voiding; sensation of incomplete voiding; and awakening at night to void. Rarely, the obstruction may progress to the development of recurrent urinary tract infections, bladder calculi, and obstruction of the upper urinary tracts with hydronephrosis and renal impairment.[16] Risks of complications with surgical intervention for BPH vary depending on the type of intervention, but can include urinary incontinence, erectile dysfunction, retrograde ejaculation, and bleeding. There is, at the present time, no clear evidence of links between BPH and prostate cancer.

While there is a general association between prostatic growth and the severity of voiding symptoms, the natural history of BPH is highly variable and poorly characterized. Enlargement of the prostate is common with aging (affecting 80% of the male population). Symptoms of prostatism are less common (30% of men) and medical complications that threaten health are rare. Therapeutic options include nonsurgical management, medical therapy (finasteride or alpha-sympathetic blocking drugs), and a variety of more invasive technologies ranging from hyperthermia to operative resection of the obstructing tissue.

Given the variability of patient reaction both to incidence and severity of present symptoms, and to assessing the likelihood and magnitude of future complications, the need for collaboration in determining appropriate medical responses to chronic or slowly progressive conditions that are relatively benign is obvious. BPH, single-vessel coronary artery disease, emphysema, cholelithiasis, and other conditions offer patent examples of why, both ethically and medically, significant patient education and participation is both desirable and necessary, if the requirements of shared decision making and informed consent are to be respected and met. Moreover, the need for shared decision making is pronounced in a second respect with regard to slowly progressive, relatively benign conditions. Significant uncertainties persist with regard to reliable outcome data about such conditions. As a result, the basis for reasonable surgical judgment is less obvious, as compared with other conditions for which such data are far more reliable, and the range of patient preferences in the light of greater certainty is better established.

Assessing the Reasonableness of the Patient's Decision in the Face of Persistent Uncertainty

The surgeon's own fair and unbiased assessment of the risks and benefits, in the face of significant uncertainty, should emphasize the patient's values as determinative of what constitutes an appropriate medical response. Although there is some evidence in the literature that patients may not wish actively to participate in decision making,[1,14] a chronic or slowly progressive condition that is relatively benign underscores the need for physicians to help patients appreciate the *crucial* function of their personally held values in determining the most appropriate therapeutic course to pursue. The patient's own values will be determinative in two key respects. First, there is a documented range in individual assessments of the risks and benefits linked with specific interventions in terms of their likely benefits and harms, relative to the assessment of the discomfort or undesirability of present symptoms.[4,14] Second, there is a documented range of variability among patients in their assessments of the relative discomforts of their present physical symptoms. In the words of Barry and his colleagues, "Patients [diagnosed with BPH] . . . need to be educated about the importance of their relative preferences for outcome states in a particular decision-making scenario before they understand the appropriateness and importance of participating in a decision."[4] This point has general application to the consent process for elective surgery.

To be sure, many patients desire significant participation in decision making. Given the emphasis in recent decades on the rights of patients, and the ideal of shared decision making, that desire is understandable and should be encouraged. Ordinarily, however, the process of informed consent also allows patients to defer to the surgeon's judgment and recommendations. Thus, in some cases, what is called "second order autonomy" is expressed by the patient's straightforward willingness to trust the doctor.[2] If that deference to the surgeon is at times appropriate (and it certainly may be in other circumstances), a relatively benign chronic or slowly progressive condition requires active patient involvement in assessing what constitutes appropriate treatment, precisely because studies of the relative benefits and risks associated with particular options remain unclear, and because the patient's own assessment of *present* symptoms and *future* consequences are central to decisions about what is both *medically* and *subjectively* desirable.

One implication of shared decision making for the surgeon, under such circumstances, is to suggest strongly that the patient should *not* defer to the surgeon in this instance, precisely because the uncertainty of outcome data cannot support a univocal recommendation. Indeed, in light of uncertain data, the surgeon should be willing to recommend that the patient solicit a second opinion from a different specialist or specialty area in a number of circumstances, for example: to corroborate the range of uncertainty associated with various treatment options in response to a particular diagnosis; to engage in a more detailed discussion with a physician whose specialty involves nonsurgical management of the patient's diagnosed condition; or more generally, to clarify, through discussion with another physician, how the values the patient has identified may best be implemented by choice of treatment. Very often, of course, the recommended second opinion may be provided by the patient's family physician, who should be familiar with the patient's health status and health-related values over a long period of time. Moreover, in the event of continuing uncertainty, the surgeon should not arbitrarily recommend a particular course simply because his or her own medical specialty is involved. In particular, the surgeon should not "recommend" surgery as the "most reasonable" option absent professional data that clearly supports that as the course of first resort.

In pursuing this education of patients, the surgeon should encourage the patient to assess a number of important aspects of diagnosis and prognosis. As we have indicated, the patient should be encouraged to evaluate his or her own affective reactions to the symptoms currently associated with his or her condition. It will also be important to compare the patient's evaluation of present symptoms,[4,14] with discrete judgments about possible states after a particular treatment option is implemented. For some patients, living with present symptoms that are either few in number or mild to moderate in severity will be preferable to opting for a range of surgical interventions that carry different risks and benefits. By contrast, for those who experience severity of present symptoms, the risk of postsurgical complications will be weighted differently. For example, in the case of BPH, the highest predictor of surgery is among those patients who describe their present symptoms as severe and assess them most negatively.[4,14] Not surprisingly, the second highest correlation from the same study links a negative evaluation of the risk, however small, of postsurgical impotence, to the decision to forgo surgery as an option in favor of the other option generally available, that of nonsurgical management.[4]

However, ongoing studies of patient preferences for surgical and nonsurgical options raise a general issue of broad relevance to chronic or slowly progressive conditions, namely, how to collaborate with the patient in determining the most appropriate option among alternatives, all of which have been recognized as therapeutic and thus clinically viable, but none (or few) of which have been subjected to randomized trials in a way that allows their relative merits to be straightforwardly compared.[4,10] For example, the typical choice for BPH in the recent literature has posed prostatectomy or nonsurgical management as the major options. But in recent years, in a pattern not unusual for elective surgery, other treatments have begun to emerge, including the administration of hormonally active drugs (e.g., finasteride) or alpha-sympathetic blockers (e.g., terazosin or doxozocin), hyperthermia, and transurethral microwave needle ablation (TUNA).[12,13] Each of these has been shown to be of therapeutic value, but their relative efficacy is not definitively known at the present time.

In a climate of uncertainty involving this range of choices, the surgeon, in the process of educating the patient, should advise the patient about what each option entails, and encourage the patient to assess all options—surgical versus nonsurgical, as well as among nonsurgical options—according to the risks tentatively identified for each and in the light of the patient's values and preferences. In such cases, the surgeon should adopt three guidelines as a general strategy:

1. Elicit the patient's own values;
2. Encourage the patient to assess alternatives for both their short- and long-term effects in light of the values identified in (1).
3. In the absence of clear data, vigilantly avoid any inappropriate discounting of the risk(s) or accenting the potential benefit(s) of each alternative, i.e., framing effects (see Chapter 2 and below).

Strategies that Encourage Greater Patient Participation in Decision Making

In addition to education, which requires a careful presentation of the data available for patients to make decisions, the surgeon should, as we have noted, encourage the patient to *participate* in decision making according to the patient's own values. Especially with slowly progressive, relatively benign conditions, the patient's own active identification of the values relevant to assessing present symptoms and to assessing future conditions after medical intervention is required. Although the surgeon can provide vital information about the expected medical benefits and risks associated with various options, the patient is uniquely situated to make judgments about the acceptability or advisability of pursuing a particular option, in light of the values that are determinative of his approach to life—both his evaluation of present symptoms and his aversion to/acceptance of varying degrees of risk associated with different possible outcomes.

One clinical issue relevant to a frank and comprehensive discussion of options, especially in light of uncertain data for slowly progressive, relatively benign conditions, may be the lengthiness of the process. As Barry and his colleagues observe, "Communicating the elements of a complex medical decision to patients, including the risks of all relevant outcomes and the nature of those outcomes, is difficult and time consuming."[14] On the one hand, of course, because the patient's own assessment is crucially determinative of what constitutes an appropriate choice among options, one might simply insist, as some commentators do, that the surgeon must accept the time-consuming nature of the process and work with the patient accordingly.[4,10,12,14] This seems especially to be the case with elective surgery because the possibilities of time trials and ongoing monitoring lessen the degree of urgency associated with more acute surgical circumstances.

Nonetheless, tools have been developed recently that may be useful as an initial step in the decision-making process regarding surgical or nonsurgical management. Barry and his colleagues have developed a "Shared Decision-Making Program" (SDP) as an alternative to the need for an extensive initial presentation of the complex and uncertain data represented by the literature.[14] Although one might question the need for such a program, in light of some ideal of time available for patient-physician conversations, a more structured and patient-driven assessment might well be preferable to less comprehensive presentations of the relevant information by physicians under pressures of time, especially in managed care settings. Indeed, the program developed by Barry et al., is designed to be shown to patients already diagnosed with symptomatic BPH after an office evaluation, who have read a brochure about options and completed a questionnaire providing information on demographics, symptoms, and the status of their overall health.

Clinical judgments in response to chronic or slowly progressive conditions might be enhanced by revising and incorporating, for specific diagnoses, elements of the shared decision-making program (SDP) developed by Barry and his colleagues for BPH. In all such circumstances, rather than being seen as a substitute for effective communication, the SDP might be better viewed as a useful part of the process that allows the patient greater latitude in thinking through the values that he or she finds decisive in choosing a particular option. However, the three general guidelines we have suggested for the surgeon should remain central to the clinical dialogue with the patient, and the SDP should remain a supplement to, not a substitute for, careful and, as necessary, time-consuming conversation between surgeon and patient.

The Framing Phenomenon

In this dialogue/discussion efforts should be made to avoid the negative effects of the "framing" phenomenon (see Chapter 2). Framing occurs when risks and benefits are couched in terms that psychologically tilt the decision to be made by the patient. Presenting only mortality data or only survival data involves a subtle form of the framing effect. To avoid this effect, the surgeon should discuss the risks in terms of *both* possible death *and* likely survival. The ethical requirement to avoid framing is especially germane to chronic or slowly progressive conditions, where the data regarding relative efficacy of treatment alternatives remain unclear, and the tendency to be unwarrantedly enthusiastic regarding one's own specialty and/or unduly pessimistic about other alternatives must be strongly resisted. In such circumstances, the surgeon should be especially vigilant against framing his or other recommendations by underplaying the risks of morbidity and reduced quality of life that might ensue from surgical management. The issue of framing is important to the process of both education of patients by physicians (the information in informed consent) and in patients' own participation in decision making (the consent aspect of informed consent), especially in identifying and applying their own values to choices among alternatives.[17]

A structured shared decision-making program, like the one developed by Barry and his colleagues, if subject to careful professional scrutiny and review, could serve as an extremely useful tool in minimizing the possibilities of framing by the surgeon, whether it is based on the surgeon's own failure to acknowledge the conflicted nature of current data or the surgeon's unsubstantiated bias toward his or her own specialty area. Indeed, as reported by Barry and his colleagues, presenting a "balanced" presentation "was critical to the underlying concept" of SDP as a pedagogical tool: "the goal was to present . . . options in a way that favored neither."[14] The SDP includes a "core segment," 22 minutes long, with several core elements: a clear outline of the basic treatment choices, including surgical and nonsurgical management; a careful depiction of the possible harms and benefits of each treatment, with the probabilities of these outcomes based on the most up-to-date findings from the professional literature and expressed both verbally and graphically; and a number of more detailed modules with information about specific sequelae of treatment, including descriptions of particular problems as experienced by actual patients. The "first-person" character of this last element offers a potentially important corrective to the "bias" other studies have found in the "educational" features of informed consent in the typical dyad of surgeon and patient.

Assessing the Reasonableness of the Patient's Decision in Cases Involving Surgical Management for a Rarely Occurring but Very Bad Outcome

As we observed in our introduction, in a second type of case, clinical judgment is complicated by the concern to avoid a very bad outcome of extremely low, but uncertain, incidence. In such cases, although the ratio of risks to benefits remains uncertain, prudential clinical judgment lends greater support to surgical management, though still not enough to warrant a univocal recommendation, given the risks of morbidity and adverse effects on the patient's quality of life.

Examples of conditions for which a general recommendation for surgical versus nonsurgical management cannot be definitively made include elective hysterectomy, radial keratectomy, parathyroidectomy, the choice between angioplasty and coronary bypass grafts, and treatment options in response to localized prostatic cancer. We will focus here on localized prostatic cancer, but our remarks are also relevant to other cases and conditions.

During the past two decades, there has been a significant increase in the recorded incidence of clinically localized prostatic cancer and the rate of surgery in response to it. Clinically localized prostate cancer occurs primarily among males over the age of fifty and is typically the object of an extended therapeutic regimen, with numerous alternatives available, including hormone therapy, surgery, radiation therapy, hyperthermia, as well as a strategy of nonoperative management. However, as one commentator notes, "rational decisions regarding treatment are compromised by the inability to predict reliably either the life expectancy of the individual host or the natural course of the particular neoplasm."[18] Moreover, uncertainties persist concerning the relative merits of particular alternatives, with regard to both the relative mortality rates of alternative approaches and the quality of life/morbidity associated with them. In a number of specific studies,[4–6,19] as well as in general reviews of the literature,[10,20] the relative results of alternative therapeutic responses to diagnosed localized prostate cancer are decidedly mixed, with the range in practice variations quite extensive, and, for many commentators, *prima facie* troubling. In one widely quoted study, Fleming and his colleagues employ extensive decision analysis to assess alternative initial treatments on quality-adjusted life expectancy for males in the 60 to 75 age group. After careful review of their findings, Fleming and his colleagues conclude that "aggressive treatment," which includes radical prostatectomy or external beam irradiation, may benefit selected patients, but that such benefits are sufficiently marginal to make nonoperative management a reasonable alternative for many such patients.[5,21] In the same vein, a literature review by Wasson et al "revealed no studies definitively supporting a benefit of aggressive treatment over nonsurgical management at 10 years following diagnosis," an "apparent[ly] equal treatment efficacy of irradiation or radical prostatectomy," as well as "greater morbidity and mortality" with surgical intervention.[10]

In the light of the increase in diagnosed prostate cancer and the indeterminate results of studies of the morbidity and mortality associated with various alternatives, the condition offers an instructive example of the crucial relevance of the patient's values in deciding what constitutes appropriate treatment. Unlike other conditions for which surgery can be clearly recommended as the preferred option, the literature suggests that surgery is generally elective in response to this condition. Thus the matter of whether or not to elect surgery, in the absence of decisive evidence in its favor, emerges under such circumstances as almost *fully* patient-driven, absent compelling medical indications in many cases.

There are a number of technical issues, relating to research design and the use of data, that are relevant to the discussion of surgical and nonsurgical options in response to localized prostatic cancer.[12,13,18,22–25] It is not our purpose here to adjudicate among these various claims in detail. Rather, it is sufficient to note that among critics of the studies suggesting parity among available alternatives, there seems a clear preference toward surgery as a first resort, even though such an advantage cannot be definitively substantiated as a general recommendation by the literature.[18,26–31] We have already mentioned the phenomenon of framing effects in relation to slowly progressive, relatively benign, conditions. Framing is obviously also a pertinent concern in cases involving a possible bad outcome of very small or uncertain incidence. Among critics of studies suggesting that current data regarding the preferability of surgery are inconclusive, an unstated assumption seems at work—namely, that the risk of mortality without surgery is the only significant factor in patient decision making. The diagnosis of malignancy itself tends to heighten the bias toward aggressive therapy that surgeons are likely to feel by dint of their own training and commitment.

Thus, when current data support the relative efficacy of surgical versus nonsurgical options, it is ethically necessary for surgeons to do three things: to guard against self-interested recommendations *that are not supported by clear evidence*; to be as unbiased and impartial in fairly describing the mixed data regarding alternatives as possible; and to emphasize the pivotal role that the patient's values and preferences will play in deciding what constitutes an appropriate response to cases that involve surgical management with a potential for rarely occurring but very bad outcome. Moreover, because both mortality and morbidity are important to the patient's assessment of alternatives, the surgeon must be especially cautious, in light of inconclusive data, to emphasize the reasonableness of interim strategies.

Responding to Inappropriate Demand for or Refusal of Surgical Management

Significant issues may arise when a patient either demands surgery deemed medically inappropriate or refuses surgery deemed medically appropriate. As discussed elsewhere in this volume (see Chapters 2 and 7), such a demand or refusal should not, even in high-risk or acute situations, be seen as evidence of a patient's diminished decision-making capacity. Rather, in most instances, noncompliance with the surgeon's recommendations will reflect failures of effective physician-patient communication during the informed consent process (see Chapter 2).

However, in the case of elective surgery, demands for or refusal of surgery are far less obviously inappropriate, for the reasons we have suggested above. First, in conditions such as BPH or localized prostatic cancer, no one option will necessarily emerge as clearly preferable according to unambiguous data. Second, absent circumstances of acute emergency or immediate high risk, strategies of nonsurgical management should be deemed appropriate choices because they protect and promote the patient's interests. Indeed, in elective circumstances, the demand *for* surgery may be more likely to emerge as inappropriate, especially if the patient's own expressed values comport with interim strategies that are less invasive. Under these circumstances, the surgeon should be willing to review those values the patient has previously identified that indicate nonsurgical management as a subjectively preferable choice. In such an instance, directive counseling by the surgeon may be ethically required.

When May the Surgeon Refuse to Perform Surgery?

The surgeon may refuse to perform elective surgery when he or she determines that the patient's own values, as clarified through a careful process of informed consent, are not being served by that choice. Surgeons are neither mere technicians nor simply servants of patient desires. Rather, surgeons have a fiduciary obligation to act in the interest of patients. In rare circumstances, the surgeon may, in good conscience, be obliged to refuse the request for surgery as a decision not in keeping with the interests previously expressed by the patient—as evidence of a lack of affective understanding. However, in such circumstances, respect for the patient's autonomy dictates the need for further discussion with the patient to identify the apparent incongruence between the patient's expressed values and his or her demand for surgery.

Under rare circumstances, the surgeon may sincerely conclude that elective surgery is not in the patient's interest, at least at the present time. In these circumstances, resources would also be wasted, injuring society's legitimate interests in conserving medical resources for those who need them. The surgeon, however, is ethically obligated not to abandon the patient and must be willing to refer the patient to another physician willing to review the case and, if required, to accept the patient.

Endorsement of a Subjective Rather Than a Reasonable Person Standard of Disclosure in Elective Surgery

It is important, in the circumstances of elective surgery, to appreciate that the ordinary "reasonable person" standard of disclosure may well be inadequate to the highly subjective nature of the patient's evaluation of alternative therapies. In light of incomplete or ambiguous data, the medical grounds for a clearly preferred course are invariably less decisive than in circumstances of acute or high risk. As we have suggested, treatment decisions in response to either of the two sorts of cases we have analyzed require that the patient be actively involved in assessing and comparing risks of mortality and morbidity in the face of uncertain data about the relative efficacy of various options. Hence what a "reasonable" person needs to know, in such circumstances, is precisely what values are central to assessing both the discomfort of present symptoms and the desirability/undesirability of certain outcome states with or without surgery.

Managing Refusal of Blood Products

Surgery in response to either of the two types of cases that we have discussed may involve significant blood loss. For example, radical prostatectomy carries an average loss of greater than one unit of blood, with loss of three to four units on some occasions. Thus, religiously based refusals of blood products may be features of the examples we have discussed, and in many other forms of elective surgery.

The context of elective surgery raises no distinctive set of issues in dealing with such refusals. However, given greater opportunity for extensive discussion with patients before scheduling elective surgery, even greater clarity can be obtained concerning the nature, scope, and bindingness of the patient's value-based objections to surgery. Moreover, in elective surgery, the use of autologous blood-conserving methods is usually an option, one that Jehovah's Witnesses may be willing to accept. Ultimately, the patient's own values will be decisive and referral to a surgeon willing to perform surgery with bloodless volume-enhancers may be necessary.

DNR Orders from Other Settings

It is estimated that only about fifty percent of hospitals currently have policies concerning the status of DNR orders from other settings in the operating room.[32,33] In circumstances when surgery is elected as the therapeutic option of choice, especially by older patients, the status of the patient's wishes regarding cardiopulmonary resuscitation in response to intrasurgical arrest should be fully explored. However, in light of the consent process that we have discussed, and the patient's own express desire for surgery as the preferred option to enhance his clinical outcome, the notion of a DNR order in the context of elective surgery makes little or no sense (see Chapter 4).

Clinical Conclusions

Elective surgical patients pose a number of interesting issues in relation to canonical understandings of the process of informed consent. By way of summary, we will stipulate answers to the four general ethical concerns that have shaped our discussion:

A fair and unbiased assessment of the risks and benefits of alternatives in the face of significant uncertainty regarding associated risks of mortality and morbidity will require the surgeon to adopt three guidelines as general strategy: (1) to elicit the patient's own values; (2) to encourage the patient to assess alternatives for both their short- and long-term effects in light of the values identified in (1); and (3) in the absence of clear data, vigilantly to avoid any inappropriate minimization of the risk(s) or promotion of benefit(s) among the available options.

An assessment of the reasonableness of the patient's decision in the face of persistent uncertainty will generally require that the patient be actively involved in weighing the risks and benefits of various options in light of the values the patient has identified as determinative. This, in effect, leads us to endorse a subjective rather than a reasonable person standard of disclosure in elective surgery.

In the face of less than definitive data, the surgeon should guard against self-interested recommendations that are not supported by clear evidence, be as unbiased as possible in describing the uncertain nature of those data, and emphasize the determinative role of the patient's values in choosing an appropriate therapeutic course. Clinical judgments in response to both sorts of cases we have analyzed might be enhanced by revising and incorporating, for specific diagnoses, elements of the shared decision making program developed by Barry and his colleagues.

In the context of elective surgery, it is critically important for the surgeon to be attentive to the values that will determine the patient's decision regarding what constitutes an appropriate response to a given diagnosis. As we have noted, the patient's own values will be decisive relative to several aspects of decisions regarding treatment options. First, the patient's values will be central to assessments of the frequency and severity of present symptoms. Second, subjective values will function centrally in judgments about the magnitude and probability of likely risks associated with surgical versus nonsurgical options. Third, the patient's values will centrally inform assessments of what constitutes an acceptable quality of life after particular interventions. Fourth, the patient's values will decisively shape differential judgments based on highly varying data regarding surgical versus nonsurgical options, as well as among nonsurgical options.

More generally, the process of informed consent, in the elective context as elsewhere, is based on an ethical understanding of the surgeon-patient encounter as a clinical partnership. Thus, informed consent is both ethically required and medically desirable. The surgeon's own ethical obligation to the patient is to provide the surgeon's clinically informed professional judgment in a way that fully respects the interests of the patient, as defined in light of the patient's values. That process requires sensitivity, patience, and the willingness to work with the patient (if necessary, over a significant period of time) to develop and monitor a therapeutic regimen that comports with the patient's interests. The elective surgical patient also has obligations in the clinical partnership: to listen carefully to the diagnosis and prognosis described by the surgeon; to ask for clarification, especially regarding the uncertainties of prognosis; to solicit the physician's advice and recommendations as needed; and to explore, fully and honestly, the personal values that will shape, and ultimately determine, the most appropriate course to pursue.

References

1. Stephen Wear, *Informed Consent: Patient Autonomy and Physician Beneficence within Clinical Medicine*. Dordrecht, The Netherlands: Kluwer Academic Publishers, 1993.

2. Tom L. Beauchamp and James F. Childress, *Principles of Biomedical Ethics*, 4th ed. New York: Oxford University Press, 1994.
3. Allen Buchanan and Dan Brock, *Deciding for Others: The Ethics of Surrogate Decisionmaking*. New York, Cambridge University Press, 1990.
4. Michael J. Barry, Albert G. Mulley, and Floyd J. Fowler, "Watchful Waiting versus Immediate Transurethral Resection for Symptomatic Prostatism: The Importance of Patients' Preferences," *Journal of the American Medical Association* 259 (1988): 3010–3017.
5. Craig Fleming, John H. Wasson, Peter C. Albertsen, et al., "A Decision Analysis of Alternative Treatment Strategies for Clinically Localized Prostate Cancer," *Journal of the American Medical Association* 269 (1993): 2650–2658.
6. Floyd Fowler, Michael J. Barry, Grace Lu-Yao, et al., "Patient-Reported Complications and Follow-Up Treatment After Radical Prostatectomy," *Urology* 42 (1993): 622–629.
7. Jan-Erik Johansson, Hans-Olov Adami, Swen-Olof Andersson, et al., "High 1-Year Survival Rate in Patients with Early, Untreated Prostatic Cancer," *Journal of the American Medical Association* 267 (1992): 2191–2196.
8. Grace L. Lu-Yao, Dale McLerran, John Wasson, et al., "An Assessment of Radical Prostatectomy: Time Trends, Geographic Variation, and Outcomes," *Journal of the American Medical Association* 269 (1993): 2633–2636.
9. Grace L. Lu-Yao, Michael J. Barry, Chiang-Hua Chang, et al., "Transurethral Resection of the Prostate Among Medicare Beneficiaries in the United States: Time Trends and Outcomes," *Urology* 44 (1994): 692–698.
10. John H. Wasson, Cynthia C. Cushman, Reginald C. Bruskewitz, et al., "A Structured Literature Review of Treatment for Localized Prostate Cancer," *Archives of Family Medicine* 2 (1993): 487–493.
11. *Canterbury v. Spence*, 464 F.2d 772, 785 (D.C. Cir. 1972).
12. James A. Eastham and Peter T. Scardino, "Radical Prostatectomy," in *Campbell's Urology*, 7th ed., Vol. 3, Patrick C. Walsh, et al., eds. Philadelphia: W.B. Saunders, 1998, pp. 2547–2564.
13. Michael W. Kattan, Mark E. Cowen, and Brian J. Miles, "A Decision Analysis for Treatment of Clinically Localized Prostate Cancer," *Journal of General Internal Medicine* 12 (1997): 288–305.
14. Michael J. Barry, Floyd J. Fowler, Albert G. Mulley, et al., "Patient Reactions to a Program Designed to Facilitate Patient Participation in Treatment Decisions for Benign Prostatic Hyperplasia," *Medical Care* 33 (1995): 771–782.
15. David J. Doukas and Laurence B. McCullough. "The Values History: The Evaluation of the Patient's Values and Advance Directives," *The Journal of Family Practice* 32 (1991): 145–151.
16. Michael Macfarlane, *Urology for the House Officer*. Baltimore: Williams and Wilkins, 1988.
17. Barbara J. McNeil, Stephen G. Pauker, Harold C. Sox, et al., "On The Elicitation of Preferences for Alternative Therapies," *New England Journal of Medicine* 306 (1982): 1259–1262.
18. Richard Williams, "Editorial Comment," Urology 42 (1993): 629.
19. Grace Lu-Yao, "In Reply," *Journal of the American Medical Association* 270 (1993): 1693–1694.
20. David Malenka, Dale McLerran, Noralou Roos, et al., "Using Administrative Data to Describe Casemix: A Comparison with the Medical Record," *Journal of Clinical Epidemiology* 47 (1994): 1027–1032.

21. Craig Fleming, "In Reply," *Journal of the American Medical Association* 270 (1993): 1693.
22. Peter C. Albertsen, Dennis G. Fryback, Barry E. Storer, et al., "Long-term Survival among Men with Conservatively Treated Localized Prostate Cancer," *Journal of the American Medical Association* 274 (1995): 626–631.
23. Gerald W. Chodak, Ronald A. Thisted, Glenn S. Gerber, et al., "Results of Conservative Management of Clinically Localized Prostate Cancer," *New England Journal of Medicine* 330 (1994): 242–248.
24. Abraham Cockett, "To the Editor," *Journal of the American Medical Association* 270 (1993): 1692–1693.
25. Willet F. Whitmore, "Management of Clinically Localized Prostate Cancer: An Unresolved Problem," *Journal of the American Medical Association* 269 (1993): 2676–2677.
26. William J. Catalona, "To the Editor," *Journal of the American Medical Association* 270 (1993): 1691–1692.
27. Abraham Cockett, "Editorial Comments," *Urology* 44 (1994): 698.
28. Martin Cohen, "To the Editor," *Journal of the American Medical Association* 270 (1993): 1693.
29. H. Logan Holtgreve, "Editorial Comments," *Urology* 44 (1994): 698–699.
30. Peter Scardino, Robert Weaver, and M'Liss A. Hudson, "Early Detection of Prostate Cancer," *Human Pathology* 23 (1992):211–222.
31. Richard Switzer, "To the Editor," *Journal of the American Medical Association* 270 (1993): 1692.
32. Cory M. Franklin and David M. Rothenberg, "Do-Not-Resuscitate Orders in the Presurgical Patient," *Journal of Clinical Anesthesia* 4 (1992): 181–184.
33. Allan L. Smith, "DNR in the OR," *Clinical Ethics Report* 8 (1994): 1–8.

9

Poor Surgical Risk Patients

AMIR HALEVY
JOHN C. BALDWIN

Patients deemed to be poor surgical risks pose special challenges to the medical care team in general, and to the surgeon in particular. These challenges result from the ambiguity that arises from the very concept of poor risk and the reality that decision making in such cases reflects the views and values of the surgeon, the referring physician, and the patient. Successfully managing such cases requires an understanding of the perspectives of the three parties involved in the determination of poor surgical risk and of the role of the informed consent process in bringing potentially diverse perspectives into a coherent decision.

Decision making in poor-risk cases requires a two-step approach. The first step is determining when surgical intervention is medically appropriate in light of the risk-benefit ratio and when the patient presents such a poor risk that the surgeon can unilaterally decide that surgery is not an option. The second question is, if surgery is deemed to be an appropriate option, how should the increased level of risk be communicated to the patient and how should this information materially affect the process of informed consent?

Potential problems stem from the initial definition of poor surgical risk and medical appropriateness. The definitions are context dependent and are contingent on the values and goals of the person defining the terms. Who defines poor surgical risk and medical appropriateness and how should they be defined? Disagreement regarding the definitions of poor surgical risk and medical appropriateness exposes potential conflicts not only between the patient and the surgeon but also among members of the health care team.

In this chapter we provide an ethical analysis of the surgeon's, the referring physician's, and the patient's perspectives on defining surgical appropriateness. In doing so, we review not only the traditional autonomy and beneficence debate but also analyze professional integrity and justice. We also explore the most commonly confronted problems, including patient or surrogate decision maker refusal of recommended surgery, requests for inappropriate surgery, patient decisions that knowingly increase the potential risk (i.e., refusal of blood products), interprofessional disagreements, and postoperative dilemmas including early pressure to "abandon hope." We also consider the case when the patient is high risk because of the potential risk of disease transmission to the surgeon. We close with a clinical summary to assist the reader facing such problems.

Ethical Analysis

Indications for Surgery and Appropriate Care

Defining appropriate surgical care, or the more frequently attempted converse of defining inappropriate surgical interventions, is a difficult problem that has been made more difficult recently as resource constraints and the concept of cost-effectiveness have entered the debate. The fundamental question is who determines appropriateness, the surgeon or the patient? Traditionally, the surgeon determines the appropriate options and offers the choice of options to the patient as part of the informed consent process. However, the recent emergence of the medical futility debate highlights the reluctance of many patients, supported by various bodies of organized medicine,[1,2] ethicists,[3] and some courts,[4,5] to allow physicians unilateral control over the therapeutic menu. Much of this reluctance grows from the dominance of the principle of patient autonomy over other ethical principles such as beneficence, integrity, and justice and the growing skepticism about the medical profession.[6]

The debate over who determines appropriateness grows directly out of the evolution of thought regarding medical decision making. Beneficence-based medical decision making was limited earlier this century by the *Schloendorff* and subsequent decisions,[7] more fully discussed in Chapter 2, which obligate physicians to respect a patient's autonomy by balancing risks and benefits from the patient's perspective. In the past two decades, numerous court decisions have been reached that allowed competent patients, or their surrogate decision makers, to refuse all forms of medical treatment, including potentially life prolonging therapy, on the basis of individual autonomy. More recently, the focus has shifted to whether patient autonomy grounds a patient's right to receive whatever therapy or treatment the patient desires. The initial court cases of this type, such as Baby K[5] and others, more fully discussed below, have limited the surgeon's ability to unilaterally limit therapy over the objections of a patient or surrogate decision maker, *even on the basis of medical inappropriateness or futility*. If patient autonomy were unlimited and the only principle of importance in medical decision making, then the concept of too high a risk is completely independent of any judgments or values other than those of the patient. Patient autonomy, however, is not unlimited. Other legitimate ethical principles should be part of the discussion regarding surgical appropriateness such as professional and institutional integrity and justice. These principles ground the surgeon's and the referring physician's role in determining surgical and medical appropriateness while autonomy continues to secure the patient's role in determining appropriateness.

The Surgeon's Perspective. An analysis of the surgeon's role in determining when surgery is an appropriate option and when the patient poses too high a risk requires an examination of the ethical basis for such a role and of the surgical definitions of too poor a risk. The principle of beneficence, or the obligation to act in such a way that the patient experiences net benefit, is based on the surgeon's value system and personal threshold for risk and benefit. Respect for autonomy, both as an ethical principle and as a legal obligation, profoundly limits the role of a beneficence-based decision as the basis for determining that a particular intervention is medically inappropriate. Beneficence, however, is not the only ethical principle that could possibly support the surgeon's right to determine which options are medically appropriate. Two other principles which must be explored are integrity and justice.

The concept of integrity has been explored by some authors[8,9] and has been cited by several court decisions but it remains a difficult concept to define. Two components of integrity need to be explored. The first is personal or intellectual integrity in the sense that the surgeon has a responsibility to master and maintain the knowledge base and clinical skills required of the profession. An important part of this fund of knowledge must be an appreciation of the limits of the profession. Personal integrity also requires the surgeon to be aware of potential self-interest in terms of mortality rates and referrals and to try to eliminate this factor from the process of determining too poor a risk. The second component is that of professional integrity: the surgeon has an obligation to use his or her talents and skills in service to patients and to the profession. While the concept of patient autonomy is clearly recognized as the basis for the prohibition against surgeons forcing unwanted medical interventions on patients, some have argued that the concept of integrity supports the surgeon's refusal to offer or provide surgically inappropriate treatment.[8]

Personal or professional integrity can ground the surgeon's refusal to provide a particular intervention. The surgeon's responsibility for individual outcomes and the right not to be forced to perform any intervention against his or her will supports such a refusal. In addition, a determination that a particular intervention is too high risk can be based on the surgeon's responsibility to the institution and peers not to perform unnecessary or inappropriate surgeries. When considering whether providing a surgical intervention would violate the surgeon's sense of integrity, the surgeon should consider whether the intervention harms the patient without any compensating benefits, results in the provision of unseemly care, or represents an inappropriate stewardship of resources discussed more fully below.[8]

Justice is an even more problematic principle to address, with multiple competing definitions and a vigorous debate as to the appropriateness of involving resource allocation decisions at the bedside.[10] However, few would argue that resources are infinite and that the surgeon need play no role as a steward of resources. These include the surgeon's individual time and effort, in that no surgeon can be at two places at once. In addition, no surgery is performed in a vacuum—that is, without utilization of significant hospital resources in terms of physical space, personnel, and material resources. In an era of limited budgets and increasingly limited resources, surgery on a patient who is an inappropriate candidate can result in delay or denial of a needed intervention for another patient.

Given the role of integrity and justice and the limited role of beneficence in making surgical judgments of poor risk, the surgeon can define too poor a risk in several ways. One is that the surgery cannot result in the desired outcome and therefore any risk is outweighed by no benefit. For example, the patient desires pain relief and there is no medical or physiologic basis to support the contention that the particular surgical intervention will address the cause of the pain. Another is that the risk of perioperative death or significant disability is extremely high. The areas of contention are obviously who defines extremes and what constitutes an acceptable definition. The surgeon must be on guard constantly to avoid the inappropriate influence of self-interest in the desire to keep mortality and morbidity rates as low as possible. The surgeon must also assess high surgical mortality in the context of the expected mortality without the procedure.

The Referring Physician's Perspective. The referring physician often determines the medical appropriateness of a particular surgical intervention because if the physician believes that surgical intervention is too high risk, the referral is usually not made and the option is never presented to the patient. However, if the option is presented to the patient, the referring physician may not be the final determiner of medical appropriateness, because he or she does not perform the procedure. The two-step nature of surgical referral raises the potential for interprofessional disagreements regarding the appropriateness of a surgical intervention, a consideration that will be discussed below.

When considering surgical referral, the referring physician can also evaluate the appropriateness of a particular intervention from the perspectives of beneficence, integrity, and justice. The referring physician has his or her personal threshold for risk and has a responsibility for the overall outcome of the patient's care and the same resource issues discussed above apply. In addition, the referring physician has a responsibility to be informed and current regarding changes in surgical practice and procedure that could change the risk and benefit profile and to be vigilant in avoiding making referral decisions on the basis of economic self-interest, which could be promoted by group practices.

The referring physician can also define poor risk as either no foreseeable benefit or extremely high risk of poor outcome. The key difference between the surgical perspective and the referring medical perspective is possibly the difference in the two cultures. The culture of medicine has been traditionally to do everything possible that a patient desires, a view reinforced by requirements that a patient, or surrogate, must consent to refuse cardiopulmonary resuscitation, even in those cases that the medical staff believe that it is futile or inappropriate. This difference has also been reinforced by the courts that have ordered attempts at resuscitation,[5] over the objections of medical personnel, while never compelling a surgeon to operate against his or her judgment.

Another potential for conflict between the referring physician's and surgeon's perspective is the dire consequence of nonsurgical alternatives, that is, when the referring physician sees death without surgery as being very likely. The referring physician may then offer surgery as a desperate hope, even though the intraoperative or postoperative risks may be very high. Such conflicts are best resolved, if possible, by the surgeon carefully explaining to the patient the risks both without and with surgery and helping the patient make a considered decision about surgery under these conditions.

The Patient's Perspective.   Unlike both the surgeon and the referring physician, the patient cannot determine the likely mortality rate or the incidence of the various complications. The patient also is not a steward of the communal resources required for his or her care. However, the patient is uniquely qualified to assess most quality-of-life and many quantity-of-life issues (see Chapters 2, 7, 8, and 10).

A very high risk patient in need of surgical intervention likely has preoperative quality-of-life limitations. While the goal of an appropriate surgical intervention is to improve and/or prolong life, the outcome from surgery is never certain. The patient must consider the potential of perioperative death or further impairment of the quality of life (e.g., a perioperative stroke). Only the patient can determine if, to him or her, a 60% chance of perioperative mortality and a not insignificant risk of worsening quality of life is worth risking in return for the possibility of some benefit in terms of either prolonged survival or improved quality of life.

Informed Consent for High-Risk Patients

The need for a strong therapeutic alliance between the patient and the surgeon is especially critical when the patient is faced with the difficult decision of agreeing to a very high risk surgery. The seriousness of the decision and the significant risk of an undesirable outcome require that the informed consent process be approached in a careful and considerate fashion. The medicolegal repercussions of the increased likelihood of serious morbidity or mortality resulting from a high-risk surgery are one reason why the patient's decision must truly be informed. A second reason is that the increased risks create a relative uncertainty as to the "correct" decision for the patient. This uncertainty requires that the surgeon present appropriate options and that an informed patient assess the potential risks and the potential benefits of the offered choices against his or her personal value system.

As with the process of informed consent in general, the disclosure of relevant clinical information by the surgeon, the understanding of the information by the patient, and the patient's decision-making process are the three interrelated elements of the informed consent process (see Chapter 2). In addition, very high risk cases require that the surgeon assess whether a particular intervention is a relevant and appropriate option to even offer to a patient. If a particular intervention is judged by the surgeon to be too high a risk and not an appropriate option, there is no obligation to offer the patient the choice of an intervention the surgeon will not perform.

The first step is for the surgeon to explain carefully to the patient the underlying diagnosis, the various potential management options (including not doing surgery and allowing the disease process to follow its natural history), and the risks and the benefits of the therapeutic options. If the surgeon believes that a particular surgical intervention is not appropriate for the patient, it would be desirable at this point in the discussion to explain to the patient why the surgeon believes that the intervention is of such high risk that it is not an option.

While the surgeon should inform the patient of his or her best opinion and recommendation regarding surgical intervention, the surgeon should present the information in such a way that allows the patient to decide without coercion. High-risk cases, by their very nature, create situations that when not guarded against can result in a coercive presentation of the medical data. The surgeon must be careful not to be too blunt or to overstate the potential risks.

Although not intervening may be associated with an extremely high mortality, the surgeon should make clear to the patient any areas of uncertainty or alternative therapies that may decrease the risk, and not merely state that the choice is "surgery or death," an inappropriate framing effect (see Chapter 2).

Another potential problem with the initial disclosure of information, not unique to high-risk cases, is the use of mortality or morbidity statistics. The surgeon should certainly use terms that the patient understands, such as risk of death, rather than mortality, and risk of adverse outcome, rather than morbidity. Beyond simple word choice, many patients may have trouble comparing various statistical likelihoods. Again, the surgeon should explain to the patient at a level that he or she can comprehend and be cognizant of any clues that a patient does not understand or is having trouble focusing on the conversation because of anxiety provoked by the disclosures.

The final potential problem with the disclosure phase of the informed consent process involves issues of morbidity. The surgeon should present the known data as clearly as possible at a level that the patient can understand. The surgeon should also avoid overstating or minimizing potential complications. Efforts should be made not to downplay the potential postoperative problems, including postoperative pain and the length of the recovery period. The surgeon should also avoid unduly influencing the patient to refuse surgery by presenting complications in such a way that it could cloud the patient's judgment. For example, stating that there exists a risk "worse than death" of becoming a "vegetable." However, in high-risk cases the dying process can be prolonged and unpleasant for the patient's family.

The second and third phases of the informed consent process, the patient's understanding of the presented information and the patient's decision-making process, also assume a greater importance in such cases because of the high risk of an undesirable outcome. The ideal disclosure by the surgeon is meaningless if the patient cannot understand the disclosed information or if he or she cannot or will not make a decision consistent with his or her values. As discussed in Chapter 2, the patient needs to listen to and absorb, retain, and recall the information the surgeon conveys. The patient must also understand that he or she is being asked to authorize or refuse a hazardous surgical intervention.

The surgeon should assess the patient's understanding and decision-making capacity at this stage of the informed consent process. Although having the patient repeat the information may be perceived as demeaning by some patients, the surgeon should inquire if the patient has sufficient understanding of the disease process, of the risks and benefits of the proposed therapy, and of the risks and benefits of the possible alternatives. As suggested in Chapter 2, the informed consent form can be used as a learning aid in this research process. The surgeon should also explore with the patient any concerns or lingering uncertainties and provide the patient with additional information as needed.

Finally, the surgeon should discuss with the patient the reasons for either agreeing to or refusing the surgical intervention. While the presumption should be that the patient has decision-making capacity and that non-agreement with the surgeon, as discussed further below, does not imply diminished decision-making capacity, exploring the patient's reasoning can reveal misunderstandings of the disclosed information or an impaired decision-making process. If such circumstances arise, the surgeon can focus on clarifying the misunderstood point or evaluating the patient's decision-making capacity.

Clinical Topics

In most cases involving the potential for a high-risk surgery, the patient, surgeon, and referring physician have reached a common conclusion based on a mutual exchange of information regarding both data and values. However, potential clinical problems emerge when disagreements over either data interpretation or values develop.

Patient/Surrogate Refusal of Recommended Surgery

Patients may refuse a recommended surgical intervention for many different reasons and refusal does not necessarily indicate diminished decision-making capacity or incompetence, especially when the surgeon, through the informed consent process, has explained to the patient that the surgery is high risk. The principle of patient autonomy, as articulated by both ethicists and the courts, holds that a competent patient may refuse unwanted medical interventions, including potentially lifesaving interventions, and that medical professionals must respect that choice even if they disagree. Thus, the principle of patient autonomy serves as the basis for a prohibition on physician-driven overtreatment.

However, respecting patient autonomy does not preclude the surgeon from further exploring the decision and the decision-making process with the patient when the surgeon believes that the intervention, although posing significant risk, has the potential to be beneficial for the patient. The presumption in such further discussions should be that the patient is competent to make such a decision and that the refusal is based on the patient holding different values.

The surgeon first needs to review the patient's understanding of his or her condition, the likely risks and benefits of the proposed intervention, and the likely outcomes if no surgical intervention is performed. As discussed above, communication of data regarding morbidity and mortality can frame the question in such a way that the patient's answer may be inappropriately influenced. In addition, many people have difficulty conceptualizing probabilities and may focus only on the high risk of the intervention while ignoring the higher risk of non-intervention. This problem is especially acute for very high risk patients. It must be made as clear as possible to the patient that the risk of surgery should not be compared to a baseline of no risk but rather to the risk of not having the surgery (which should be higher if the surgery is indicated and appropriate). The surgeon should also determine if other factors are unduly influencing the patient's decision. Such factors include, but are not limited to, fear and mistrust of the medical profession, depression, excessive anxiety, and undue external influences such as family and friends with strong views, pro or con, about the surgery. If, after carefully reviewing with the patient the above points, the surgeon concludes that the patient's decision-making capacity is intact, the surgeon should explore other options with the patient such as a time- or symptom-limited trial of non-surgical therapy. If such a course is pursued, the patient and surgeon need to develop together a clear understanding of what constitutes medical failure and what circumstances would warrant surgical intervention. If the patient remains adamant in refusing surgical intervention, the surgeon should respect the decision of a competent patient.

If, however, the surgeon believes that the patient's decision-making capacity is limited or impaired, the surgeon has an obligation to define the limitation in decision-making capacity and to assess the need for obtaining a surrogate decision maker for the patient. Competence determination when the surgery is high risk but potentially life-prolonging can be difficult. The decision-making capacity required to consider a potentially life-prolonging therapy is greater than the decision-making capacity required to consent to a minor invasive procedure and a sliding scale of competence has been proposed to deal with such problems.[11]

A useful first step is to involve a consulting psychiatrist in the case. The goals of the consultation should be to assess the patient's decision-making capacity and to consider possible interventions to restore or improve that capacity, if possible. If the patient is determined to not have decision-making capacity and there is no likelihood that he or she will regain it, even transiently, then the surgeon must turn to a surrogate decision maker to speak for the patient. The order of surrogacy varies from state to state but in most cases the nearest relatives are the default surrogates if the patient has not specified a particular surrogate decision maker.

The surrogate decision maker can make any and all necessary decisions on behalf of the incompetent patient. The surgeon should explain to the surrogate the same information that would be required under informed consent and the same care should be taken to minimize framing or bias. The surrogate may decide to consent to or refuse the recommended intervention, based on either knowledge of what the patient would have wanted if known, "substituted judgment," or what is in the "best interests" of the patient[12] (see Chapter 2).

Requests for Inappropriate Surgery

Demands for interventions that the surgeon believes are surgically inappropriate because they are too high risk present a difficult challenge. Although such demands are currently a relatively uncommon problem, the nonsurgical literature on persistent requests for futile or medically inappropriate treatment is growing rapidly.[8,13,14] Such cases are examples of patient-driven overtreatment and resolution of this type of case in a way that acknowledges the all-too-real limits of medical interventions requires consideration of ethical principles other than just patient autonomy. Although having the surgeon unilaterally declare he or she will not perform the unwarranted intervention is certainly appealing and emotionally satisfying to physicians, the resolution of this type of problem is not so simple. As mentioned above, the major problem is determining who defines appropriateness and too high a risk.

There is a major division in the United States between those who believe that it is always the patient's right to determine what is medically appropriate for each particular patient and that the physician never has the right to unilaterally determine that an intervention is inappropriate and those who believe that physicians have a right to determine what are legitimate medical choices. Those who are opposed to any physician role in the ultimate determination of medical appropriateness ground their opposition on the principle of patient autonomy. They argue that because nothing in medicine is absolute and that no surgeon can determine, with 100% certainty prospectively, that an intervention will not have a desired outcome, any limitation of the patient's right to choose is based on indefensible value judgments.[3] Defenders of the concept of medical futility, or the physician's role in determining appropriate treatments, counter that holding patient autonomy paramount in all situations is also a value judgment that in some circumstances is indefensible in that it always values autonomy over other important principles such as provider integrity and social justice.[8]

Even among proponents of the concept of futility, there is no agreement as to the definition of medically futile or inappropriate treatment. Four different conceptions of futility have been proposed in the literature.[15] Some have argued that there is no obligation to provide treatment that is *physiologically futile*.[16] Others have drawn the line at *imminent demise futility*, arguing that if there is no likelihood of patient survival to discharge, the physician has no obligation to provide the treatment.[13] A third concept of futility is that of *lethal condition futility*: the patient may survive for a short while but the underlying condition will result in death in the not too distant future.[15] The final conception proposed for futility is that of *qualitative futility*, the resultant quality of life is so poor that a reasonable person would not choose the treatment.[13] Problems exist for any single definition of futility, and some, including the American Medical Association,[17] have concluded that it cannot be meaningfully defined but that a process-based approach to resolving conflicts between patients and physicians be adopted. This lack of agreement and the competing but mutually exclusive futility definitions are problematic for surgeons and other physicians dealing with such high-risk cases because even if the intervention were futile under one definition, the patient or surrogate can retort that it is not futile under other, equally valid, definitions.

The courts are usually relied on for guidance in resolving such conflicts but there exists considerable uncertainty regarding the subject. In the case of Baby K,[5] an anencephalic infant whose mother demanded aggressive support, a Federal District judge denied a hospital's request to discontinue aggressive treatments on the basis of futility as a violation of several federal statutes. The decision was upheld on appeal to the Fourth Circuit Court of Appeals. However, in the only known case to go to trial after the intervention was actually denied and the patient died, a Massachusetts jury found that although the woman had requested the intervention, the hospital was not obligated to provide futile treatment.[18]

Given the current ethical and legal confusion, what is a surgeon to do when faced with a demand for an intervention that he or she believes to be medically inappropriate because it is too high risk? When presented with such a request, the surgeon should discuss carefully with the patient or the surrogate decision maker the nature of the ailment, the various therapeutic options, and the reasons why the requested intervention is medically inappropriate. The surgeon should also recommend obtaining an independent second opinion. If there is still no agreement, the surgeon should utilize the assistance of the most trusted institutional resources, such as patient care representatives, chaplains, or an ethics committee in an attempt to resolve the conflict. Another option is to transfer the care of the patient to a surgeon who believes that the requested intervention is appropriate or who is at least willing to provide it. In the rare case that the disagreement is not resolved at this point, the surgeon must decide if providing the intervention violates his or her sense of integrity. If so, the surgeon should turn to the relevant institutional policies to resolve the dispute. A growing number of hospitals and institutions have developed policies to deal with demands for futile or inappropriate treatments,[14] a trend likely to be reinforced by developments in the field.[19]

Refusal of Blood Products

A potential problem area for surgeons is the patient who consents to surgery but imposes a limitation that potentially increases the risk of the intervention and thus transforms a low- to moderate-risk surgery into a high-risk surgery. The standard example is the Jehovah's Witness who consents to all medical interventions but refuses blood and blood product transfusions.

Jehovah's Witnesses evolved from a small group founded by Charles Russell in the nineteenth century into a sect with several million adherents worldwide. A 1945 church decision banning transfusions is the source of the conflict between patients and physicians. This position can affect surgical practice and patient care in two ways. First, in the setting of acute blood loss, transfusion therapy may be life-prolonging. Second, in the case of operative intervention, the refusal of blood products can significantly increase the risk of a poor outcome. The courts have consistently held that a competent Jehovah's Witness who is not pregnant has the right to refuse blood transfusions, even if the transfusion were life-prolonging. The general caveat is that while adults are free to make martyrs of themselves, they cannot martyr their dependent children.[20] Thus, the surgeon cannot compel an adult, competent patient who is not pregnant to accept the transfusion.

The surgeon, however, does have options when confronted with a patient who refuses perioperative blood product support. First of all, the surgeon should speak to the patient in private and assure the patient of the confidentiality of the medical records. Even though few minds may be changed, this private conversation is important to confirm that the patient is making an autonomous choice and is not unduly influenced by family and friends. If the surgeon believes that continued refusal constitutes such a high risk that the surgery is no longer appropriate, then the surgeon should approach the problem as he or she would a request for a medically inappropriate intervention, which is discussed above. If there is still no resolution of the difference of opinions, then the surgeon should transfer the patient to a surgeon willing to operate within the patient-imposed constraints. If he or she believes that the surgery is still appropriate, despite the added risk, then the surgeon should work with the patient and focus on perioperative management that attempts to minimize the increased risk.[21] Efforts should be focused at minimizing blood loss, maximizing hematopoiesis, and maximizing oxygen delivery and transport. Restricting phlebotomy to only small volumes for essential lab work and using cell savers and hemodilution are examples of minimizing blood loss. The use of erythropoietin and pharmacologic clotting enhancement are also usually acceptable. Although these measures have made some bloodless surgeries safer, they cannot transform all such surgeries into a low-risk class. Overall plans should be coordinated with nonsurgical colleagues who may have downstream responsibility for the patient's care.

Interprofessional Disagreements

Medical decision making is not an exact science and it is well known that clinical judgment varies among competent clinicians (see Chapters 15 and 16). This disagreement or variation of opinion occurs at a not infrequent rate within the same specialty and even more often between different specialties. Given the usual surgical situation that involves a referring physician and the surgeon, there exist potential disagreements resulting from differences in opinions regarding the appropriateness of surgery.

The disagreement can take one of two forms. One scenario is the surgeon's concluding that surgery is too high a risk or not appropriate for the particular case. The second scenario is the referring physician's concluding that the proposed operation is not appropriate or too great a risk. The latter circumstance is less likely to result in disagreement about the necessity for surgery than with the particular choice of procedure. These differences may be a result of the differences in the cultures of the various specialties but it may also be a result of individual variation regarding the valuation of risks and benefits, with one physician focusing on a particular morbidity while the other focuses on mortality.

Regardless of the reasons for the disagreement, both the surgeon and the referring physician must collaborate in order to protect the patient's interests. The surgeon and the referring physician should discuss their opinions and review available data that could resolve the disagreement. If no resolution is reached, the surgeon and/or the referring physician should review objectively and comprehensively with the patient the differing opinions and the supporting evidence and criticisms of the various positions. If after a thorough discussion, the patient and referring physician still desire to pursue a surgical option that the surgeon does not believe to be appropriate, the case should be referred to another surgeon for consideration. If the patient decides that surgery is not an appropriate option, medical management or a time trial of observation should be pursued as the patient prefers.

The Postoperative Period

In those very high risk situations where the surgeon, the referring physician, and the patient all agree that despite the risk, a surgical intervention is the prudent course, the potential ethical issues do not end at the conclusion of the surgery. The postoperative period in a poor surgical risk case can also expose ethical conflicts and tensions. High-risk patients, when they survive the initial surgery, often have prolonged and difficult postoperative courses. Two potentially interrelated problems may arise. The first is identifying the appropriate surrogate decision maker in those cases in which the patient does not quickly regain decision-making capacity. The second is reassessing the appropriateness and desirability of continued aggressive support.

Ideally, the patient regains his or her decision-making capacity soon after the surgery and long before any major decisions need to be made. However, the potential for a prolonged period of diminished decision-making capacity should be considered in most major surgeries and in all cases that involve poor surgical risk. The surgeon should discuss preoperatively with the patient, as part of a comprehensive informed consent discussion, the possibility of a temporary loss of decision-making capability in the postoperative period. Although most states have established procedures for surrogate decision making that rely on next of kin when the patient has not clearly named a surrogate decision maker, these default policies, while obviating the need for a court-appointed guardian, may result in the decisional authority being vested in someone other than the patient's first choice. Rather than relying on such policies, the surgeon should explore with the high-risk patient whom he or she would choose to make decisions if the patient lacks decision-making capacity. If the chosen surrogate differs from the surrogate specified by the default mechanism, the patient should be encouraged to execute a durable power of attorney for health care to ensure that his or her wishes are followed[22] (see Chapter 4).

The second possible dilemma, reassessing the appropriateness and desirability of continued aggressive interventions, is much more problematic. In those cases where there are complications and/or a prolonged postoperative course, both the surgeon and the patient, or surrogate decision maker, must continually assess the situation in light of the patient's goals and the capabilities and limits of surgery. The surgeon needs to be wary of both the problem of early termination of treatment and of overtreatment.

The pressure for early termination of treatment is a relatively new phenomenon that has emerged in the wake of new societal emphasis on death with dignity and fear of physician-driven overtreatment.[23] This pressure can come from a variety of sources, ranging from family members who believe that their loved one is suffering excessively in the surgical intensive care unit to other members of the health care team who may have different perceptions of the ongoing care and different understandings of the goals of therapy.[24]

While the surrogate decision maker of a patient with diminished decision-making capacity may refuse on behalf of the patient any unwanted intervention, including potentially life-prolonging interventions, the surgeon should carefully review the medical situation and assess the likely outcomes with the surrogate. Both parties must remember that patients who pose a poor surgical risk are often very sick preoperatively and that a "normal" postoperative course for such patients is rare. Attention should be focused on the likelihood of attaining the patient's previously stated goals in regard to the treatment. One option for the surgeon to offer, which can bridge the differing opinions, is a trial of continued management with clear stopping rules if the patient does not respond to continued support (see Chapter 10). If the surrogate and the surgeon conclude that continued aggressive treatment is not what the patient would have wanted nor in the patient's best interests, then the treatment plan should focus on palliative care. If after carefully discussing the situation with the surrogate, however, the surgeon believes that it would be premature to withdraw support and that such a decision is not in the patient's best interests nor is the surrogate willing to consider an appropriate time trial, he or she should refer the case to the hospital's ethics committee or dispute-resolution mechanism for review and advice. Given the very strong ethical and legal consensus that competent patients have the right to refuse unwanted therapy, the surgeon who chooses this route must be prepared to provide data supporting the position that continued therapy would result in significant benefit for the patient and that the surrogate is not acting in the patient's best interests.

While the surgeon must be vigilant in guarding against premature termination of treatment in the name of "death with dignity," he or she must also be willing to recognize evidence that the condition of the patient is deteriorating and that the likelihood of attaining the desired outcome is diminishing (see Chapter 10). The surgeon must remember that there is no ethical or legal distinction between withholding medical treatment and withdrawing unwanted or ineffective therapies. If the patient's condition deteriorates to the point that the surgeon believes that continued treatment is of questionable or no benefit, the surgeon should inform the surrogate decision maker of the changes in the patient's status and discuss the various alternative therapeutic approaches and levels of care. The surgeon should consider this discussion as an extension of the informed consent process and not merely ask "what do you want me to do?" or "should we resuscitate him if his heart and lungs were to stop?" The surgeon should provide the surrogate with his or her opinion regarding the appropriate level of care and the reasons for the opinion. In most cases where there has been good communication regarding the patient's postoperative course, the surrogate and surgeon agree on the appropriate level of care. In those cases where there is no agreement after a thorough discussion of the medical issues, and the surgeon believes that continued aggressive support is medically inappropriate, the surgeon should initiate a review under an institutional policy on medical futility, if such a policy exists, or refer to the institutional ethics committee.

Risk of Disease Transmission to the Surgeon

The concept of a high-risk patient, as discussed above, is framed in terms of a high risk of a poor outcome for the patient. However, the discussion can also be framed in terms of a risk of a poor outcome for the surgeon. Intraoperative disease transmission to the surgeon would clearly be such a poor outcome. While the risk of transmission of hepatitis B has existed for many years, the emergence of the human immunodeficiency virus (HIV) has focused much attention on this subject.

Occupationally acquired HIV infection has been documented in a number of cases, the majority being in nonsurgical health care workers. Based on several studies, the estimated risk of acquiring the infection from a percutaneous exposure to a seropositive patient is 1 in 330.[25] Concern regarding this risk has resulted in vigorous discussion regarding a surgeon's (or any other health professional's) determining that the risk of disease transmission to the surgeon was grounds for determining that surgery was inappropriate. While reports of overt refusal to treat HIV-infected patients are rare, evidence of covert decisions to deny an intervention are not. Whether one agrees with such responses or not, one must acknowledge, given the lethality of HIV infection, the legitimacy of the concern. A thorough analysis of this potential problem requires evaluation of both ethical and legal principles.

The initial response by organized medicine and various ethicists was to focus on the ethical basis of a claim that a surgeon must assume some risk. Some argued that there was a professional responsibility, akin to that of firefighters and police officers, to accept some risk as part of the profession.[26] Others based the duty to treat on general ethical principles.[27] The AMA[28] and the American College of Physicians[1] argued that physicians could not refuse to treat on the basis of HIV infection. While no one argues that surgeons, or any other professionals for that matter, have an obligation to assume unreasonable or significant risk, the basic argument relies on the acceptance of some risk.

Despite ethical pleadings and the public pronouncements of organized medicine, it was suggested that "thousands of physicians may be systematically avoiding or refusing to care for AIDS patients."[29] Because of the legal doctrine of the "no duty rule," individual physicians had no obligation to treat individuals who were not their patients and thus there was no legal basis, aside from malpractice claims, to compel physicians to treat HIV-infected individuals.[12]

In response to this concern and a general concern that existing federal protections for the disabled were inadequate, Congress extended civil rights protections to HIV-infected individuals, among others, with the passage of the Americans with Disabilities Act,[30] which banned discrimination "on the basis of disability" in places of public accommodation. The Act specifically includes the "professional office of a health care provider, hospital, or other similar service establishment" as a place of public accommodation. Thus, Federal law now requires the surgeon, as well as other health care professionals, to treat an HIV-infected patient as he or she would any other non-infected patient and does not allow the surgeon to unilaterally determine that the patient is too high risk because of the possibility of infecting the surgeon. A surgeon refusing treatment on such a basis could be subject to an injunction or civil penalties under action brought by either the patient or the U.S. Attorney General.[31]

This prohibition is not, at least in theory, unlimited. The Act carved out an exception to discrimination in those cases when the ". . . individual poses a direct threat to the health and safety of others. The term 'direct threat' means a significant risk to the health and safety of others that cannot be eliminated by a modification of policies, practices, or procedures or by the provision of auxiliary aids or services."[30] However, the fact that the AMA and others state that the risk to caregivers who follow required universal precautions is not significant essentially eliminates the use of this exception as a defense for not treating infected individuals.[32]

Such cases also reinforce the role of the surgeon as a steward of hospital resources in that the decision to perform the procedure also involves many other hospital personnel. The Act's inclusion of hospitals as places of public accommodation also obligates the institution to provide the necessary resources, including the staff.

Clinical Conclusions

The determination of the surgical appropriateness, or inappropriateness, of a particular intervention in light of poor risk is potentially problematic because of the different values, risk thresholds, and goals of the participants in the decision-making process, namely the patient, the surgeon, and the referring physician. The three-way nature of the discussion exposes potential conflicts not only between the surgeon and the patient but also among health care professionals.

When the patient refuses surgically appropriate interventions, the surgeon should review the indications and risks for surgery and further explore the patient's concerns and reasons for refusal. The surgeon should also consider and offer, when possible, negotiated solutions such as time trials. The presumption should be that the patient possesses decision-making capacity and that patient autonomy grounds the right of a competent patient to refuse unwanted but potentially life-prolonging interventions. In those cases in which the patient lacks decision-making capacity, the surgeon should turn to the appropriate surrogate decision maker for either consent or refusal of surgery.

A patient's demand for a medically inappropriate procedure requires the surgeon to thoroughly explain the reasons why the procedure is not indicated in a particular case. If the patient persists in demanding the intervention, the surgeon should turn to institutional policies to deal with such problems or urge the creation of such policies in institutions that have not addressed the issue. The virtue of integrity could ground the surgeon's decision not to perform any medically inappropriate procedures.

Refusal of blood products, or other patient requests that increase surgical risk, should cause the surgeon to explore options that minimize the potential for problems. These include new techniques and interventions to minimize blood loss and maximize oxygen-carrying capacity; these also include referral to colleagues with greater experience in such techniques.

Interprofessional disagreements require good communication between the surgeon and referring physician and also between the professionals and the patient. Such disagreements should be resolved in favor of protecting the patient's best interests.

The problems of decision making in the postoperative period can be minimized by advanced planning for possible loss of decision making capacity as part of the informed consent process. Also, the surgeon and the patient must constantly reassess the goals of therapy and the capabilities of medicine in light of changing conditions. Time trials can be appropriate ways to bridge disagreements between the surgeon and the patient or surrogate decision maker.

The potential transmission of disease from the patient to the surgeon should not affect the decision regarding the appropriateness of a particular intervention. A risk of disease transmission to the surgeon does not alter the surgeon's responsibilities to the patient.

The poor surgical risk patient poses special but not insurmountable problems for the surgeon. The high risk of an undesirable outcome necessitates careful consideration of the medical appropriateness of any surgical intervention and highlights the importance of a thorough process of informed consent. Such cases are best handled by good communication and a strong therapeutic alliance between the surgeon and the patient.

References

1. "American College of Physicians Ethics Manual," *Annals of Internal Medicine* 117 (1992):947–60.
2. American Medical Association, Council on Ethical and Judicial Affairs, "Guidelines for the Appropriate Use of Do-Not-Resuscitate Orders," *Journal of the American Medical Association* 265 (1991):1868–71.
3. Robert D. Truog, Allan S. Brett, and Joel Frader, "The Problem with Futility," *New England Medical Journal* 326 (1992):1560–64.
4. *In re Wanglie*, No. PX91–288 (Prob. Ct., Hennepin Co., MN, 1991).
5. *In the Matter of Baby K*, 16 F.3d 590 (4th Cir. 1994).
6. Julia E. Connelly and Courtney Campbell, "Patients Who Refuse Treatment in Medical Offices," *Archives of Internal Medicine* 147 (1987): 1829–1833.
7. *Schloendorff v. Society of New York Hospital*, 211 N.Y. 125, 126, 105 N.E. 92, 93 (1914).
8. Amir Halevy and Baruch A. Brody, "A Multi-Institution Policy on Medical Futility," *Journal of the American Medical Association* 276 (1996):571–4.
9. Laurence B. McCullough, "Preventive Ethics, Professional Integrity, and Boundary Setting: The Clinical Management of Moral Uncertainty," *Journal of Medicine and Philosophy* 20 (1995): 1–11.
10. Peter A. Ubel and Robert M. Arnold, "The Unbearable Rightness of Bedside Rationing," *Archives of Internal Medicine* 155 (1995): 1837–1842.
11. James F. Drane, "Competency to Give an Informed Consent," *Journal of the American Medical Association* 252 (1984): 925–927.

12. George J. Annas, "Reconciling Quinlan and Saikewicz: Decision Making for the Terminally Ill Incompetent," *American Journal of Law and Medicine* 4 (1979): 367–396.

13. Larry J. Schneiderman, Nancy S. Jecker, and Albert R. Jonsen, "Medical Futility: Its Meaning and Ethical Implications," *Annals of Internal Medicine* 112 (1990): 949–954.

14. Tom Tomlinson and Diane Czlonka, "Futility and Hospital Policy," *Hastings Center Report* 25 (1995): 28–35.

15. Baruch A. Brody and Amir Halevy, "Is Futility a Futile Concept?" *Journal of Medicine and Philosophy* 20 (1995): 123–144.

16. The Hastings Center, *Guidelines on the Termination of Life-Sustaining Treatment and the Care of the Dying*. Bloomington: Indiana University Press, 1987.

17. American Medical Association, Council on Ethical and Judicial Affairs, *Code of Medical Ethics 1994 Edition*. Chicago: American Medical Association, 1994.

18. Gina Kolata, "Withholding Care From Patients: Boston Case Asks, Who Decides?" *New York Times* April 3, 1995.

19. George D. Lundberg, "United States Health Care Reform: An Era of Shared Responsibility Begins," *JAMA* 271 (1994): 1530–1533.

20. *Prince v. Commonwealth of Massachusetts*, 321 U.S. 158 (1944).

21. Marianne C. Mann, John Votto, Joseph Kambe, et al., "Management of the Severely Anemic Patient Who Refuses Transfusion: Lessons Learned during the Care of a Jehovah's Witness," *Annals of Internal Medicine* 117 (1992): 1042–1048.

22. D. A. Peters, "Advanced Directives. The Case for the Durable Power of Attorney for Health Care," *Journal of Legal Medicine* 8 (1987): 437–464.

23. Herbert Hendin, "Selling Death and Dignity," *Hastings Center Report* 25 (1995): 19–23.

24. D. Caswell and H. G. Cryer, "Case Study: When the Nurse and the Physician Don't Agree," *Journal of Cardiovascular Nursing* 9 (1995): 30–42.

25. Bernard Lo and Robert Steinbrook, "Health Care Workers Infected with the Human Immunodeficiency Virus," *JAMA* 267 (1992): 1100–1105.

26. Ronald Bayer, "AIDS and the Duty To Treat: Risk, Responsibility, and Health Care Workers," *Bulletin of the New York Academy of Medicine* 64 (1988): 498–505.

27. Edmund D. Pellegrino, "HIV Infection and the Ethics of Clinical Care," *Journal of Legal Medicine* 10 (1989): 29–46.

28. American Medical Association, Council on Ethical and Judicial Affairs, *Code of Medical Ethics, Annotated Opinions of the Council on Ethical and Judicial Affairs of the American Medical Association*. Chicago: American Medical Association, 1992.

29. Oscar W. Clark and R. B. Conley, "The Duty to 'Attend Upon the Sick'," *JAMA* 266 (1991): 2876–2877.

30. *The Americans With Disabilities Act of 1990*. Pub L No. 101–336, 104 Stat 327.

31. Amir Halevy and Baruch A. Brody, "Acquired Immunodeficiency Syndrome and The Americans With Disabilities Act: A Legal Duty to Treat," *The American Journal of Medicine* 96 (1994): 282–288.

32. George J. Annas, "Legal Risks and Responsibilities in the AIDS Epidemic," *Hastings Center Report* 18 (1988):26–32.

10

Care of Dying Patients

STEPHEN WEAR
ROBERT MILCH
W. LYNN WEAVER

Most adults in the United States die in institutional settings, and most of those deaths occur under medical or surgical care. Surgeons tend not to like death, especially after an operation. As a consequence of the first factor, surgeons cannot avoid dying patients and, as a consequence of the second factor, surgeons tend not to speak candidly and specifically to dying patients about their situation and prospects. Nonetheless, dying patients confront surgeons with a number of ethical challenges, in no small measure because of these two factors and their consequences, to which we address this chapter.

Proper care of dying patients would seem to turn on when to make the clinical judgment that any particular patient is, in fact, dying. Prior to such a judgment, aggressive medical and/or surgical interventions can be offered. Conversely, once such a judgment is appropriately made, aggressive interventions can be withheld or withdrawn, palliation pursued, and the patient and/or family assisted to respond to the many facets of terminal illness.

Surgical practice predisposes surgeons to binary thinking. *However, this common binary way of managing gravely ill surgical patients dooms such efforts to broad failure.* If the surgeon waits until it is clear that the patient is dying, many patients will end up being overtreated, their suffering will have been inadequately addressed, and attempts to help such patients and families come to terms with the patient's mortality will be too little, too late, and jarring. The problem is that long before the patient's mortality is clear to the surgeon, a substantial number of patients can be known, *statistically*, to be irreversibly dying.[1]

If uncertainty regarding which patients are actually dying is the root problem, then an anticipatory form of management for potentially dying patients is, we will argue, the ethically justified response to grave illness. Dying patients do not fall within a narrow clinical definition. Rather they exist along a clinical spectrum from those at significant risk of dying (10% mortality upward), through those at high risk of dying (50% or greater risk of mortality), to those whose diseases have become clearly and irreversibly lethal. In this chapter, we provide an ethical analysis of these three points on the clinical spectrum that delineate subpopulations of dying patients. We recommend that such patients, including the many who will be legitimate surgical candidates, should be concurrently approached as potentially unsalvageable. This concurrent approach begins by including the fact that they may be dying in their differential diagnosis. As the probability of any such patient's death increases, the surgeon's obligations to that patient will change in clinically and ethically significant ways. Such a strategy may seem unduly pessimistic to many surgeons. But it is essential to clinically appropriate and ethically sound management of the spectrum of dying patients defined and addressed in this chapter.

Ethical Analysis: The Ethical Challenge of Dying Patients

An anecdotal sense of the ethical challenges of caring for dying patients is readily detailed, and in two basic senses. One sense regards the common, inappropriately high expectation of patients and/or their families that aggressive surgical response will save the patient. This expectation is not only *not* grounded in reality, and often quite difficult to dislodge, but equally overlooks the morbidity such aggressive management can involve and the adverse effects of that morbidity on a patient's quality of life. The family member, particularly, who says to the surgeon, "Do everything that you can do," simply does not appreciate the price in iatrogenic morbidity and lost quality of life that may be paid for pursuing an unrealistic outcome that may not materialize. Surgical deaths in this present time of high technology are neither rapid nor without suffering for the family as well as the patient and surgeon.

In sharp contrast to the preceding, perhaps because of this lack of understanding, tales of the overtreatment of patients, and of the poor quality of life that can result from the surgeon's efforts are widespread. Increasingly patients and/or their loved ones are reporting such stories, coupled with a reluctance to proceed with clinical interventions that often are clearly indicated and even involve some of the most effective developments of the art. Many patients and families have had some close friend or loved one who suffered from overtreatment that resulted in a series of complications, when the fact of his or her dying might have been accepted. The scenarios here range from patients who remained connected to myriad machines in a surgical intensive care unit (SICU), to those left to languish on some back ward. Thus, a second basic challenge of the dying patient to the surgeon is the growing, ambivalent public perception of what occurs to people in hospitals.

This tendency of many patients and/or families to be either unrealistically optimistic, or ambivalent to the point of pessimism, can certainly complicate any attempt to prudently manage serious illness. Adding fuel to this fire, these two potentially contradictory perspectives are often mirrored in clinical practice and the bioethics literature by similar contrasting views.

On the one hand, typical surgical behavior often accepts the optimistic patient or family and seeks to minimize pessimism. On the other hand, the clinical literature, particularly that of bioethics, tends in the opposite direction. Empirical research indicates that enormous health care resources are expended on "dying" patients—those who, it turned out, were in their last six months of life.[1] Numerous authors then proceed to conclude that many dying patients inappropriately received aggressive medical management. It is also documented that limitations of treatment, especially DNR, are seldom in place until the very end of the dying course[2]; clinicians are often unaware of patients' wishes regarding treatment limits, and sometimes do not honor them even if they are[3]; and many of these patients suffer substantial but poorly managed pain.[4,5] Various antidotes are then offered—for example, living wills, designated proxies, and the unilateral withholding of futile treatment, as well as more effective communication and candor between doctor and patient. In parallel, pessimistic sentiments are growing about all this as may be seen in various movements, including attempts to legalize active euthanasia, as well as the sentiment that such patients might be better off not going into hospitals in the first place. As Annas recently suggested: "If dying patients want to retain some control over their dying process, they must get out of the hospital they are in and stay out of the hospital if they are out."[6]

Annas' recommendation works, of course, only if the fact that a patient is dying is readily determinable in some clear fashion early on. Otherwise, either many dying patients will still come in for trial interventions in the hope that they are not dying, and then many will receive the "needless care" that they fear; or potentially salvageable patients will give up the chance of being saved for the sake of avoiding the aggressive treatment that might have helped them. This is hardly an attractive (or necessary) way to frame the decision such patients face, particularly those who have grave illness, who may well die regardless of clinical response, but before receiving it are just as appropriately seen as treatable. Annas' argument succeeds only by ignoring the uncertainty at the core of medicine.

The absence of an early, clear, unambiguous sense of which patients are dying is the case and the problem. The alternatives of optimism or pessimism are both thus simply unrealistic for the class of seriously ill patients prior to such patients having declared themselves clinically. And that we are not dealing with readily solvable problems, but profound dilemmas, is suggested by a recent major study where much of the new wisdom of bioethics was arguably instituted and failed to produce the desired and expected results.

The SUPPORT Study: Adding Insult to Injury

The SUPPORT study involved a large, 4-year multicenter study of 9,105 patients and was directed toward improving "end-of-life decision making and reducing the frequency of a mechanically supported, painful and prolonged process of dying."[2] SUPPORT refers to "The Study to Understand Prognoses and Preferences for Outcomes and Risks of Treatments." SUPPORT involved "a two year prospective observational study (Phase I) of 4301 patients followed by a two year controlled clinical trial (Phase II) with patients and their physicians randomized by specialty group to the intervention group (n=2652) or control group (n=2152)."[2] One inclusion criterion was that subjects have at least a 50% chance of dying in 6 months. The study included patients with chronic obstructive pulmonary disease, congestive heart failure, cirrhosis of the liver, acute respiratory failure and coma, as well as patients with terminal malignancies and multi-organ failure.

The observational and intervention outcomes to be measured were "physician patient communication," "incidence and timing of DNR orders," "physicians' knowledge of patients' preferences not to be resuscitated," "number of days spent in an ICU, receiving mechanical ventilation or comatose before death," "level of reported pain," and "use of hospital resources." The intervention was "physicians in the intervention group received estimates of the likelihood of 6-month survival for every day up to six months, outcomes of cardiopulmonary resuscitation (CPR), and functional disability at 2 months. A specially trained nurse had multiple contacts with the patient, family, physician, and hospital staff to elicit preferences, improve understanding of outcomes, encourage attention to pain control, and facilitate advance care planning and physician-patient communication."[2]

The results of the data collection in Phase I of this study mirrored the public perception of the fate of dying patients in hospitals (e.g. overtreatment and unrelieved suffering), and about half of the included patients (47%) did die within 6 months, with most deaths in hospital. *The result after the Phase II intervention was, simply and starkly, that there was no statistically significant change in the outcomes studied*: there was no change in the "timing of DNR orders," "physician-patient agreement about DNR orders," "number of undesirable days," "prevalence of pain," or "resources consumed."

The Clinical Significance of the SUPPORT Study

The SUPPORT study investigators responded to this lack of results by suggesting that "greater individual and societal commitment and more proactive and forceful measures may be needed" to change the outcomes at issue.[2] But they provided no detail as to what such commitment and measures should be. At most, such a lack of results counsels that no quick fixes are available and that some of the "current wisdom" of bioethics at least needs more clinical sophistication to be effective in practice.

The surgeon reader may object here that the SUPPORT study was basically focused on medical patients and thus lacks relevance to the practice of surgery. We respond. The results reported quite accurately reproduce our own experience from years of the practice and observation of surgery. The type of patients studied (e.g., those with congestive heart failure, terminal malignancies, multi-organ failure, or coma) are as prevalent in SICUs, and any reference to the myriad outcome studies available show similar ranges of good and bad outcomes.[1] We see no reason to think that the interventions the SUPPORT study instituted would be any more effective in SICUs than MICUs; if anything, internists often have more time than surgeons to develop the sort of relationships where any such communication and counseling might be effective. Nor do we see any greater commitment to such realistic communication and counseling among surgeons than internists. We would predict that the end points that the SUPPORT study attempted to influence would be the same in the surgical milieu and that no better results would have occurred from any such attempt to change them.

The study may be criticized as flawed because the "intervening" nurses were not members of the treating teams and a physician might have been more effective; the nurses gave prognosis data only to the clinicians, not to the patients and or families, so it is not surprising their preferences did not change, or become more clinically realistic; the 50% death rate inclusion criterion leaves 50% who might well not die and for whom treatment might well be vigorously preferred by all involved (i.e., patients, families and physicians)—in effect, the study was *not* dealing with patients who were dying in any unambiguous way; and the futility of further aggressive treatment may well only have become clear in the last few days for the bulk of these patients, so the fact that DNR orders were enacted only in the last days for both groups of patients may well have been appropriate. Our basic point at this juncture, however, is that this study in no way dictates pessimism regarding the enterprise of responding to the "challenge" of "dying" patients.[7]

Nonetheless, the SUPPORT study performs the crucial service of showing that it will not suffice simply to redouble our efforts regarding such patients and their families. This is because in this population, though 50% of its members are dying, most patients will either be not clearly dying or probably salvageable. The "optimistic" binary approach to grave illness—be optimistic until the patient becomes clearly unsalvageable—is thus as clinically unrealistic as Annas' injunction to avoid hospitals altogether. We will argue for a middle, clinically more realistic ground between these dichotomous views by holding that *all* of these patients need to be approached, *partially*, as if they were dying, even though aggressive surgical management will usually be chosen at the same time.

Surgical Management of the Dying Patient

We recommend that the class of dying patients be broadened to include all those who have a significant chance of dying regardless of surgical response. This has several important implications. The class of dying patients becomes a *spectrum* that extends from those who have a significant chance of dying to those who are clearly terminal regardless of therapeutic response. (The SUPPORT study's "50% or greater mortality" population thus occupies a roughly middle ground in this spectrum.) Once the patient's differential diagnosis includes the possibility of dying, certain tasks will be indicated depending on the circumstances of the case at hand, including, when ethically justified, a fully aggressive surgical response. The patient with a resectable lung cancer, for example, should still be assisted to appreciate that surgical intervention may not succeed and some discussion should be initiated about what such a result might mean to the patient, as well as what his or her views and wishes regarding such a result may be. There will rarely be a magic "objective point" in this spectrum where medical science and art can unilaterally say: "this is a terminal patient for whom all aggressive treatment should be abated." What a patient will be willing to risk and suffer for the sake of cure or life extension will vary substantially from patient to patient. Only within the quite small subpopulation of patients for whom all aggressive treatment will be clearly futile will surgeons be able to declare futility unilaterally (see Chapter 9). Only rarely, therefore, will unilaterally declaring futility and discontinuing aggressive management be options in the overall population of dying patients.

Defining the "Dying" Patient

We are suggesting a 10% chance of dying, even with full therapeutic response, as the threshold for placing the diagnosis of "dying" in a patient's differential diagnosis. We admit that this is somewhat arbitrary but, in our judgment, many surgeons, as well as patients and families, would judge significant the possibility of death as one out of ten. We also recommend this threshold because we think there are certain anticipatory tasks for the surgeon to address with any such patient early on. Given that we are *not* suggesting that a 10% mortality indicates that treatment should be abated, the real issue is not where we place the threshold, but what we propose should be done once the threshold is reached. Beyond this point, our task will be to identify what other issues emerge as the probability that a given patient is dying increases (e.g., as we get into the population addressed by the SUPPORT study), and what management should be once the diagnosis of "dying" becomes primary within the differential. In what follows, we will offer our basic management recommendations, first regarding what it generically means to include the diagnosis of "dying" within the differential of a patient, and then regarding the three main subsets of this class of patients.

General Ethical Management of the "Dying" Patient: Putting Everyone on the Same Page

The one complaint that we believe can be legitimately lodged, without appealing to hindsight, regarding the usual management of this general population of dying patients, is that they usually lack a *comprehensive* plan of management. These patients are often managed only partially, and without paying sufficient attention to the possibility that they may die regardless of whatever the surgeon does. Further, as their mortality becomes more probable, their management, if anything, becomes even more abstract, haphazard, and unconnected with clinical realities. This problem becomes compounded when clinicians continue to be hopeful of outcome and encourage (false) hope in patients and families, regarding high-mortality patients, such as those studied by SUPPORT. Not to begin to anticipate and plan for the morbidity and mortality of patients in this population simply courts disaster and, in doing so, tends to produce the ambivalence and bad feelings previously noted.

Lack of prior planning and anticipation leads to management that is harmfully unheedful of clinical realities and options. The surgical team, whose threshold for abating treatment has been reached, then attempts to "get the DNR" from the patient and/or his or her family. The common result, particularly in SICUs, is the following. First, given that there usually has been little real anticipation of the patient's morbidity and mortality by the patient and/or family, the attempt is quite jarring. Many patients and families thus respond unrealistically, having been given no chance to prepare for such an eventuality. Second, given that a DNR dictates only non-response to cardiopulmonary arrest, all of those things that one might well do short of arrest, from fluid pushes, central lines, intubation, and further surgery, to appropriate response to pain and suffering, or maximizing remaining quality of life, remain unaddressed and undecided. Good clinical management is in the details and, particularly in SICUs, these details are too often, in our judgment, addressed quite vaguely if at all when surgeons wait too long in recognizing that the patient is dying.

To attempt to specify management when cure is no longer anticipated requires, therefore, not just detailed response once this is clear and accepted, but earlier, ongoing activities by way of preparation (see Chapters 2 and 4). These tools of preventive ethics are at the heart of the concurrent activities that we recommend for all patients in this population.

Informed Consent: Presentation and Consideration of a Regimen of Care

Informed consent, in the care of dying patients as we define this population, should aim at an elaboration of the *essential regimen of treatment and care* being proposed to the patient. This is *not* the same as the specific, content-rich informed consent process that appropriately occurs for a specific intervention within a broader course of management (e.g., insertion of a central line). Rather, we are calling for a candid, to the point of bluntness, *explanation of the totality of the patient's basic situation and prospects, with and without treatment, and a clear sense of the potential downsides and limitations of the course of therapy being proposed*. Such a presentation would thus eschew the detail that the legally motivated consent offers in favor of what Brody refers to as a presentation that makes "transparent" to the patient what the surgeon's hopes, plans, *and* fears are for him or her,[8] and seeks to produce a true acceptance of an overall course of care based on a broadly realistic sense of the patient's situation and prospects.[9]

Such an informed consent would differ markedly from the typical, legally motivated informed consent. In fact, we recommend that the two be pursued quite separately. The differences would be roughly as follows. This consent to a regimen of care would eschew extensive detail about multiple risks, or potential complications, in favor of an essential presentation of what the surgeon is especially hopeful of and worried about regarding the whole course of management. This approach converts the traditional paternalistic concern to maintain a patient's hope to the *challenge* of generating and sustaining *realistic hope* in a patient who either may not do well or, at least, may end up having to go through more than expected and with less benefit than was hoped for. This approach should be intentionally *interactive*, as described in Chapters 2 and 4, in contrast to the typical "legal" consent that aims only at the provision of information and all too often does not even attempt to ascertain whether actual understanding is achieved in the patient. The appropriate tactic for this interactive consent process, after the surgeon first presents a generic view of the regimen of care being recommended, is to ask the patient to tell the surgeon what he or she now understands his or her conditions and prospects to be. This report can then be evaluated by the surgeon and corrected as necessary, addressing misunderstanding of negative factors such as risks and complications, and by encouraging and frankly answering questions that the patient may have. The surgeon should also be attentive to and discuss areas of doubt or hesitation. Such a discussion might well occur as a process, or dialogue, that occurs over time, but it should from the outset seek as much insight as possible[9] and sets the stage for further discussion as treatment proceeds and the patient's clinical course unfolds.

This sort of presentation is often not made to patients at the threshold of this diagnosis or further on, particularly in the sense that real candor is offered. Nor is a serious attempt often made to assess and enhance both the patient's actual understanding of his or her situation, prospects, and the regimen of care that is being offered and to obtain an authentic "buying-in" to these realities. As has been argued elsewhere, such a candid and interactive approach can yield major dividends in patient compliance and satisfaction, and tends to cut down treatment refusals or disputes based on vague fears, feelings of powerlessness, and the simple lack of a relationship between surgeons and patients and their families.[9] In fact, if a therapeutic relationship is as important as we believe, one would wonder what better and more efficient way there is to generate one. We recognize, as studies of informed consent repeatedly document,[9,10] that many patients only grasp so much, and often are just waiting for the surgeon's recommendation. But these do not justify failing to attempt to generate an initial insight on the patient's part and then more substantial insight as treatment and further discussions proceed. Equally, we would suggest that such a candid approach can generate trust and some sense of security in patients and their families that their goals and preferences will be taken into account.

This preventive ethics approach should diminish the following complications: the patient or family who tends to make hindsight complaints of overtreatment because no real attempt was afforded them to gain *foresight* about what was proposed; the patient or family who balk at continuing or augmenting therapy when complications occur or less than optimal progress is made, or refuse to accept recommendations to abate treatment (such problems frequently arise because patients and families were not prepared for other than optimal results); and the disputes and dissatisfaction that arise, leading sometimes to law suits or disruptions within the regimen of treatment, from those who can legitimately say, after the fact, that they were not adequately informed.

A final suggestion regarding this consent to a regimen of treatment should be made here: we commend the tactic of involving patients' families in such interactions from the beginning. One is thus both engaging persons who may have to assume decision-making roles later on, as well as involving those who may well be able to help the patient gain understanding (or be able to notice when the patient does not adequately understand or accept what is going on). Such family involvement, of course, must be agreed to by the patient, but we recommend that the surgeon strongly encourage it.

Identification and Discussion of the Patient's End of Life Preferences

Chapter 4 discusses the usage of advance directives in detail, so we will mainly direct the reader there. There are two types of advance directives: those that specifically note certain situations in which the patient does or does not want some specific treatment (e.g., if they end up in a vegetative or clearly terminal state): and advance directives that, however much they may also include statements of the first type, appoint decision-making surrogates to speak for the patients if and when they lose decision-making capacity. Solicitation of advance directives from dying patients (as we have defined the population) should be done early on. Certainly it is fair and credible to no one to approach an acutely hypoxic patient regarding whether he or she wishes to be intubated. But there is an old Spanish saying that should make us less than enthusiastic about soliciting patients' views about situations that they are not yet in and may not have previously experienced: "as one moves from the stands to the arena, the aspect of the bull changes."

Following this suggestion, the issue becomes what should be solicited, by way of prior statements, from patients. We suggest that the appointment of a health care proxy as the preferred strategy for two main reasons. First, there are significant numbers of patients for whom such a proxy designation is preferable, given their personal situations. One example of such a patient would be one who is known to be estranged from the person(s) who would be approached for consent as his or her legal next-of-kin if he or she lacked capacity or became incompetent. Another example would be the HIV-infected homosexual male patient, who may well have a lover with whom he may have discussed his views; but, absent a proxy designation for that person, his parents, who may not only be unaware of his wishes but also his diagnosis and orientation, would have to be approached as decision makers. Second, to broaden this category of patients who should be encouraged to designate health care proxies, we will simply report that, via our own informal polling of many different groups of people, as well as the actual solicitation of proxy designations from many patients, it appears that about *a third of people would designate someone other than their legally primary next of kin if asked*. The reasons here range from "he would not be able to let me go," to "I would not want to burden him," to "my sister, the nurse, would probably make the best decision," to "my friend knows me better than any of my family." To us, this rough third of patients is sufficient to indicate the need for strong encouragement to *all* such patients to make such a designation; we thus recommend that the surgeon strongly encourage all "dying" patients to designate a health care proxy.

We anticipate that this recommendation to solicit health care proxies from all patients in this population will be met with the objection that this is just a "New York State thing," where inflexible and quite restrictive laws regarding abating treatment obtain, and such proxies are one way around them. We respond: the arguments in the text relate to any patient, not just patients in New York State; and given the legal climate in New York in this area, we were initially forced to solicit all sorts of prior specific patient directives subsequent to various restrictive Cruzan-like precedents in the courts; the health care proxy law should be appreciated, in large part, as a later legal option created to address the shortcomings and problems with specific prior statements, including vagueness, as well as overspecificity. Our experience of the many patients who change their mind when they get into the arena also added to this further development. In summary, we would suggest, our experience in New York State has forced us, much more than those in more flexible jurisdictions, to aggressively seek specific prior patient statements and this search has instructed us that such statements often create more problems than they solve.

As to the solicitation of patients' specific wishes early on, we will simply report a certain ambivalent nervousness here. On the one hand, most living wills seem to focus on clearly end-stage scenarios (e.g., permanent vegetative state or eminently terminal illness). We have no difficulty with patients ruling out aggressive treatment in such arenas, even if they have not been in them, and in some states the law seems to require such prior statements for certain treatments to be abated, even if a health care proxy has been designated.[11] Patients' prior statements, written or verbal, regarding other, less extreme "arenas" are more problematic to us. We are increasingly encountering patients who have made prior verbal statements that rule out potentially valuable therapeutic responses. Most common is the patient who says that he or she would never want to be placed on a "breathing machine." But this rules out a trial intervention of ventilatory support for a potentially treatable but otherwise lethal infiltrate (e.g., pneumonia in a patient with chronic obstructive pulmonary disease in the postoperative period). Equally, it rules out ventilatory support where a legitimate surgical exploration is indicated (e.g., surgical exploration of a bleed in the abdomen). We will report in this regard, simply, that the roughly four dozen patients whom we have encountered who had made such prior statements *all* opted for ventilatory support once they understood the "acute, potentially treatable infiltrate" scenario. Similar changes of mind have occurred fairly routinely with gravely ill surgical patients; we sense this is a common experience of all surgeons. In addition, written living wills, as long as they relate only to clearly end-stage scenarios, are not problematic and may well be helpful. Finally, part of the surgeon's assessment of any such patient, from the beginning, should address whether the patient has made any ill-advised or vague prior statements regarding potentially useful therapies, which would cause difficulties of interpretation later.

Managing Patients within the Three Subpopulations of this Diagnosis

We turn now to the issue of how the surgeon should respond to the possibility of withholding or withdrawing aggressive surgical management in the population of dying patients. Our experience is that most of the patients in this total population will tend to opt for aggressive surgical management, even a fair number of those in the probably lethal disease category, particularly once they appreciate the options and reassurances that the preceding discussions should contain. That this is everyone's experience, and hope, with most patients at the threshold of this diagnosis is clear. Regarding the middle group of this population (i.e., those with 50% or greater mortality), the SUPPORT study and our own experience suggest the same general preference. At most, one encounters better-informed patients who initially may balk because they are worried about having a difficult dying process. Most of these tend to elect aggressive management once it is portrayed as a trial intervention of specific duration that will be abated if the chance of benefit evaporates, or if that benefit comes to pale in the face of extended and substantial morbidity. This strategy minimizes the risk of overtreatment. In addition, this strategy minimizes the risk of undertreatment. By contrast, continued insistence by surgeons on the "optimistic-binary" approach to such patients may lead directly to more sympathy for Annas' pessimistic approach and the unjustified undertreatment it would produce.

As to patients in the "probably lethal disease" category, even they will have some tendency to opt for low-yield interventions, particularly if they have some hope that they will not have to pay too much for the attempt in terms of increased morbidity and decreased quality of life. Further, even those who have an absolutely lethal condition may opt for aggressive surgical intervention if it offers the hope of significantly extending their lives, particularly if the life thus extended has a real chance of containing qualities that the patient values. The patient with a newly diagnosed metastatic pancreatic carcinoma, for example, though certainly in the "probably lethal disease" category, at point of diagnosis may still have an immediate mortality of 10% or less, and aggressive surgical intervention may offer real hope of extending a life that is not yet seriously symptomatic. The clinical ethical challenge here is to help the patient assess carefully the aggressive pursuit of such quality-of-life possibilities in the context of the potentially long and unpleasant character of some terminal illnesses (e.g., lung cancer), where attempts at life-extension may well yield an excess of burden and suffering over benefit. Here, as anywhere, trial interventions, coupled with hard-nosed clinical realism, may appropriately balance the possibilities, for good or ill, at hand.

We believe that the SUPPORT study and much of bioethics has been based on the assumption that many dying patients would reject aggressive therapy if only given the chance. Our experience, and the results of the SUPPORT study, suggest the contrary. But our experience also makes clear that treatment refusals can occur throughout the continuum of dying patients. The general approach and deportment of the surgeon to dying patients needs to take this clinical variability into account. We do so for each of the three subpopulations identified earlier.

Managing Patients at the Threshold of this Diagnosis

Patients with approximately 10% mortality will usually opt for aggressive therapy and it is surely reasonable for the surgeon to recommend and encourage this. Nonaggressive management should be identified and discussed as an alternative. The primary concurrent approach to this category of patients has thus already been spelled out, namely, the ongoing consent to a regimen of care must be provided, and patients' views regarding end of life scenarios solicited and evaluated. In most cases, the dividends of such activities will accrue later in the management of such patients, although this activity can certainly yield valuable results in enhancing patient compliance, alleviating unreasoned fears, and so forth.[9] The surgeon must, however, be ready to respond effectively to the uncommon patient who does not wish aggressive management even in such a relatively optimistic situation. This possibility raises the one major variable regarding the concurrent approach to this subgroup, and the various sources of such refusals merit identification and analysis.

Treatment Refusals Based on Quality of Life Factors. Consider an elderly female patient, who steadfastly refused surgical resection of a probably discrete, eminently resectable tumor. In response to encouragement to consent to major surgery, she made clear that although she was not "about to jump out of the window," she had no interest in doing anything to "stick around" because "I'm stuck in a nursing home, my friends and family are mostly dead and the others don't come to see me, and I'm just bored to death with my life." This case suggests a type of patient, even at the threshold of the continuum of dying patients, for whom surgeons should be prepared, namely, patients who though their surgical mortality is low, still do not wish aggressive surgical management. Such patients also come in the form of those with concurrent chronic and devastating illness that will remain even if the surgery is successful (e.g., advanced multiple sclerosis or paraplegia). Or they may be like our lady in the sense that though physiological life can be extended, existentially they see it as approaching its end. Functional or quality-of-life deficits may well indicate that even low-risk, high-yield surgery may not be appropriate from the patient's point of view.

Treatment Refusals Based on Clinically Treatable Depression or Other Remediable Factors. Matters are often not so simple, however. Some patients suffer from clinically treatable depression, where a workup and treatment, not false respect for autonomy, are appropriate. Their refusal may be based on other *remediable* factors that could be addressed; this could include transferring the patient to a different living situation, or attempting to produce a rapprochement with absent family members or friends.

Treatment Refusals Based on Knowledge Deficits. Some of the strongest treatment refusals can come from patients who refuse consent to therapy because an acquaintance or loved one suffered a death that was worsened by surgery in what they see as an analogous situation. One such patient, diagnosed with a resectable bowel tumor, steadfastly refused surgical intervention. This refusal, it turned out, was strongly influenced by the patient's experience of his sister, who was diagnosed with metastatic pancreatic cancer and treated aggressively and optimistically, only to suffer long and needlessly. A great deal of counseling and reassurance was needed to get him to accept that he was not in his sister's "shoes," and he accepted surgical resection only after specific written assurance that all aggressive treatment would be abated if his prognosis changed substantially for the worse. For such patients the consent process justifiably becomes more demanding, including negotiating with them to abate treatment if initial optimistic estimates of their situation and prospects prove inaccurate.

Knowledge deficits can also result from denial of the seriousness of the patient's illness, requiring further counseling and encouragement. Conversely, patients who are tending to emphasize the severity of the effects of their illness, and fail to appreciate the rehabilitative possibilities beyond surgery, fall into a similar category. The classic bioethics case of the otherwise healthy patient who refuses amputation of a dead extremity symbolizes this category, and merits the same response as the patient in denial. With all due respect for patient autonomy and the right to refuse treatment, such a patient should be approached as operating out of a serious knowledge deficit: the belief that life would not be worth living without one's leg focuses only on what will be lost and does not take into account how rehabilitation can supplement the loss and thus help protect the patient's quality of life. In summary, we support the surgical perspective of aggressive surgical response to patients at the threshold of dying, with the caveat that the surgeon must be prepared to respond to ambivalence with counseling, reassurance, and negotiation—and to refusal with accepting the wishes of the patient who, for quality-of-life reasons beyond the immediate clinical situation, does not wish aggressive response.

Managing Patients Whose Mortality Has Become a Substantial Probability

We believe that this subpopulation of dying patients, exemplified by the SUP-PORT study's 50% or more mortality population, is often *mismanaged* as follows. Clinicians tend to view such patients as salvageable and communicate this view, with little or no qualification, to patients and/or families. This view then endures, well beyond what the facts justify, because of factors such as the clinician's own discomfort, the sense of death as a failure, legal concerns or misconceptions, and the culture of health care institutions. (See our discussion of "barriers to effective 'end of life' management" below.) This delay can then engender at least an equivalent delay in insight on the part of patients and/or their families, who receive such belated information in ambiguous bits and pieces, or in some unanticipated and thus jarring fashion. Because of the factors mentioned, and these delays, the option of timely readjustment of such patients' management is raised too late if at all, and with little or no clear vision about or commitment to it. Patients and families later speak of being "taken for a ride," and wish they had somehow avoided the whole process. "If only the doctors had been honest with us, Daddy would not have suffered so much."

The pivotal clinical ethical difference with this subpopulation is that the patient's situation and prospects have become less ambiguous, and more negative; the risk-benefit ratio for this subpopulation of patients is much more problematic. At the threshold of this diagnosis, nine out of ten patients will at least get life extension if not cure from the regimen of treatment. Move to the SUPPORT study's population and five out of ten will be subject to the burden of aggressive management without its benefit. Unalloyed optimism and reassurance are no longer indicated. The surgeon should thus seriously raise the possibility of not proceeding aggressively in such cases with patients and their families. Equally, the discussion of negative end-stage scenarios should become more specific, because such outcomes are both more likely and predictable in their specifics.

The presentation of the regimen of care should thus proceed as if abatement of aggressive treatment is a legitimate possibility. In other words, the surgeon should *not* simply proceed by making a recommendation for aggressive management, *even if he or she personally believes it is indicated.* Aggressive surgical management, as well as its alternatives, should be presented to the patient and family for their serious consideration. This approach explicitly addresses the oft-heard complaint by patients that they were not given the chance to opt out of what later became regrettable. But its more positive goal is a true, knowledgeable buying-in to a regimen of care.

Though we believe that a firm recommendation for aggressive management may still be legitimately offered for such patients, we do insist that such a recommendation must be accompanied by a discussion of advanced planning for poor outcomes. The surgeon should take this approach so that patients and families have the opportunity to consider the actual pros and cons and reach a considered judgment about them. Patients and families will, we suspect, often still choose aggressive management. The goal is to give them the opportunity to see what is really at stake. Patients and families who are just "waiting for the punch line" or "hoping against hope" should be challenged explicitly to appreciate that all things may not work out as they hope. With such individuals, the surgeon might especially consider temporarily withholding a recommendation for aggressive response, so that the complications, limitations, and extended burden of aggressive response can be adequately addressed by the patient and his or her family.

There are other management issues that arise more urgently with this particular patient population. Symptom management is surely one of the most important. One way to make the benefit versus burden calculation more favorable is to diminish the burden of pain and suffering on the patient as one concurrently pursues the benefit of aggressive intervention. Trade-offs regarding quality of life as treatment proceeds may also merit discussion—for example, whether treatment should be provided on an outpatient basis even if in-hospital management would be medically optimal. There may be ways to avoid sacrificing the patient's remaining good time while the benefit of aggressive, but relatively low-yield, treatment is pursued.

In summary, the bias of the surgeon for aggressive response in the threshold subpopulation of dying patients is simply out of place, but not because most patients and/or families will not choose aggressive response; they probably will, in our experience. But the much lower yield, higher risks and greater morbidity of this middle-spectrum patient counsel that this is a very personal and perilous decision. For the surgeon to believe or act as if he or she "knows best" for such patients, without the patients' own knowledgeable reaction, involves confusion as to what the clinical knowledge does and does not contain.

Managing Patients Whose Mortality is Probable

If we reverse our threshold subpopulation (i.e., to those patients for whom substantial life extension if not cure is at best 10%), it would seem we have our third subset of this diagnosis. But even if such a definition is accepted, we do not see that it has any necessarily clear implications for management. That only one in ten may "profit" from the intervention, in the sense of life-extension, does not necessarily indicate that it should not be offered by the surgeon. It may well be that one discrete, though low-yield, intervention is all that is necessary to determine whether the patient is the one who will profit, or among the nine who will not. Equally, the patient might still elect such an intervention given that without it he or she has no chance at all. The core decision in such instances should relate more to the burden, duration, and limitations of aggressive treatment than the simple chance of success or failure. In essence, the dialogue should focus on what the patient will have to pay in morbidity, pain, suffering, lost quality of life, and earlier death for attempting to gain therapeutic benefit in a statistically low-yield situation.

Management of the probably dying patient thus does not necessarily have to be nonsurgical. Other important values might well be gained by surgical management within the context of a clearly lethal illness. The majority of patients and families would probably tend to opt for nonsurgical management in many such situations, but this remains somewhat conjectural prior to full disclosure and discussions with them. We further submit that the consent process be equally wide-ranging and not assume that any particular conclusion to this process is preferable. The difference will be that, contrary to the other two points on our spectrum, a recommendation for aggressive surgical response in such instances would be completely out of place. Only the patient who is willing to pay the price for such a limited benefit should be the one to select it. So actual understanding approaches being a necessary condition for aggressive response here, and may merit candor to the point of bluntness. Conversely, for the patient who is eminently terminal, and for whom the chance to do "last things," or spend more quality time with loved ones, approaches zero, a strong recommendation to opt for nonoperative management by the surgeon may well be indicated.

Clinical Topics

The Basic Principles of Nonoperative Surgical Management

As noted, the practice of "getting the DNR" leaves clinical management abstract and most of its ensuing issues, short of cardiopulmonary arrest, indeterminate; whether management short of arrest will be aggressive, or otherwise, is not determined. In effect, this is not management, but the absence of it. The prudent clinical question, especially when management falters or is absent, is "what are the goals of care?" Once one elects to forgo aggressive surgical management, we submit, there are four basic goals: (1) to not prolong the process of dying needlessly, (2) to keep the patient as comfortable as possible, (3) to secure whatever positive opportunities and quality of life that are still possible for the patient, and (4) to proceed with all this with patients and/or their families having as full an understanding of and input into this regimen of care as possible.

A little reflection on each point should commend them. Not to prolong the process of dying needlessly seems simple enough; why do anything that satisfies no need? Further, as with the second goal of maximizing patient comfort, this first goal incorporates the time-honored adage of "first do no harm." If no needs can be met, in effect, then only burdens and harms are possible. Equally, tradition is seconded by the basic clinical principle that one should have good reasons for doing anything. The third point recognizes that even within nonoperative management the patient may have other interests beyond simply getting through the dying process as rapidly and comfortably as possible. Doing last things and spending time with loved ones obviously qualify here. And the final point about continuing to pursue needed patient and family insight and input into the regimen of care simply continues the same focus that has been operative throughout our approach to dying patients. Slight this last goal and the other three may well be undermined or derailed. Equally, part of what it will mean to keep the patient comfortable, as well as support the remaining positive quality of life, involves the patient trusting that he or she will continue to be cared for in a humane fashion and not be abandoned or end up suffering needlessly. Before spelling all these goals out further then, we should reflect on why such management is not readily instituted or comprehensively pursued.

Barriers to Effective Nonoperative Management

Denial of Death. Numerous commentators, particularly those reflecting on the lack of improved results in the SUPPORT study, have tended to emphasize the death-denying culture of contemporary society and particularly of health care institutions as barriers.[7] Hence Annas recommends that dying persons just stay out (or get out) of hospitals. We have suggested that matters are not this simple (nor so simply rectified), but we do agree that some of the root causes lie in these arenas. These are often reflected in the law, to which we now turn.

Legal Barriers to Effective Nonoperative Management. Living and practicing in the State of New York, we are prone to be inordinately impressed with the negative role of the law in managing dying patients, because in New York abating treatment is complicated by the legal requirement that clear and convincing prior statements by the patient are the only legal ground upon which such abatement can be justified.[11] Such a rule then runs afoul of the fact that many dying patients can no longer speak competently to treatment issues, nor have they usually done so beforehand with any specificity. The fact that all parties, clinicians and family members, may be in agreement about the appropriateness of abating treatment is thus legally irrelevant; no one has the legal right to opt for abatement without clear and convincing prior statements from the patient.

We believe, however, that the negative effects of the law, even in New York State, on the management of dying patients, is much overexaggerated and, in the end, a red herring. We take this view, in part, on the basis of the fact that most of the institutions in the SUPPORT study exist in localities where the law is much more accepting and facilitative of abating treatment. We also take this view as we also practice in the VA health care system, where the regulations in this area are quite facilitative, and the same negative results reported by the SUPPORT study tend to occur. In summary, even when the law and policy are facilitative of abating treatment, the negative factors addressed by the SUPPORT study continue to occur. Why? Our strong belief is that even if the law were more facilitative of abating treatment, the problems would remain, because surgeons, patients, and families are reticent to take such a course. We submit that this belief is strongly supported by the SUPPORT study itself.

Such reticence, in turn, produces not just complaints that the law is being obstructive but supports, if not generates, a number of basic misconceptions about what the law, in fact, requires, allows, or forbids. The misconceptions have been well stated by Meisel: "There are a number of myths about what the law permits concerning the termination of life support, some of which spring from a fundamental misconception of what law is. A serious misunderstanding of the law can lead to tragic results for physicians, health care institutions, patients, and families. The misunderstandings are: (1) anything that is not specifically permitted by law is prohibited; (2) termination of life support is murder or suicide; (3) a patient must be terminally ill for life support to be terminated; (4) it is permissible to terminate extraordinary treatments, but not ordinary ones; (5) it is permissible to withhold treatment, but once started, it must be continued; (6) stopping tube feeding is legally different from stopping other treatment; (7) termination of life support requires going to court; (8) living wills are not legal."[12]

Institutional and Professional Barriers to Effective Nonoperative Management. Whence come such misconceptions, if not from the law itself? Our suggestions are (1) from the reticence and discomfort of surgeons, patients, and families, particularly when they are dealing with the ambiguous 50% or greater mortality population of the SUPPORT study, and (2) from the nonfacilitative, often obstructive culture of our hospitals, where institutional support of abating treatment is often lacking, if not hostile, and where the "safe" legal course, "informed" by the previously noted legal myths, is often parroted by institutional leaders. Add to this reticent, nonfacilitative culture the tendency to see death as not only a failure, but something that needs defending (as if the known statistics did not exist), and it is no wonder that the SUPPORT study failed to alter outcomes.

The remaining, and more basic, culprits here are the reticence of surgeons, patients, and families who are unprepared or unwilling to opt for effective nonoperative management when the appropriate time comes. The purpose of the approach proposed in this chapter is to assist all parties to be better prepared for such a transition when the time comes. The extent to which staff have surmounted such barriers is, we believe, the key to changing the culture of health care institutions. We can think of no better antidote to such in-hospital barriers than to proceed to spell out, individually, what the guiding principles and tactics of effective nonoperative management are.

The Ordinary versus Extraordinary Treatment Distinction: Its Clinical Inappropriateness. Much has been made in recent years of the supposed distinction between ordinary and extraordinary treatment, the latter being elective and thus abatable (e.g., ventilatory support), the former being mandatory (e.g., artificial feeding and hydration). Regarding the theoretical incoherence of this distinction, we can do no better than simply offer McCormick's basic point that what makes a treatment extraordinary is *not the nature of the treatment, but the nature of the patient*.[13] One would hardly abate intubation in an otherwise healthy patient who has a life-threatening but eminently treatable (with ventilatory support) infiltrate. This is not extraordinary treatment; surgeons do it all the time. Equally, to keep a moribund or vegetative patient alive with an intravenous line or a nasogastric tube, often also strapping him or her down to a bed because he or she keeps trying to remove it, is a profound and obvious example of something extraordinary in the sense that really should be at issue: it places a profound burden on the patient without affording that patient any substantial benefit. As to the use of antibiotics, an older wisdom, which physicians used to honor, held that pneumonia might appropriately be allowed to be the "old man's friend," the idea being that when one has reached the end of his or her life, nonaggressive management provides an exit from a life of profound debility and suffering that, as we know so well, tends to follow from aggressive management. So intravenous lines and nasogastric or PEG tubes, as well as antibiotics, are not always, in and of themselves, obligatory. They should be used only when they advance some specific patient wish or interests. Often, in fact, as we shall describe below, such "ordinary" interventions are not only not justified by any specific patient need, but they are, in fact, harmful to the patient—for example, when the view that one must always hydrate a patient results only in an increase in suffering via pulmonary edema for a patient in the end-stages of lung cancer. In sum, whether or not any treatment is offered to a patient, its only justification lies in its ability to advance some patient interest. And, to proceed, one such alleged interest (i.e., in life itself), turns out to quite problematic.

Vitalism: Its Clinical Inappropriateness.   The view that life itself is a benefit, whatever profound diminishments or burdens that sustaining life involves, is a view held by few if any *for themselves* and is simply contrary to the ethical traditions of the medical profession. The Hippocratic texts, for example, are quite clear that treatment should not be offered to patients who are "over-mastered" by their disease. This caveat is as useful as any in capturing the point of the earlier rehearsed complaints about overtreatment of dying patients and surely fuels the widespread practice of generating advance directives as well as the (we believe misguided) attempt to legalize physician-assisted suicide. The latter may thus be seen as an extreme attempt to counter extremism on the part of some clinicians and families. Neither is prudent.

The ethical point about vitalism is that life should be seen as a *condition* for the possibility of being benefited, not as an absolute benefit or end in itself. Continued existence can be solely and profoundly a situation of burden and suffering. The surgeon who espouses vitalism may certainly indicate this by prior statements (i.e., that he or she would want to be sustained at all costs). We would suggest only that he or she does not foist this view on those placed under his or her care because few will hold such a view. In summary, if treatment cannot be justified by direct appeal to specific, nonvitalist interests of one's patients, then that treatment is contraindicated.

The Distinction Between Withholding and Withdrawing Treatment: Its Clinical Inappropriateness. Many clinicians, and some patients and/or families, seem to subscribe to this distinction. But this distinction is clinically incoherent and potentially quite damaging. To be reticent or unwilling to withdraw aggressive treatment (e.g., ventilatory support) tends to make one opt for management that is simply inappropriate. This can occur in two basic forms. If treatment is already instituted, one will tend not to withdraw it even though the clinical justification for it has evaporated; then patients who are overmastered and burdened by disease and treatment are maintained in states beyond what most rational people would value; treatment thus continues in the absence of any rationale. Discomfort about withdrawal can result in the tendency to withhold trials of therapy that may well be in the patient's interest. Here the scenario of asking the acutely short-of-breath patient with severe chronic obstructive pulmonary disease whether he or she wants the "breathing machine" is as good an example as any. Prior to a therapeutic trial, it may well be quite unclear as to whether this is a treatable infiltrate or not. But what is clinically preferable here: not to intubate a patient who may or may not have a treatable infiltrate or to intubate a patient who may be treatable and, if he or she is not, abate what turns out to be no-longer-beneficial treatment? The appropriate answer here is that one should make treatment decisions on the basis of knowledge, not discomfort and uncertainty, and treatment can be elected while one still limits the scope of the potential burden by being fully willing and able to abate such a trial intervention when the patient's interests are no longer served by it. In summary, it is better to determine that the patient is, in fact, overmastered by disease after a reasonable therapeutic trial, than to turn that possibility into a death sentence by default.

Specific Components and Tactics of Nonoperative Surgical Management

Institutional change can be slow and difficult, but one surely can surmount such myths and barriers in one's own practice. The surgeon can then focus on the previously noted basic goals of nonoperative management.

Not Prolonging the Process of Dying Needlessly. In a fair number of cases (e.g., with the dying patient who is unresponsive), nonoperative management may be quite simple. All treatment that prolongs the dying process should be withheld or withdrawn and "nature allowed to take its course." To maintain any therapy, even intravenous hydration, that retards this process serves no substantive patient interest and only extends the indignity and devastation for others of dying. Equally, the eminently dying patient will usually benefit from just being kept comfortable and avoiding what only prolongs the dying process. Even if we speak only of air-hunger, it should be clear that substantial suffering can occur in a few minutes of continued existence, so treatments that solely burden the patient, either in themselves (e.g., hydration that produces pulmonary edema) or by retarding the process of dying (e.g., cardiac medications for hypotension), should be seen, unequivocally, as contraindicated.

Treatments That Add to the Burden of Dying. Beyond merely prolonging suffering and the process of dying, some treatments also compound pain and suffering by their physiologic effect and are thus doubly contraindicated. Various "ordinary" treatments come particularly to mind here, but especially artificial feeding and hydration. Numerous studies have documented that "many patients who do receive artificial nutrition and hydration are observed to develop distressing and serious side effects such as nausea, vomiting, diarrhea, congestive heart failure, peripheral edema, pulmonary congestion, and aspiration pneumonia."[14] In hospice programs, where "patient comfort and patient-determined intake of foods and fluids" are emphasized, however, "observers have noted that terminal patients in varying degrees of dehydration and starvation are not uncomfortable."[14] "Ordinary" treatments can thus become profoundly extraordinary and thus may be as contraindicated as anything in surgery.

Symptom Management. Most patients do not immediately and conveniently exit even when all agree it is "time to go" and life extension serves no substantive interest. The clinical challenge is to keep them comfortable in the interim as well as not prolong that interim or do something that adds burden to it. But this may be insufficient and positive steps may be required (i.e., active symptom management). Now, as already mentioned, pain management has been documented as often woefully inadequate in the dying patient.[1,2,4,5] Why this is so even when their dying is accepted remains a mystery only if one ignores the previous discussion of barriers to effective nonoperative management. The same discomfort and ambivalence that fuel notions of the obligation to provide "ordinary" treatment, or to not withdraw no longer indicated life support, also affect approaches to symptom management.

Perhaps the clearest instance of such thinking is when someone objects to the continuation or augmentation of narcotic analgesia for a dying patient on the ground that the patient will become addicted to it. Surely powerful, and irrational, forces are operative when the commonsense notion that addiction is hardly a concern in a patient who is about to die becomes short-circuited. As it turns out, addiction has been found to be quite rare in such patients. In one study of patients who regularly received opium for pain control over a 3-month period, the frequency was four patients out of twelve thousand.[15]

Again, certain myths and barriers seem to be operative. We all know colleagues who have been called on the carpet, either by their institution or, worse, by outside regulating bodies, for overmedicating patients. The classic instance where this legitimate concern arises to thwart adequate symptom control is with the short-of-breath patient for whom morphine would be palliative but may also depress respiratory drive. The concern is thus not just with hindsight regulation and sanction, but also with the justified aversion to doing something that may kill one's patient.

Much of this is, however, factually inaccurate. Assuming one increases analgesia incrementally, all one is doing is responding to the known acclimation of the patient to it, and such acclimation is not just to its analgesic effect but also its tendency to depress respiration. Second, incremental increases of analgesia can reach quite high doses without, by themselves, precipitating respiratory depression. Patients who proceed to respiratory depression and arrest in such instances do so essentially because of other clinical factors—for example, severe pulmonary or cardiac insufficiency from tumor or chronic obstructive disease. Is it still accurate to say in such patients that analgesia killed the patient, that at least the patient might have survived a bit longer absent one's analgesic efforts? Perhaps the latter, but this hardly constitutes a killing. The problem here lies in preferring to be swayed by an unknown and conjectural clinical factor, and in the process accepting that the price of this is increased patient suffering—suffering that by definition can be alleviated. Again, attention to traditional notions may be helpful here. The traditional doctrine of double effect—that is, that one can with ethical justification give analgesia that may depress respirations, or even contribute to the patient dying, without intending to do so—is available; the intention is to alleviate suffering, often the only clinical benefit the surgeon has to offer the patient.

Aside from this, we will simply report that we know of no instances where clinicians have been successfully sued or sanctioned for responding aggressively and incrementally to documented discomfort in the dying patient. And again, the patient and/or family who have been assisted and encouraged to have insight and input into the "regimen of care" is probably the best barrier to any threat to the clinician who seeks to be conscientious about this. Add to all this the fact that death will be primarily attributable to factors other than the analgesia (e.g., cardiogenic shock), and one should not be ethically or legally uncomfortable in giving clearly indicated care.

Securing Whatever Positive Opportunities and Quality of Life that Remain for the Patient. For some patients, particularly if they are unresponsive or no longer communicative, simply allowing their death to occur as soon as possible may be the only reasonable solution. Others, however, may have needs or desires that indicate something other than symptom management and the abatement of all life support. Doing last things may be needful, whether it is getting one's affairs in order, waiting for a distant loved one to arrive, or attempting to find spiritual equanimity. So the four principles of nonoperative management enunciated here must be integrated into a plan of care.

If death is not imminent, various issues arise to complicate future management. Whether the patient will spend his or her remaining time in the hospital or in the community is perhaps the most basic issue. If he or she is to be sent out into the community, various allied issues will need to be addressed, including who will care for the patient, whether appropriate standing orders limiting treatment exist if the patient has to return to hospital for either respite or end-stage care, and whether trade-offs must be discussed, for example, short term response to acute, potentially treatable problems for the sake of life extension, or lessened analgesia for the sake of more alertness. All such matters should be basic foci for discharge planning. Here the complexity of management can rival anything that aggressive treatment can involve, and the surgeon should make a referral for hospice care, which has been designed especially to comprehensively address such management issues.

The Hospice Alternative: Its Wisdom and Limitations

In earlier drafts of this chapter we tended to refer to nonoperative care as conservative management, or palliative care. We ended up avoiding either term because both tend to have a passive connotation that is exactly the opposite of what we believe to be clinically and ethically indicated for the dying patient who has refused aggressive management. The World Health Organization's statement of the principles of palliative care captures the essence here:

> the active, total care of a person whose condition may or may not respond to curative treatment. That care encompasses physical, psychological, social, and spiritual aspects of suffering, and aims at reducing suffering and enhancing quality of life. It offers a support system to provide continuity of caring to the patient, and support systems to help families cope with illness and bereavement.[5]

Now, the hospice movement, with its unique philosophy and approach to the dying patient, has long carried this particular banner. For all its merits, however—candor with patients and families, aggressive symptom response, and comprehensive management of all facets of a dying patient's life—we should also note that separate hospice response will not prove much more effective for a population like that of the SUPPORT study than the use of medical futility judgments. This is so as only a portion of this population will be unambiguously unsalvageable. The bulk of this population will present with varying degrees of "dying" (or "salvageability") and appropriately be considered for (and desire) interventions. In this regard, Miller and Fins recently suggested that hospice beds be integrated into hospitals near ICUs,[6] thereby rendering the transition from aggressive to hospice management easier, more seamless. But, as we have argued above in detail, it is not the physical distance from ICU to hospice bed that creates the problem here, nor even the absence of the hospice philosophy. Rather it is the uncertainty regarding which sort of bed any of these patients should actually be in at any given time. Presently, hospice receives the more unambiguous cases and we all have much to learn from its approach to them. But the bulk of the SUPPORT study's population is no more in need of a hospice bed than Annas' panacea of just staying out of the hospital.

The comprehensive approach that hospice has evolved, as found in the WHO statement, particularly with its emphasis on care in the community, ongoing attention to symptom management, anticipation of and provision for problems that arise in the community (e.g., respite care), as well as provision for end-stage management in a facility or environment that it manages, addresses and supports the four goals mentioned above. We therefore strongly recommend that our reader make connections with local hospice programs. Beyond this, there is a broad, quite detailed knowledge base that any such program would likely be able to readily offer. It is as much a specialty as any other and merits detailed familiarity by other clinicians, not just for patient referral, but for what it can offer the surgeon regarding dying patients who remain under his or her care. If the entire argument of this chapter produces nothing else, we would hope that it generates a strong tendency to hear one's hospice colleagues out in detail.

Specifying Further Management and Remaining Engaged

The last general consideration regarding nonoperative management regards the role of the surgeon in fashioning that management and his or her subsequent involvement with the case. Two basic caveats merit emphasis here. It is clearly the treating team and attending surgeon who should assist the patient and/or family to fashion the specific details of a nonoperative plan of management, whether or not any of them will be the actual providers of that management. It should be apparent at this juncture that simply making the dying patient a DNR and transferring him or her to the floor, or discharging him or her to the community, is inadequate and inappropriate. The team who has gone through all that has led up to the decision to opt for nonoperative management, informed by the experiences, insights, and relationships thus developed, remains an essential resource for developing the plan of care. To do otherwise is unwise and unfair to all concerned, including the strangers who will take over care. To do so is tantamount to abandonment. The surgeon should therefore remain engaged with the further process of the dying patient's care even if he or she in no way provides that care. The surgeon should at least let the patient or family know that he or she is available if problems arise. This can be a crucial reassurance and source of comfort even when all proceeds according to plan. Beyond this, simply to check in occasionally on the patient and the patient's family, physically or at least by phone, can satisfy the same needs and monitoring function. It would seem appropriate to attribute a significant part of hospice's success to the trust and reassurance that patients and families feel that they will not be abandoned, and that they will be cared for in all senses of the term by dedicated professionals to the very end. The surgeon who continues to be engaged in such a fashion can contribute substantially to such feelings with a minimum of effort.

Clinical Conclusions

Our recommendations regarding how the surgeon's approach to dying patients should be modified may seem a very tall order. So be it. It is difficult not to be affected by the culture of the society and institutions in which surgeons practice. And most commentators are very impressed with how robust the barriers to major change are. In this regard, Fins and Miller offer the somewhat reassuring point that the management of childbirth has successfully undergone just such a radical change over the past few decades[6]; so we might hope for something similar in the clinical approach to the dying.

However optimistic one may or may not feel, it should at least be seen that the approach for which we have argued in this chapter enjoys basic support from common sense, the traditions of medicine and surgery, empirical research, and basic principles of good surgical practice. To obtain adequate informed consent for trials of surgical management, to abate those that no longer clinically benefit the patient, not to prolong needlessly either suffering or dying, to keep people as comfortable as possible and focus on what positive benefits may still be available to them, and to avoid anything that does not commend itself on the basis of specific patient wishes or needs, are goals that may be simply and unequivocally stated. The opposition can only hide away so long in obfuscation, myths, and behaviors that will not bear analysis. The 20/20 nature of clinical hindsight, as long as it is judiciously appreciated and applied, can be a formidable ally, as we hope to have demonstrated.

We are moved to note that some current wisdom holds the problem to be that our technology has outpaced our ethical skill and wisdom. We reject this analysis. Rather, we have allowed this technology to bewitch us out of a traditional, commonsense orientation to dying patients that is still available and adequate to the tasks and issues at hand. To "do no harm," not to seek to treat those who are "overmastered" by their disease, to provide comfort and seek to maintain a patient's dignity, to protect whatever possibilities that remain within a life that may be severely limited and at its ending—*these are all principles that require no new ethical epiphany.*

All that needs be new here is that given that the lethality of a disease can now be thwarted, we need to install appropriate anticipatory tactics to make sure this is done in a timely and comprehensive fashion, and in ways that are supported and understood by the parties involved. To do such, and to recognize the broad population of "dying" patients upfront, one can avoid throwing the "baby" of medical progress out with the bathwater as Annas proposes, while still responding systematically to the fears of countless patients and families. In summary, *we are simply talking about what should, on well-informed ethical reflection, constitute good surgical outcomes in the care of seriously ill patients.*

References

1. William Knaus, Frank Harrell, Joanne Lynn, et al. "The SUPPORT Prognostic Model: Objective Estimates of Survival for Seriously Ill Hospitalized Adults," *Annals of Internal Medicine* 122 (1995): 191–203.
2. The SUPPORT Principal Investigators; "A Controlled Trial To Improve Care for Seriously Ill Hospitalized Patients: The Study to Understand Prognoses and Preferences for Outcomes and Risks of Treatments (SUPPORT)," *Journal of the American Medical Association* 274 (1995): 1591–1598.
3. Nancy King, *Making Sense of Advance Directives*. Dordrecht, The Netherlands: Kluwer Academic Publishers, 1994.
4. Charles Cleland, René Gonin, Alan Hatfield, et al., "Pain and Its Treatment in Outpatients with Metastatic Cancer," *New England Journal of Medicine*, 330 (1994): 592–6.
5. World Health Organization, "Cancer Pain Relief and Palliative Care", *Technical Reports Series 804*, Geneva: World Health Organization, 1990.
6. Franklin Miller and Joseph Fins, "A Proposal to Restructure Hospital Care for Dying Patients," *New England Journal of Medicine* 334 (1996): 1740–1742.
7. Daniel Callahan. "Once Again, Reality: Now Where Do We Go?," *Hastings Center Report* 25 (1995): S33–36.
8. Howard Brody, "Transparency: Informed Consent in Primary Care," *Hastings Center Report* 19 (1989): 5–9.
9. Stephen Wear, *Informed Consent: Patient Autonomy and Physician Beneficence in Clinical Medicine*. Dordrecht, The Netherlands: Kluwer Academic Publishers, 1993.
10. Alan Meisel and Loren Roth, "What We Do and Do Not Know about Informed Consent," *Journal of the American Medical Association* 246 (1981): 2473–2477.
11. New York Public Health Law: 1991, "Orders not to Resuscitate Act" #2960–2978 and "Health Care Proxy Act" #2980–2994 (*McKinney Supp. 1991*).
12. Alan Meisel, "Legal Myths About Terminating Life Support," *Archives of Internal Medicine* 151 (1991): 1497–1502.
13. Richard McCormick, "To Save or Let Die: The Dilemma of Modern Medicine," *Journal of the American Medical Association* 229 (1974): 172–76.
14. William Nelson, Shirley Ann Smith, et al., *Hospice Ethics*. Washington, D.C.: Veterans Health Administration, 1995.
15. John Porter, "Addiction Rare in Patients Treated with Narcotics," *New England Journal of Medicine* 302 (1980): 123.

11

Patients Who Are Family Members, Friends, Colleagues, Family Members of Colleagues

JONATHAN D. MORENO
FRANK E. LUCENTE

Mixing the Ethics of the Surgeon-Patient Relationship with Marriage, Kinship, Collegiality, or Friendship

The provision of surgical or medical care to those with whom one shares bonds of marriage, kinship, collegiality, or friendship seems to raise issues that distinguish such patient care from caring for patients with whom one is not otherwise associated. These issues are both ethical and psychodynamic in nature and have long been recognized as such. In general, while ethical traditions counsel caution in such practices, they also stress that doctors have a special obligation to make their skills available to those in need, perhaps especially those close to them, an obligation that is often couched in terms of duties of professional courtesy. Because of the ambiguity inherent in traditions of medical ethics on these issues, a more finely tuned analysis that speaks to various sets of circumstances is required.

A common justification for the decision to undertake the care of those toward whom one feels a deep sense of personal obligation is that one would not want to entrust the care of that individual to another surgeon. Clearly, a strong measure of self-confidence is admirable and perhaps essential in the psychological makeup of a successful surgeon. However, self-confidence should not be permitted to substitute for a reasoned evaluation of the pros and cons of this decision, and it is rarely true that the surgeon in question is the only qualified prac-

198

titioner in a given case. As we shall elaborate, the same factors that motivate this "take charge" impulse weigh heavily against succumbing to it, especially when those in need of surgical care are intimates. On the whole, we argue that the surgeon who would provide surgical care for family, friends, or colleagues assumes a burden of proof. The weight of this burden varies from one sort of relationship to another, with the performance of surgery on a close relative requiring an especially high level of justification.[1] But in each case the ethical basis of the surgeon-patient relationship requires justification for surgeons who would care for those to whom one is otherwise related.

Historical Context

Discussions of these issues are of ancient origin, especially with regard to the care of colleagues and their family members. The Hippocratic admonition to treat one's teachers and their families as if they were relatives is taken to be the classical source of the doctor's commitment to professional solidarity:

> To hold him who has taught me this art as equal to my parents and to live my life in partnership with him . . . and to regard his offspring as equal to my brothers in male lineage and to teach them this art—if they desire to learn it—without fee and covenant. . . .[2]

It appears from this passage that the writer or writers advised both taking care of colleagues' sons as though they were one's own and also waiving tuition for training their sons in the medical arts. For those who subscribed to this view, it seems to have followed that the medical care of these offspring should also be provided without fee, which obviously presupposes that it is legitimate to provide care to those to whom one is so related in the first place.

Two thousand years later, in his classic 1803 text *Medical Ethics*, Percival also approves the propriety of care for colleagues and their families, but he supplements the rationale of professional solidarity with a practical concern about the health of such persons if free services were not available.

> All members of the profession, including apothecaries as well as physicians and surgeons, together with their wives and children, should be attended gratuitously, by any one or more of the faculty residing near them, whose assistance may be required. For as solicitude obscures judgment, and is accompanied by timidity and irresolution, medical men, under the pressure of sickness, either as affecting themselves or their families, are peculiarly dependent upon each other. Distant members of the faculty, when they request attendance, should be expected to defray the costs of traveling. And if their circumstances be affluent, a pecuniary acknowledgement should not be declined. For no obligation ought to be imposed, which the party would rather compensate than contract.[3]

Percival's concern about doctors and their families receiving inferior care is one to which we shall return later in this chapter. His view that the affluent should pay for care rendered by their colleagues places him at odds with the fraternal Hippocratic tradition. The 1847 American Medical Association (AMA) Code of Ethics reiterated Percival's view in nearly the same language, and it appeared in the 1949 code essentially unchanged.

> As a general rule, a physician should not attempt to treat members of his family or himself. Consequently, a physician should cheerfully and without recompense give his professional services to physicians or their dependents if they are in his vicinity.[4]

According to this view the combination of financial costs of care and the temptation to self-treat or treat one's family is dangerous. To avoid the temptation that would follow, it is best that colleagues provide free care. Underlying this position is a drastically different assessment of the propriety of taking care of family members than that inherent in the Hippocratic tradition, that under these circumstances doctors' judgment may be "obscured," and they may be too "timid and irresolute."

In recent years code passages that referred to treating family members have tended to be regarded as outdated. Neither the drastically revised and shortened 1957 AMA Code of Ethics nor the 1980 version mentions either treatment of the family or professional courtesy.[5] The AMA Council on Ethical and Judicial Affairs dropped an opinion in its *Opinions and Reports* on physicians' treatment of their own family members as an "anachronism," though guidelines on professional courtesy were retained and insurance benefits were viewed as acceptable.[6] In 1989 Medicare barred payments to physicians for the care of "immediate family members" in order to avoid financial abuse.[7] Four years later, the AMA Council itself concluded that self-treatment or treatment of immediate family members is inappropriate except for emergencies or for minor medical needs.[8]

Thus, a distinction seems to be drawn between the suitability of treating family members on one hand and colleagues or their relatives on the other. A rationale for this distinction can perhaps be expressed as follows. The bonds of affection that tie physicians and surgeons to family members (and, by analogy, to close friends) can cloud clinical judgment. Not only is this not the case with respect to colleagues and their family members, but professional solidarity and other considerations support the proposition that professional courtesy deserves to continue in some fashion. In the remainder of this chapter we will examine whether the rationale for an ethical distinction between family treatment and professional courtesy can be sustained.

Empirical Studies of American Practices

Empirical studies have been conducted on the prevalence of physicians' treatment of their own family members as well as on their provision of professional courtesy. These studies include surgeons and surgical procedures among their subjects. Although the studies were conducted with different sample populations, they generally indicate that while professional courtesy is almost always extended by a broad range of practitioners, including surgeons, the incidence of family treatment seems to vary with the degree of invasiveness of the intervention, among other factors.

A 1991 study of Oregon physicians' care for relatives conducted by Reagan et al. ranked responses to 17 procedures according to a relative frequency scale ranging from "never" to "often." The mode response to all but the top two services was "never." The first two services were minor prescribing (e.g., colds, flu, allergies) and prescribing oral antibiotics, both of which had a mode response frequency of "sometimes." Further down the list were minor surgery, gynecological care, assisting in surgery, and major surgery. Reagan et al. also studied the self- reported comfort level of respondents who did care for their relatives, from "very comfortable" to "very uncomfortable." The highest comfort level was with treating one's own child, followed in this order by niece or nephew, spouse, grandchild, sibling, sibling-in-law, parent-in-law, parent, and grandparent. The mode response for treating a child was "comfortable," for a niece or nephew "neutral," and "uncomfortable" for all others. Convenience was the main reason given for family treatment, followed by the fact that a request had been made, and saving a relative some money. Many respondents offered anecdotes and reflections on the issue. The authors conclude that treating family members is rare apart from minor prescribing, but that when it does occur, it takes many forms and is a source of discomfort for doctors.[9]

A study of Iowa physicians' treatment of their own children was conducted by Dusdieker et al. in 1990. Seventy-four percent of respondents said that they usually treated their own children for an afebrile acute illness, with 36% of those responding stating that they rarely or never contacted the child's primary physician under such circumstances. However, 88% said they usually contacted their child's physician if the child was ill with a fever, and 55% reported that they would rarely or never treat their febrile child without the physician's advice. Among the other interesting findings, 65% reported prescribing antibiotics for their children at least sometimes. Cost was the least prominent reason for treatment of their own children, convenience the most. Of concern to this study's authors was the apparent result that physicians are taking care of their children regardless of their level of training or specialty.[10]

In their 1990 study of physicians' treatment of their own families, LaPuma et al. surveyed all members of the medical staff of a large suburban community teaching hospital. Ninety-nine percent of the respondents reported requests from family members for medical advice. Eighty-three percent of these had prescribed medication, 80% had diagnosed medical illnesses, 72% had performed physical examinations, and 15% had acted as a family member's primary attending physician in the hospital. Concerning surgical procedures, 9% had performed elective surgery on a family member and 4% emergency surgery. A few respondents specified the "most important" procedures they had performed on family members, including cardiothoracic, cosmetic, dermatologic, general, obstetric-gynecologic, ophthalmologic, and orthopedic surgery. Of these, dermatologic procedures were the most common, followed by obstetric-gynecologic.[11]

As mentioned above, a modern rationale for professional courtesy has been to reduce the temptation among physicians to give self-care or to treat their family members. If treating family members is indeed infrequent or limited to relatively minor illnesses and interventions, data suggest that professional courtesy remains a widespread phenomenon and one surprisingly recalcitrant to changes in the way that health care is financed or to the cost of care. Three surveys conducted between 1958 and 1966 showed that free or discounted care was provided by at least 90% of physicians. A 1991 study of randomly selected AMA members again found that over 90% of doctors in all fields (except psychiatry at 80%) offered free or discounted care to physicians or their families; general surgeons were reported at 98% and surgical subspecialists at 99%. The proportion of physicians providing professional courtesy was significantly lower than in 1966 (94% vs. 88%), but the absolute change in proportion was still small. Ninety-two percent of respondents agreed with the statement, "I consider it an honor to care for other physicians," 79% agreed that "professional courtesy solidifies bonds between physicians," and 62% that "giving professional courtesy is sound business practice." Only 15% agreed that "professional courtesy discourages physicians from appropriately seeking care," and only 14% that "professional courtesy interferes with the formation of an appropriate physician-patient relationship."[7]

Ethical Analysis: Concerns in Clinical Judgment and Practice

Challenges to Clinical Judgment

All of the surveys of doctors' treatment of their family members provide reason for concern both about the problems this can create for physicians and the quality of the care provided. One respondent to the Reagan et al. study worried about lack of proper assessment, and others reported that school forms were filled out without an examination.[9] The Duisdieker et al. survey indicated that children were diagnosed and treated despite their physician parents' lack of pediatric training.[9] LaPuma et al. found that 72% of those who refused to treat family members did so because the complaint was outside his or her area of expertise, but 10% who felt uncomfortable with the request for this reason treated anyway.[11] Taken together, these results identify the family members of physicians as a group at risk for substandard medical care.

There is ample anecdotal evidence that clinical judgment and objectivity are impaired by affective bonds. Some of this evidence emerges in the studies summarized above, others in communications by doctors to medical journals. For example, a physician reported attributing his son's abdominal discomfort to test anxiety, but at his wife's insistence the boy was seen by another physician, who found acute appendicitis.[12] While there are those who contend that love and concern can have offsetting benefits,[9] the surveys strongly suggest that the discomfort caused by treating close relatives is one reason that most, but not all, physicians decline to treat them for any but the most minor complaints.

Challenges to Confidentiality

Caring for the medical or surgical needs of family members appropriately requires not only access to the usual historic and physical intimacies associated with medical care, but also the ability to keep the confidences of one's relative and patient (see Chapter 3). It requires little imagination to recognize the conflicts this can pose for a doctor caring for an otherwise self-determining married son or daughter, for example, when both the physician's spouse and in-laws have a legitimate concern about his or her condition. In caring for a fellow physician confidentiality may be at hazard if he or she is a colleague in the same health care facility, especially if casual consultation with colleagues is the norm. Friends of colleagues, while more distant in their independent connection with a treating physician, may nevertheless be at high risk for loss of confidentiality to the extent that the colleague is confused about his or her own role and expects to be consulted by the treating physician.

Challenges to the Informed Consent Process

The psychological content of personal relationships can jeopardize what is already a complex and subtle set of communications that take place between a surgeon and a patient, as described in Chapter 2. Because the preferred informed consent encounter is a two-way communication, both parties can be affected: the surgeon, in attempting to convey information, and the patient, in attempting to understand and evaluate the significance of the information and in expressing preferences to the surgeon. Moreover, the surgeon's obligation to communicate bad news to the patient, an unpleasant task under the best of circumstances, can be made more burdensome when affective bonds are present.

To be sure, there are some apparent advantages in having a standing relationship with a patient. For instance, it could be argued that communications can be enhanced by familiarity with how a person processes important information, and what values that individual holds about health care and important life decisions. Yet it is also true that the surgeon is as susceptible as anyone else to error and self-deception about the perceptions of someone who is close to him or her. Therefore, in spite of the seeming benefits associated with historic connections to the person one is treating, the psychological intricacies of a personal relationship can interfere with those insights, especially when serious medical matters are involved.

Professional Courtesy and Challenges to Integrity in Business Practices

As compared with taking care of family members or friends, these psychological issues may seem less prominent in the treatment of colleagues or their relatives. Yet, depending on the precise circumstances and history of a collegial relationship, the same comments may apply in individual cases. Even where this is not the case—and most of the AMA members surveyed in 1991 did not think the practice interferes with appropriate physician-patient relationships[2]—professional courtesy raises other ethical issues, as well as some legal ones. Thus some have suggested that though intended to remove an obstacle to physicians' seeking care from colleagues rather than making the mistake of treating themselves or their family members, professional courtesy may rather have resulted in physicians' seeking too much treatment.[13] An objection to professional courtesy that is both principled and practical is that it inappropriately insulates doctors and their families from the costs of health care, thus discouraging their active support of health care reform.[7,13]

As fee-for-service practice has dwindled, professional courtesy is often exercised through the waiving of copayments. But surgeons who bill a third-party payer may have a contractual obligation to bill the patient for any copayment. The failure to do so is a form of overbilling the third-party payer, since the actual charge for the service has been lessened, and is unethical. Moreover, forgiveness of copayment is illegal in at least one state, Colorado.[7]

Proponents of the spirit of professional courtesy argue that it plays a humanizing role in an increasingly depersonalized health care system. They suggest that there may be other, less objectionable ways to preserve it. For example, special scheduling efforts may be made for colleagues, as well as keeping in close touch with them to avoid the hazards of self-treatment.[14] Such suggestions would be easier to justify if more was known about the risks of self-care and care of family members by physicians, and whether professional courtesy really does significantly reduce these risks. As we have seen, in spite of the continued practice of professional courtesy in a modern form, surgeons do sometimes provide care to their family members.

An Ethical Framework for the Care of Family Members, Colleagues, or Friends

In the previous sections we have discussed various issues mainly in empirical and historical terms. In this section we bring these considerations together in an ethical framework that will form the basis of our subsequent arguments and recommendations.

LaPuma and Priest have developed a series of seven questions that clinicians should ask themselves before providing non-emergency care or treatment for other than minor illnesses to their family members:[15]

1. Am I trained to meet my relative's medical needs?
2. Am I too close to probe my relative's intimate history and physical being and to cope with bearing bad news if need be?
3. Can I be objective enough to avoid giving too much, too little, or inappropriate care?
4. Is medical involvement likely to provoke or intensify intrafamilial conflicts?
5. Will my relatives comply more readily with medical care delivered by an unrelated physician?
6. Will I allow the physician to whom I refer my relative to attend him or her?
7. Am I willing to be accountable to my peers and to the public for this care?[7]

To these well-considered questions we add two more of a specifically ethical nature:

8. Can I maintain the confidentiality of my relative?
9. Can I engage in a consent process that is respectful of my relative's rights and interests?

All of these questions can be adapted to situations involving colleagues and friends, as well as relatives. A qualified answer to any one of them should be enough to persuade a doctor to help the prospective patient find a suitable alternative caregiver.

Embedded in these questions are three ethical obligations governing the physician-patient relationship that, taken together, constitute a framework that can be applied to the problems we address in this chapter. Each obligation articulates an element in the ethical basis of the physician-patient relationship. In this chapter we cannot engage in the important process of philosophical justification of the principles underlying these obligations, but we believe that all are widely accepted and justifiable from various philosophical perspectives.

The first of these obligations is respect for and promotion of patient self-determination, or autonomy. The surgeon contemplating involvement in the care of a person with whom he or she has an independent relationship may have emotional or other connections to the individual that compromise the ability to recognize and implement the patient's preferences. Since respect for and promotion of self-determination requires that the patient be given the information about his or her condition and reasonable treatment alternatives needed to make an informed decision, disclosure is a critical feature of this obligation.

The second obligation that we highlight is the surgeon's fiduciary responsibility to protect and promote the patient's interests. At first this obligation may seem easier to satisfy in the kinds of relationships we are discussing in this chapter than in professional relationships with others. But a moment's reflection reveals that we may harbor other motives even—and perhaps especially—with those with whom we have strong affective ties. Often these motives are not conscious, and certainly they may not be venal, but they may nevertheless interfere with the obligation to protect and promote the patient's interests. For example, the surgeon may have an emotional need to demonstrate his or her ability to take care of loved ones, a need that competes with the patient's interests when the surgeon's ability to serve these interests may not be clinically adequate. Thus, a surgeon contemplating an intervention with his or her own child may not be familiar with pediatric surgical technique and thus risk injury to the patient's interest in adequate and, ideally, optimal surgical management.

Now consider whose conception of the patient's interests should predominate. According to the obligation to respect and promote self-determination or autonomy, the patient should be the one who defines his or her own interests. But, again, close personal ties can make it difficult for one to accept the judgment of another about his or her own interests. Almost by definition, close personal relationships involve an emotional "investment" in what one party regards as the interests of the other party. This obligation can be compromised either by inadvertently substituting one's conception of the other's interests, or by an open conflict between the competing conceptions of the other's interests.

The third obligation is that of maintaining patient confidentiality. Not only the dynamics of families, but also those of professional units and friendship networks, can gravely infringe on the likelihood and practical ability of the surgeon to preserve confidentiality. Further, like the other two sorts of obligations, *the surgeon should avoid situations in which confidentiality could foreseeably be compromised*, because the consequences for the individual can be serious and irreparable. With this understanding, the third obligation alone puts a significant burden of justification on one who contemplates the surgical care of a relative, colleague, or friend.

Taken together, these obligations imply that the surgical care of family members, close friends and colleagues can raise serious ethical concerns. Although they do not rule out such patient care in all cases, they make it clear that careful management is required.

Clinical Topics

Disclosure of Questionable Quality of Care by Previous Physician

Sometimes in the course of providing care for a family member, colleague, or friend, the surgeon will identify a history of questionable or substandard management on the part of another physician. The patient may also raise this concern independently. Physicians appear generally to be reluctant to disclose questionable previous care to their patients. Professional solidarity and a reluctance to speak with confidence about the conditions under which previous treatment took place are probably among the reasons for this reluctance.

Avoiding such an awkward position is likely to be more difficult when the affected party is a close family member or friend, or a colleague. Emotional bonds in the first two cases, and collegial regard in the third, could easily outweigh traditional fraternal sentiments, whether rightly or not. This is a possible result that the surgeon contemplating care for family members, friends, or colleagues should consider in advance.

When the topic of previous care does arise, it seems appropriate to acknowledge that there are many alternative forms of therapy (as well as diagnostic techniques when the question involves over- or undertesting), and that there is frequently disagreement on which treatment or test is preferable. Even questionable techniques of traditional Western medicine may have some basis in alternative therapy plans and this may have been what the other physician had in mind. Moreover, what seems "questionable" to one physician may not seem that way to others. It is important to distinguish between care that is "wrong" and care that is not common practice.

Sometimes, however, it is apparent that care provided would be seen by the overwhelming majority of one's colleagues as inappropriate under the circumstances. It may be important to distinguish between the quality of the person doing the act and the merit of the act itself, because even "good" people can make mistakes. In rare instances there could be a suspicion of adverse intent on the part of the previous physician (greed, a desire to harm the patient, negligence, etc.), but it would be irresponsible and potentially dangerous to all parties to voice such a suspicion to the patient. Indeed, in all such conversations it is important to listen very carefully to the verbal and nonverbal communications of a patient who may have been subjected to "questionable" quality of care and reflect carefully on the content and impact of one's answer before responding.

In the final analysis, one's response should be geared mainly to the information that the patient should have, to make an informed decision about future treatment. If that information necessarily involves the judgment that previous care was inappropriate, then that judgment should be offered in the context of planning the next steps and without unhelpful speculation about the circumstances of the care. The obligations to respect and promote patient self-determination, as well as to advance the patient's interests, seem both to require this course of action.

When there is a well-founded suspicion of inappropriate care, this properly engages concern about protecting the interests of other patients under that physician's care. It is best to use collegial techniques to explore the issue with the physician who rendered the inappropriate treatment. Remind him or her that there is a Continuous Quality Improvement (CQI) system that is designed to be helpful to all. It is always wise to consider whether the questionable care resulted from physician impairment due to drugs, alcohol, ignorance, a neurological disorder, and so forth. Above all, one should be honest (but not sanctimonious) with a colleague, realizing that, in the long run, questionable care affects all of us because it diminishes the value of the health care system and can be harmful to the individual patient.

Curbside Consults

Surgeons whose colleagues seek personal medical advice on a casual basis are in danger of allowing themselves to be drawn into a *de facto* therapeutic relationship without the continuity and context this relationship requires. The normal framework of such a relationship includes formal elements that are in the interests of both parties, including consent processes and billing practices. In the absence of these elements there is ample room for role confusion and misunderstanding.

As soon as a curbside consult is requested the "consultant" must determine:

1. Who is consulting me? (The speaker on behalf of himself, the speaker as a surrogate, a disinterested observer asking about a medical principle or practice, someone asking about a previous personal experience, someone who is angry and has another agenda, etc., or some combination of these?)
2. What is the message I am hearing?
3. What is the motivation for this consult? (To acquire information, make a judgment, save a "real visit," or get free advice?)

A typical communication of this kind might take the following form:

MD1: "What do you think about giving A for condition X? What do you do for condition Y? Is there any role for B?"

MD2 (Bad Answer): "Never! Always do C!"

MD2 (Better Answer): "Tell me more about the patient. Tell me more about the setting, the previous history" and so forth.

The goal of the better answer is gradually to turn a "curbside" into a "deskside" until all necessary facts are known. By conducting this process slowly one demonstrates to the person asking for the consultation that a "curbside" answer is not possible or prudent. At a certain point one might say something like

MD2: "This is clearly a complex issue and I cannot give you the solid answer *that you deserve* without more exploration of the situation. Why not stop over at my office at your convenience?" (Or, if appropriate, "Why not bring in/send in the patient?")

The basic message here is "Don't ask me to do less for you as a consultant than you as an equally good doctor would want to do for me, given the opportunity." In other words, there is a settled view of the obligations of a consultant, and curbside consults violate those obligations.

Unsolicited Medical Advice

Like all who are trained in health care, surgeons are often able to assess potential medical problems at an early stage simply through casual observation. Some risky behaviors, such as tobacco use and excessive drinking, are relatively easy to identify in this way, whereas others, like moles that seem to be changing color, are less so. In either case, when close relatives, friends or colleagues are involved it can be hard to suppress both personal concern and the professional determination to prevent suffering—nor is it at all clear that such feelings *should* be suppressed. When one is concerned about the well-being of someone to whom one is close, the wisest course for the surgeon would seem to be to urge that person to seek an independent opinion, and to offer to help find an appropriate consultant.

When dealing with someone who has *received* unsolicited medical advice, one should try to discern its appropriateness and accuracy. When the advice is incorrect it should be corrected and an effort should be made to allay any anger toward the source of the unsolicited medical advice. Like the curbside consultation problem, this issue calls attention to communication within the medical profession as well as with patients.

The Poor Medical Care of Physicians and Surgeons and Their Family Members

As suggested earlier, there is reason to believe that physicians and their family members often receive substandard medical care. Indeed, it is one of the great clichés of medicine that those most vulnerable to poor care are the rich, the famous, and physicians' families. The main problem seems to be a failure of physicians and family members to respect the definition and importance of the physician-patient relationship and to assume the appropriate role.

Inadequate care can occur in the form of overtreatment and undertreatment, such as in the case of a physician who accidentally gave her daughter four times the correct dose of an antihistamine, which led to an emergency room visit; she attributed the error to her lack of objectivity. In other cases, it has been noted that the children of physicians may have physical examination forms filled in by their parents without having actually been examined.[9]

As a matter of policy, the historical, empirical, and ethical considerations in this chapter weigh heavily against surgical care of family members. This conclusion is framed so as not to exclude all possible interventions of this kind but to place the burden of justification for exceptions to our recommended policy on the circumstances of the individual case. Exceptions would be those that present only a remote possibility of compromising the relevant ethical obligations of the surgeon-patient relationship, and with regard to which the questions listed above could all be answered without serious reservations.

Clinical Conclusions

The study by Reagan et al. suggests that surgical treatment of family members is extremely rare, and that when it does occur the practitioner experiences varying degrees of discomfort.[9] These results are consistent with the psychological complexities of such procedures, and also with the philosophical implications of the surgeon's obligations to his or her patients. The patient's self-determination, the satisfaction of the patient's interests as he or she understands them, and the patient's confidentiality are indeed at hazard under these conditions. They are even more at hazard when the family member is an adolescent. The surgeon's reported psychological discomfort is an index of the looming ethical difficulties. Taken together, the empirical data and the ethical analysis support the conclusion that except for extreme or emergent situations, surgeons should not operate on family members. As suggested earlier, the surgical treatment of family members requires a rather heavy burden of justification.

Being both surgeon and friend seems, on its face, less likely to cause confusion than being both surgeon and relative. Yet in a culture in which friendships are often closer than family ties, this cannot be assumed. Further, recall the old adage that we choose our friends but not our relatives. The patient who chooses a friend to take care of his or her surgical needs can too easily confuse the basis of one relationship with another, so that the surgeon who has historically been a stalwart friend may seem cold and distant when assuming a professional demeanor. Thus the patient may be seriously disappointed and even angered when the surgeon-friend does not behave as expected.

Perhaps the best advice for the surgeon contemplating the care of a friend is first to consider whether this arrangement can pass the following test: Would I be prepared to lose my friendship with this person or (more likely) for the character of our relationship to be irrevocably changed? If the answer is no, then the friend should be referred to another. Because a change in the nature of the relationship is likely, and considering the potential psychological difficulties for the patient-friend, the wisest policy seems to be one that discourages the surgical care of friends. Exceptions to this policy would, again, have to satisfy the conditions and ethical obligations reviewed earlier.

Even when it has been decided that an exception to this rule may be made because the chances that it may lead to violation of the surgeon's ethical obligations are remote, the utmost care must be exercised to ensure that the friend is clear about the professional role of the surgeon and how it may differ and even conflict with his or her role as friend. The potential patient should also be challenged to consider whether he or she would be prepared to have this friendship end or change, rather than to seek care from another surgeon.

Here we need to distinguish between "colleagues" in the general sense of membership in the same profession (a professional colleague), and in the sense of membership in the same department, staff, or other institutional unit as well as the same profession (an institutional colleague). Colleagues in the latter group raise a special concern that is considered later in this chapter, namely confidentiality. First, however, we will consider treating colleagues in the latter group— those who are members of the same profession but not necessarily the same institutional unit.

While doctors may decide not to seek the skills of an institutional colleague when surgery is indicated, they cannot avoid consulting a professional colleague at such times. To be sought and chosen by a professional colleague to provide surgical care is a great compliment. However, there are some features of the relationship to which the surgeon should be alert. For example, the surgeon may be inclined to suppose that the colleague knows more about his or her condition and about alternative approaches to treatment than is the case. When assuming responsibility for the care of another physician, it is best to assume that this patient's intellectual and emotional preparedness is similar to that of other patients. Otherwise, one may fail to address important needs for information and support.

We have already discussed the status of professional courtesy, which may be justified as an expression of professional solidarity. Whether the practice of extending professional courtesy tends actually to improve the health care of doctors is harder to say, but it seems unlikely that the practice will end altogether. In any case, surgeons should be aware that waiving copayments may be in technical violation of contractual arrangements. Even if the financial aspect known as professional courtesy does not survive, it seems likely that, in the future, efforts will still be made to give some special consideration to the colleague who is a patient. So long as these efforts do not compromise the care of others they do not seem to be objectionable and may indeed reinforce a sense of professionalism.

The emotional distance between surgeons and family members of their colleagues does not appear to present as great a problem as the other relationships we have been considering. However, the colleague whose family member is a patient could present a distinct management issue. For example, some colleagues may presume that they are a virtual consultant on a case involving their relative, and the surgeon may (and should) come to feel uncomfortable with this presumption due to the colleague's emotional involvement. Nonetheless, especially in matters that directly affect the care of the patient, the norms of confidentiality and informed consent should not be abrogated at the colleague's insistence, but only with the explicit permission of the decisionally capable patient. In order to avoid confusion, it is prudent at the outset to be clear with both parties about one's respective obligations to the colleague and his or her relative. Especially troubling are circumstances in which the colleague gives information or advice to his or her family member that conflicts with that given by the surgeon. While these problems cannot always be avoided, clarity about roles can reduce their misunderstanding.

We will concern ourselves only with confidentiality in the care of relatives, friends or colleagues, or their family members. Chapter 3 contains a more detailed discussion of confidentiality in surgeon-patient relationships.

A continuing concern in this chapter has been the need for special discretion when providing care for those with whom one has an additional relationship. So accustomed are surgeons to sharing information about relatives, friends, and colleagues in their interpersonal networks that the need for special discretion can pose greater difficulties than are immediately apparent. As we have noted, because confidentiality is one of the few universally accepted elements of the doctor-patient relationship, doubt about one's ability to maintain confidentiality in a surgical case is a good reason to decline involvement and recommend another source of care.

In some instances confidentiality is justifiably—and even necessarily—waived, as, for example, when the patient suffers from an infectious disease reportable to public health authorities. The surgeon who faces such a dilemma when working up a relative, friend, colleague or colleague's relative for a surgical intervention may be put in a delicate and sometimes embarrassing position. Because it is rarely ethically acceptable for a surgeon to violate the law (the exception being instances in which the law is at odds with ethical obligations), and because all doctors have a duty to protect the public health, the condition must be reported in accordance with the law. Indeed, with required reporting of some stigmatizing diseases, like HIV/AIDS, the social consequences for the patient can be serious, despite legal protection against discrimination. Possible circumstances such as these should give the surgeon pause in accepting as patients those whose social well-being is of personal concern.

If the informed consent process is accepted as an essential part of the ethical practice of surgery, then modifications of, or exceptions to, that process must be subjected to close scrutiny and rigorous justification. Informed consent generally includes the disclosure of information about the patient's condition, risks and benefits of the recommended treatment and of both surgical and nonsurgical alternatives, including no treatment; assurances that the patient understands the information and appreciates the implications of the alternatives for his or her own life; and a voluntary decision by the patient (see Chapter 2). Modifications and exceptions can be justified, as in the case of emergency surgery (see Chapter 5), and most often involve the interests of patients, sometimes called beneficence-based judgments. Such judgments are usually made when patients are not competent or there is no reliable information about the patient's wishes. The traditional therapeutic exception or therapeutic privilege, according to which one could withhold information that was seen to be potentially counter-therapeutic, is no longer viewed as applicable in any but the most extreme cases (a patient with a history of clinical depression facing a terminal diagnosis, for example). Even then eventual disclosure is considered ethically obligatory.

Deviations from the practice of informed consent due merely to the fact of a preexisting personal relationship are unacceptable, and only the highest standards of practice are to be tolerated. Similarly, in advising family members, friends, colleagues, or their family members who are to undergo surgery, one must not participate in or condone any deviations.

In the surgical care of those with whom one has close personal attachments, especially family members and friends, the understandable reluctance to disclose information, such as a grim prognosis or the risks of surgery itself, is a great obstacle to the informed consent process. More insidious is the equally unfortunate tendency to assume that one knows more about the patient's ultimate wishes than is warranted, particularly in the case of intimates.

Less close relationships, such as those with colleagues or their family members, are presumably less likely to be subject to these psychological complexities on the part of the surgeon. However, one may find it hard to resist making assumptions about the colleague's level of understanding of his or her medical situation, assumptions that one may not make with a layperson and that may not be warranted.

Unlike much primary care practice, which may directly involve only the treating physician and the patient, decisions made by a surgeon commonly involve the resources and personnel of medical centers themselves. A surgeon's decision to accept a relative, friend, or colleague as a patient can have special implications for institutional interests. We have seen that both minor and major surgical procedures are sometimes performed on relatives. This is also the category with respect to which we have urged the utmost caution, a view evidently shared by medical tradition, professional codes, and those who have been surveyed on the question.

It seems prudent, at least, for appropriate institutional officials, such as medical directors and chiefs of surgical departments, to consider whether a policy concerning surgical treatment of family members should be developed. Policies can be guided by the relevant ethical obligations discussed in this chapter. Assistance in formulating a policy suitable for the institution's local situation could be obtained from members of the institutional Ethics Committee. Policies might justifiably include constraints, or at least guidelines, on the surgical care of colleagues and friends. But the way that these cases are handled might best be left to local judgment, depending on the circumstances and values of the community that is being served. For example, institutions with relatively few surgeons may not find it feasible to impose strict conditions on these kinds of relationships.

Sound policies are important because it is often easier for institutions to make rules based on good medical practice than to cope with individuals on a case-by-case basis and still achieve medical goals. In general, institutional policy development is an educational process based on all participants' recognizing the importance of the issues, looking at their own role within the institution (including an understanding of the meaning of "institution"), understanding the principles according to which decisions are to be made, and making decisions that do not compromise principle. In this way sound policies can help to prevent ethical problems that can arise when surgeons treat family members, friends, colleagues, or colleagues' family members.

References

1. William B. Spaulding, "Should You Operate on Your Own Mother?" *Pharos* 55 (1992): 23–26.
2. Hippocrates, "The Oath," in *Ancient Medicine: Selected Papers of Ludwig Edelstein*, Owsei and C. Lilien Temkin, eds. Baltimore, Md.: Johns Hopkins University Press, 1967, p. 6.
3. Thomas Percival, *Medical Ethics*. Birmingham, AL: The Classics of Medicine Library, 1985. (Originally published in 1803.)
4. American Medical Association, *American Medical Association Principles of Medical Ethics*. Chicago, IL: American Medical Association, 1949.
5. Rena A. Gorlin, ed., *Codes of Professional Responsibility*, 2nd ed. (Washington, D.C.: BNA Books, 1990).
6. American Medical Association. Council on Ethical and Judicial Affairs, *Opinions and Reports of the American Medical Association Judicial Council*. Chicago, IL: American Medical Association, 1977.

7. Mark A. Levy, Robert M. Arnold, Michael J. Fine, et al., "Professional Courtesy—Current Practices and Attitudes," *The New England Journal of Medicine* 329 (1993): 1627–1631.
8. American Medical Association, Council on Ethical and Judicial Affairs, *Opinions and Reports of the American Medical Association Judicial Council*. Chicago, IL: American Medical Association, 1993.
9. Bonnie Reagan, Peter Reagan and Ann Sinclair, "'Common Sense and a Thick Hide': Physicians Providing Care to Their Own Family Members," *Archives of Family Medicine* 3 (1994): 599–604.
10. Lois B. Dusdieker, Jody R. Murph, William E. Murph, et al., "Physicians Treating Their Own Children," *American Journal of Diseases in Children* 147 (1993): 146–149.
11. John LaPuma, Carol B. Stocking, Dan LaVoie, et al., "When Physicians Treat Members of Their Own Families," *New England Journal of Medicine* 325 (1991): 1290–1294.
12. Edward E. Rosenbaum, "When Physicians Treat Their Own Families," *The New England Journal of Medicine* 326 (1992): 895. (letter)
13. Robert Steinbrook, "Rethinking Professional Courtesy," *The New England Journal of Medicine* 329 (1993): 1652–1653.
14. Jeffrey Algazy and Mark Lachs, "Professional Courtesy Then and Now," *Archives of Internal Medicine* 154 (1994): 257–261.
15. John LaPuma and E. Rush Priest, "Is There a Doctor in the House? An Analysis of the Practice of Physicians' Treating Their Own Families," *Journal of the American Medical Association* 267 (1992): 1810–1812.

12

Research and Innovation in Surgery

JOEL E. FRADER
DONNA A. CANIANO

The art and craft, as well as the science, of surgery create challenges for those who want to systematically evaluate surgical outcomes and progress. Even on the same day, with similar patients, a single surgeon may perform "the same" procedure somewhat differently, due to anatomic or physiologic differences among patients or for other reasons. If one patient has a better result, the surgeon may want to try to reproduce what he or she did with that patient when next performing the operation. At some point these adaptations become "innovation." How much change has to occur to constitute an innovative approach and call forth an open and unbiased effort to assess the effectiveness of the new treatment?

Surgeons have frequently resisted such evaluative questions, citing the difficulties, discussed below, of adequately judging their work. Even as mundane, not to mention novel, medical therapies and diagnostic technologies have been increasingly subjected to audit regarding their efficacy, effectiveness, and cost/benefit ratios, surgeons have not been held similarly accountable as they continue to employ procedures of uncertain worth or invent new operations. But the era of limitations on health care expenditures and renewed concern about the human burden of unproven medical interventions may herald a sea change in attitudes toward surgery. It is likely that surgeons will more and more need to demonstrate that their preferred approach has solid justification and that new

216

techniques actually accomplish what they are designed to do. Whether greater examination of surgical practice will involve formal research protocols or hospital/insurance company/managed care organization "quality assessment" measures, surgeons need to consider the risks and benefits of adopting what is new, whether it is employing "minimally invasive" versus open techniques or devising and starting unique treatments, such as bio-artificial organ replacement. This chapter reviews the ethical issues and some of the methodologic concerns prompted by innovation and research in surgery.

Ethical Analysis: Issues in the Protection of Human Research Subjects

A Brief History

Ever since the widespread recognition that disease and disability, on the one hand, and interventions to ameliorate and/or cure medical disorders, on the other hand, follow patterns discernable by science, people have attempted to apply systematic research to medicine. And, no matter what steps may come first, medical investigations must ultimately be put to the test with human subjects. The moral import of the risks this might entail did not escape early scientific researchers, who often volunteered as the first subjects of their own experiments. Nevertheless, no general pressure developed for publicly articulated social controls on medical and surgical research on humans in the United States until the revelations of the Nazi medical experiments, the Nuremberg war crimes trials, and the subsequent generation of the Nuremberg Code.[1]

Even then, relatively little happened in the United States until 1966. In that year Henry Beecher, a highly regarded medical researcher, published an "exposé" of what, in his view, constituted risky clinical research, some of it involving surgery, done in prestigious U.S. medical institutions without appropriate patient or surrogate permission or other ethical safeguards.[2] At that point, National Institutes of Health authorities accelerated efforts, already under way, to regulate human experimentation funded by the federal government.[3] Indeed, according to one historian, ". . . the events [including Beecher's publication] accomplished what the Nuremberg trials had not: to bring the ethics of medical experimentation into the public domain and to make apparent the consequences of leaving decisions about clinical research exclusively to the individual investigator."[3]

Thus, beginning in 1966, the Public Health Service required all research it supported to have "institutional review to assure ethical acceptability."[4] Further guidelines were then proposed and final regulations on various aspects of human protection issued by the Department of Health, Education, and Welfare/Health and Human Services in 1971, 1973, 1974. These have been revised subsequently on several occasions; collectively they constitute a segment of the Code of Federal Regulations, Title 45, Part 46 (known as 45 CFR 46).[5]

An important development in the federal government's regulation of clinical research was the formation of the National Commission for the Protection of Human Subjects of Biomedical and Behavioral Research. Established by Congress with the National Research Act of 1974, the Commission brought together a distinguished group of scientists and clinicians with experts in law, religion, and ethics to review the "basic principles that should underlie the conduct of biomedical and behavior research involving human subjects and to develop guidelines which should be followed to assure that such research is conducted in accordance with those principles."[6] The Commission issued a highly influential summative statement, known as the Belmont Report, in 1979 that laid out the foundation for many of the changes in federal regulations that took effect in the 1980s and remain in force today. Of special importance to the surgical community, the report noted that "major innovation[s]" or "radically new procedures," while not automatically research, in the sense that the innovator intends immediate patient benefit rather than the generation of new knowledge, "should, however, be made the object of formal research at an early stage in order to determine whether they are safe and effective."[6]

The Belmont Report also affirmed the critical role that the informed consent of research subjects should play before investigation can proceed. The standards for research consent, the Commission noted, need to be higher than standards for consent in medical practice (for these standards, see Chapter 2) because one cannot presume that participation in a scientific endeavor benefits the subject. Another distinctive feature of the Belmont Report was the statement that special care needs to be taken when considering research on classes of persons one might consider vulnerable—for example, children, prisoners, members of minority groups, those with mental illness, or the economically disadvantaged. This last notion has especial importance when one recognizes that just such groups constituted a large proportion of those subjected to both the Nazi medical experiments and the research projects Beecher wrote about in 1966.[7]

In 1978, the U. S. Congress created the President's Commission for the Study of Ethical Problems in Medicine and Biomedical and Behavioral Research to explore further, among other matters, problems pertaining to the way the federal government had responded to the recommendations of the earlier National Commission. The President's Commission encouraged the consolidation of somewhat conflicting and confusing differences in federal protections for research subjects promulgated by different agencies within the U.S. government and spurred the issuance of special regulations regarding particular populations (e.g., children).

The major result of this activity at the federal level of government was the establishment of a system of local social control over medical research that is only in a loose sense overseen by the federal government. That is, our history has led us to place a large share of the responsibility for the ethical conduct of clinical investigation on the shoulders of researchers' close peers who sit on institutional review boards (IRBs) in hospitals, medical schools, universities, and independent research centers. These bodies are accountable to the federal regulatory apparatus, embodied in the Office for Protection from Research Risks at the Department of Health and Human Services (DHSS), and to the Food and Drug Administration through documents known as Multiple Project Assurances (MPAs) that pledge that the institution will follow federal guidelines designed to protect the interests of human subjects of biomedical and behavioral research.

Most IRBs, at least those in academia, promise to apply the same ethical standards to *all* proposed research, regardless of whether the federal government or another source supports the investigation. Though we cannot fully explore this topic here, we should note the paucity of data to bolster the widely held assumption that IRBs truly do what they are designed to do.[8] Indeed, some empirical research and at least one commentator have offered substantial reasons, chief among them conflicts of interest for IRB members, to doubt the effectiveness of the IRB system.[9–13]

Ethical and Legal Foundations

The Belmont Report and actual federal regulations, reflecting the history of the abuse of human subjects of medical research in the mid-twentieth century, emphasized the importance of informed consent in protecting human subjects. The doctrine of informed consent is, of course, derivative of a more basic ethical notion: that individuals with adequate decision-making capacity or, if lacking such capacity, those most able and likely to speak on their behalf deserve deep respect. The traditions of law and medical ethics in the United States place great weight on the view that those who are capable of understanding their circumstances, who have sufficient information to appreciate the consequences of alternative decisions, and who can freely (i.e., without undue pressure from others) express a preference should have the liberty to choose among reasonably available courses of action (see Chapter 2). In medical research, where, again, one cannot assume that participation in investigation is likely to benefit the research subject, this emphasis on personal freedom or autonomy assumes paramount importance. The prospective research subject, generally speaking, has no immediate obligation to participate in any proposed investigation.

We should note two cautions here. First, many would argue that persons, as members of a community from which each of us derives some benefits, have some measure of obligation to place themselves at risk as research subjects in order to further the common good. Just how far any individual must take on such a responsibility, however, is far from clear. Second, and much more practically important, in some clinical research prospective subjects may, in fact, stand to benefit from participation. Indeed, in circumstances where no known effective treatment exists, the only prospect for benefit may come through enrolling in a clinical trial where at least a proportion of the research subjects will receive interventions hoped and/or believed to have promise.

The issue of the risks and benefits of so-called "therapeutic research" has received voluminous attention in the medical literature. Recently Shimm and Spece summarized the problem this way: the clinician has a fiduciary responsibility to his or her patient and the clinical investigator has *additional* (and at least potentially conflictual) responsibilities to the scientific enterprise (i.e., to science itself, to society, to those who support the research, and to the institution[s] where the investigation takes place).[14] In any given circumstance, it may be very difficult to tell where the investigator's primary loyalty does or should lie. Those who value generation of knowledge as a transcendent good will, of course, claim the primacy of the research project. Where the "ordinary" therapeutic researcher stands is not so clear. Perhaps, as Lantos claims, "Real clinical investigators generally act primarily to benefit their patients . . . Research is a way of testing their intuitions."[15] A test question should be whether the researcher would, under similar circumstances, refuse to enroll himself or herself or a relative.

Enrolling individuals in clinical research also turns out to be problematic because many subjects in clinical trials, despite presumably adequate efforts to provide thorough informed consent, believe that the clinical researcher who directs their care does so according to "purely" patient-centered criteria, rather than adherence to one or more scientific protocols. For example, in one study of a psychiatric research unit where investigators made considerable efforts to explain the experimental nature of the treatment:

> . . . the patients seemed to have substantial difficulty in distinguishing research from treatment. In general, they found it hard to believe that the staff was not acting in their best interests in all circumstances. They seemed to have difficulty in understanding the systematic features of the research design and the ways in which these affected the staff's decisions about how to treat them."[16]

A host of conflicting interests, as well as myriad psychological and social influences, may complicate the ethical landscape when clinical research becomes (inevitably) conflated with treatment. Nevertheless, almost everyone agrees on the need for such investigations. The history of medicine and surgery clearly demonstrates the harms done in the name of "treatments" of unproven worth. Surgical examples include routine episiotomy; internal mammary artery ligation for angina; gastric freezing for peptic ulcer disease; initial attempts with implantable devices to provide artificial support of circulation; indiscriminate adoption of endoscopic, especially laparoscopic, surgery; and various operations for disparate forms of cancer. The presumption of benefit in the purely clinical doctor-patient relationship is, in fact, *only* a presumption often accompanied by little or no empirical support. One well-known sociologist of medicine and surgery has commented that the belief in the beneficial power of new clinical interventions amounts to "scientific magic."[17]

Research Design Issues

If one accepts the need for research on the value of new surgical techniques, then one faces the question of acceptable and appropriate research strategies. While we cannot here address all of the ethical issues surrounding formal clinical trials, we can at least attempt to touch on some pertinent concerns.

Concern about how to make progress in surgical knowledge is, of course, not new. Barnes, one of the editors and authors of a seminal book in the field, refers to an 1889 address by a Boston surgeon in which the main message is that one will only know, with time, what does and does not work.[18] Presumably, this perspective sees little place for concurrent comparison of one treatment with another. This view survives in a not too different version into the modern era: ". . . new operations are introduced tentatively . . . Technics are refined . . . A randomized clinical trial conducted during such an evolutionary phase will often be invalidated. . . ."[19] Seen this way, time-related phenomena, such as the surgeon's experience with a procedure and the refining of operative details, make too much difference for surgery to be subjected to the same testing methods used in the rest of medicine. A related argument says that in evaluating operations, as compared to medications, therapeutic trials do not occur "at a comparable stage in [the treatment's] development."[20]

These criticisms have been addressed by surgical investigators. In a recent text on research in surgery, the authors of a chapter entitled "Ethical Principles in Research" state that

> If the achievement of good medicine [and surgery] is an ethical imperative, it must exert . . . the *constructive force* of an invocation to comprehending and voluntary collaboration in constantly redesigning the standards of good medicine . . . rigorous testing is ethically mandatory for the protection of individual patients and the just use of limited resources.[21] (emphasis in original)

These authors and others clearly recognize the inadequacy of case series and historical comparisons under most circumstances.[22,23] Most agree to one important set of exceptions, namely, those situations in which patients face near certain death or devastating disability, no known interventions have worked, and a new operation—or other therapy—seems to hold a reasonable prospect of benefit. Of course, these situations leave hopeless patients most vulnerable to pressure to accept unproven interventions.

Reports using case series and historical controls cannot account for a variety of confounding variables, such as bias in the selection of those being treated or reported (or the nonreporting of failures), for substantive changes in the overall effectiveness of care from one period to another, and for inadequate knowledge about the "natural history" of the disease in the absence of the intervention of interest. Moreover, to the extent that uncontrolled reports favor an operation and an accumulation of such reports contributes to a (possibly mistaken) view that the surgery provides benefits, conducting more definitive trials becomes more and more difficult, even subject to claims of being "unethical."[24,25]

Responses to the problems of surgical learning curves and variances in the level of experience of surgeons who might be involved in a trial are, admittedly, more difficult. As Chalmers has asserted, "The only way to avoid the distorting influences of uncontrolled pilot trials is to begin randomization with the first patient. . . . The possibility that the new treatment may turn out to be worse than the old makes randomization a most ethical procedure."[26] Nevertheless, skill performing a procedure does tend to improve with experience and the results for the first one, dozen, or hundred patients may not be fully comparable with the results for patients 250 through 350. Note, however, that this problem applies to *all* interventions requiring mechanical skill and the same level of objection has not generally been heard with respect to trials involving, say, endoscopy or various cardiac catheterization procedures. Even medical treatments (principally drugs, but also those involving devices—e.g., ventilators—and clinician-patient interactions) change and sometimes improve with experience, whether through learning the best time of day to give a medication to avoid side effects, the optimal ratio of the inspiratory to the exhalatory phase of the respirator's cycle, or the most effective words to encourage adherence with the regimen specified in an investigative protocol. Such difficulties in designing and implementing clinical trials do not bring a halt to all therapeutic research.

In addition, one can, at least in principle, make statistical adjustments (e.g., through the use of stratification) to control for operative skill and experience. Another approach, of course, is to have the same surgeon do all the cases in a trial. This surely limits the number of patients who can be enrolled and one cannot completely control for any unconscious bias the surgeon may have for or against one or another procedure or for the difference in experience that a single surgeon has with each operation, but it does reduce the difficulty of variations in operative skill. Other strategies have been proposed, including one using a run-in or prerandomization period for surgeons to practice new techniques and a phased-trial system, analogous to that used with medications.[27,28]

Control Strategies: Randomization, Placebos, Blinding, and Adaptive Designs

We have already alluded to the issue of randomization several times but must address the basic ethical concerns about its use. Several reviews[22,23,25,29] of reported clinical trials in surgery have noted that surgical research may underuse such designs: "Although there is agreement that randomized controlled trials (RCT) are the best trial design for assessing treatment effectiveness, it is perceived that surgical therapies are usually not tested by this experimental design."[30] There may be several reasons for this phenomenon, including the conviction that other methods of data collection have sufficient "evidentiary strength,"[31] the view that RCTs invariably create non-representative populations of patients and thus the results are not adequately generalizable,[31] the idea that RCTs are unnecessarily expensive and cumbersome to complete, especially when they lock patients and surgeons into inflexible protocols made obsolete by evolving new information,[19] and other arguments. But the fundamental moral criticism of RCTs is that they deprive surgeons and patients of the opportunity to make choices based on the surgeon's clinical intuitions, skill, and experience and the patient's preferences. That is, RCTs undermine the fundamental obligation of the doctor to try to help the patient accept what the surgeon believes is best, under the circumstances.

While we cannot respond to this objection completely here, it should be clear that the above view is based on assumptions about the adequacy of general surgical knowledge or the specific knowledge and abilities of a particular surgeon. As we noted earlier, doctors typically know less about what actually works and doesn't work than they (and their patients) believe to be the case. Fashion, economic self-interest, and human psychology can also influence the recommendations doctors make.

> It may be good for the sense of wellbeing of both surgeon and patient after successful surgery to assume that, but for their courageous partnership, the patient would by now be dead or disabled. But an uncomfortable lesson that formal trials often teach is how surprisingly well patients in the control group fare without surgery.[31]

The ethical problem then should probably be restated, as Schaffner has done: "When is it ethical to start a trial?"[32] The answer must depend a great deal on the context: the clinical condition, the state of the art of various treatments, the speed with which knowledge and technology relevant to the condition and the treatment are evolving, as well as the features and design adequacy of any specific proposed randomized trial. To the extent that an RCT truly limits physician or patient autonomy, that is, when the doctor cannot offer nor the patient obtain a particular therapy except through enrolling in the study, this may raise serious questions about unjust restraints on clinical action. But when we remember the harms done through unnecessary or unnecessarily disfiguring or disabling surgical treatments believed to offer great benefit, we have to wonder whether individual freedom should always trump valid attempts to gain the most knowledge.

Surgical trials clearly do face some unique challenges. The first has to do with placebos. There are two problems here. First, any surgical procedure, even one designed to have a particular effect, in and of itself may exert a powerful "placebo effect." That is, the simple fact of having surgery, independent of whether the operation achieved its specific aims, may result in symptom relief and functional improvement, as demonstrated by relief of angina from internal mammary artery ligation.[1,21] This phenomenon, while complicating the assessment of an operation's efficacy, lends credence to the importance of using a comparative research design. Presumably, when one compares two or more surgical approaches to the same disorder, the placebo effect will be more or less balanced and not confound the analysis of what works better.

The second problem with placebos concerns the common approach to demonstrating the worth of new treatments, typically drugs, and involves comparisons in the form of concurrent "dummy" or placebo control arms of a research protocol. The need for such an approach in appraising the value of a surgical procedure has been summarized by Barsamian:

> . . . effectiveness is a distant fourth as the basis for the early popularity of an operation. Although responsible surgeons obviously care if their patients are improved postoperatively, all too often the assessment following an operation is difficult and subjective. If an 'authority' states that an operation is effective . . . then this judgment is apt to be accepted, especially if the operation is also simple and safe.[1]

Thus, what is new, especially when endorsed by influential members of the surgical community, stands a good chance of being adopted before its usefulness has been demonstrated adequately. In the case of internal mammary ligation for angina, two separate surgical groups in the late 1950s conducted studies employing random patient assignment to identical procedures, save that one group of patients had their mammary arteries ligated after exposure and the other patients had no ligation done.[33,34] The research showed no statistically greater improvement in signs or symptoms in the ligated group in comparison to that in the sham procedure group (some patients in each group had subjective reduction in their angina).

The ethical problem here involves how much risk (i.e., from the anesthetic, from surgical accidents, from wound infections, etc.) one can legitimately ask even fully informed and cooperative patients to assume, knowing that a proportion of them will submit to an operation that can only work—and perhaps only temporarily—through its placebo effect. To be sure, asking patients to submit to allegedly therapeutic surgery that has not been shown to work also raises profound moral questions. Beecher, writing about mammary artery ligation, noted that in one case series of 24 patients, three patients had intraoperative hypotension and one developed a pneumothorax and an anteroseptal infarction—all this in a simple and believed-to-be-safe operation.[35] He goes on to comment, "It is, therefore, essential for the surgeon to be on his guard, lest he deceive himself, and others, in perpetrating costly, dangerous, even fatal operations whose effectiveness is only that of a placebo."[35]

One can find only a few supporters, in the mid-1990s, for placebo or what have been called sham controls in surgical research. One text states baldly ". . . sham operations are ethically unjustifiable and would not be considered today."[21] Another group states a similar position, "The only true placebo is a sham operation which is unethical. Surgical trials cannot, therefore, be fully placebo controlled."[36] Clearly, invasive sham treatment remains controversial, though some protocols, with IRB approval, continue to employ it—for example, in arthroscopic knee repair and fetal tissue transplant for Parkinson's disease. Presumably the acceptability of placebo surgical controls depends on finding adequately informed volunteers willing to assume the relevant risks and minimizing the invasiveness of the sham procedure, in order to (altruistically) demonstrate the efficacy of a new or even a "standard" operation.

Similar ethical concerns have been raised about blinding procedures in the evaluation of operations. In the classical, double-blind randomized controlled trial of medications, neither investigator nor patient knows which intervention the patient-subject receives—placebo, new agent, "standard" treatment, or some variation on these. Naturally, blinding is much more difficult to accomplish in surgery. The person who operates knows what he or she has done. The patient, however, need not know precisely which operation has been done and, again assuming an informed volunteer, some patient-subjects may indeed be indifferent to technical details which they, in any case, may not be able to discern beneath the healed incision. In those cases, at least, single blind studies are possible.[23]

One typically wants a blinded design in order to avoid the bias observers (patients, surgeons, other evaluators of outcome) might have based on explicit or unconscious allegiances or antagonisms for some arm or arms of a study. One way to avoid such bias in the evaluation of the results is to have independent observers who are themselves unaware of how any given patient has been treated. This often can be accomplished using objective, functional outcome measures that do not depend on the precise treatment being revealed in the process of obtaining the information (e.g., biochemical indicators of intestinal function for patients who have had gut surgery, such as bowel lengthening or the creation of intestinal "valves," or electrocardiographic findings in patients who have had various procedures to improve coronary artery blood flow, such as percutaneous balloon dilatation or stent placement versus grafting with autologous arteries or veins). As one text puts it, ". . . blindness is an important strengthening feature and should be used wherever possible. For example, histologic slides, x-rays, or laboratory tests can be read by a physician blinded to the patient's treatment allocation."[37]

The final research strategy issue that we will address briefly concerns "deviations" from the classical randomized controlled trial, collectively known as "adaptive designs." There is a large technical, especially statistical, literature on this matter, as well as a growing body of commentary from the ethics community. The major question, which has both scientific and ethical import, concerns how much departure from the "standard" design is tolerable. Too much "compromise" in statistical power or the ability to reach confident conclusions about the validity of the results clearly runs the risk of undermining trust in the research and one's ability to feel ethically comfortable about enrolling patients in a nonstandard project.

Various alterations in design other than strict standardization with pure random assignment of patients have been proposed and used. One approach allows some degree of individualization of treatment within different arms of a study rather than having rigid treatment protocols.[38] So, for example, the physician might adjust drug doses in order to achieve some physiologic result, such as blood pressure control or serum glucose level. In a surgical trial this could involve the operating surgeon exercising judgment about the amount of bowel to be removed for intractable Crohn's disease or around a localized cancer.

Experimental studies involving single subjects ("n-of-1 randomized controlled trials") have also been suggested and employed.[39] These involve sequential trials of pairs of treatment, each of which has some currency in the therapeutic community caring for persons with a specific, usually relatively stable, chronic illness. While this might not as readily apply to surgery as to medications or the use of some devices, it could, in theory be used with surgical procedures that are relatively simple and of low risk, as well as reversible, such as enterostomy.

Another technique involves so-called prerandomization. In this scheme, randomization to standard therapy or the experimental arm of the study occurs prior to seeking patient or surrogate permission to be enrolled in research and only those who are assigned to the experimental arm are asked to give consent to participate in research. A key reason to attempt this approach is to get around the ethical and/or psychological discomfort some physicians have with not being able to inform potential subjects which treatment they would receive or which treatment they believe to be best. If physician comfort increases, recruitment into the study may increase. Additionally, patients may be more willing to enroll if they know which intervention will be applied to them, also increasing patient accrual.[40] Such a design also has ethical merit because it more quickly and more efficiently answers study question(s) and adds to scientific and clinical knowledge.

Some have responded with ethical objections. The major argument has been clearly explained by Marquis in the following manner: because some conventional randomized trials can be and have been finished within a reasonable period, prerandomization to speed up the completion of a trial is not *always* necessary. When it is needed, it involves weakening of the research consent process—and may, in fact, mean that study patients assigned to conventional treatment never really agree to be research subjects at all—and this involves a violation of medical ethics. "It follows that for any given trial prerandomization is either unnecessary or unethical."[41] We will not resolve this debate here. Clinician-investigators have used prerandomization and discussions of this experience suggest adaptive designs may be useful in the face of strong convictions about which treatments are better and why.[42-44]

To a large degree the discussions above have addressed the issue of innovation occurring without formal protocols. That is, to the extent that one claims that we simply cannot know adequately whether a new intervention will, in the long run, turn out to be more beneficial than harmful, anything new *ought* to be subjected to formal research scrutiny at the earliest possible stage. From this perspective, there should be no innovation without protocols. Others say that physicians, surgeons or otherwise, have a positive obligation to use their clinical knowledge and skill to do what they can for patients, even under conditions of uncertainty about the "true" value of an operation, a device, a drug, or some other treatment. This claim is made all the more strongly, as we have noted, when the clinical situation is desperate, when past approaches have not been helpful, and when the clinician believes he or she has some especially promising innovation to address the problem at hand.

Practically speaking, new ideas come along at a furious pace and many obstacles exist, including time, money, and bureaucracy, that inhibit or discourage the conversion of innovative ideas into formal research protocols. Besides, surgeons (and others) will surely remind us that each case is, in some sense, unique and one is "always" innovating midstream in an operation or other course of therapy. The difficult questions are, again, what level of deviation from the standard approach—which, we must remember, may itself have not been adequately proven in the scientific arena—creates a moral obligation for a test by research criteria and under what circumstances. Perhaps if the change is "minor" and the stakes are low, informal innovation shouldn't get us all that excited.

Lantos has suggested that we get into trouble thinking about these issues because of the different goals of research and practice. Research aims at knowledge, practice—innovative or not—aims at helping patients. These conceptions have led to suspicion that patient benefit may be sacrificed—and risk substantially increased—via the research route, which, in turn, has led to regulation of research. By contrast, innovation, in the name of treatment, receives relatively little scrutiny, even though the actual risk may be quite high.[15] One could add that great economic, academic, and psychological rewards may come to the innovator, well before he or she shows a new technique to have definite worth.

Citing the example of assertive AIDS patients eager to have access to innovative approaches to their terrible disease, Lantos suggested that we should revise our thinking. Perhaps we should appreciate that research does not automatically "create greater hazards for patients than they face from the loyalty of a compassionate but uncurious clinician" and that when given an opportunity to participate in decisions about how to proceed with innovations (i.e., have a role in the "design and evaluation" of treatment programs), patients-subjects will accept a formalized research approach to innovation.[15] Thus, one way to finesse the research/innovation dilemma is to draw those most affected by concerns (i.e., the scientists, clinicians, and community of patients and their loved ones) into a collaboration designed to minimize, if not eliminate, the difference between the two approaches and allow the development of protocols when innovation is contemplated. Such an approach, of course, requires a willingness of all parties to "lighten up" on their strongly held (but often unvalidated) beliefs and preferences about both specific strategies for progress and the value of particular interventions. As Lantos and Frader noted

> With regard to . . . innovative therapies, a desire for rigid rules and for a clear demarcation between standard and experimental therapy may be unwise and unrealistic. Instead, virtue may lie in acknowledging that a degree of uncertainty is the price we have to pay in order not to sacrifice other important ethical values.[43]

Special Populations

As mentioned above, certain populations may be at increased risk for exploitation when proposed as subjects in research: those who lack decision-making capacity—children, the mentally ill, the elderly with cognitive impairments, and so forth—and those who don't have complete freedom to accept or reject participation in research—prisoners, those in the military, patients receiving "charity" care, and so on. The main issues are (1) those lacking capacity cannot adequately evaluate the potential risks and benefits of participation and thus cannot make ethically valid expressions of their preferences to become or not become research subjects and (2) captive populations may not have sufficient freedom to make truly voluntary, uncoerced choices. Prisoners may feel that opting-in to a research program may or even should earn them special consideration for institutional privileges or parole, in which case enrolling might be considered to take place under conditions of undue inducement while refusal may result in reprisals. Similar concerns, especially about the withholding of rewards or services to "nonvolunteers" apply to those in the military or those receiving treatment at the "mercy" of uncompensated institutions or individuals.

Although these considerations have validity, our society certainly has not ruled out research, and should not do so, involving these populations. To categorically forbid research on those lacking certain mental capacities would at least diminish, if not preclude, potential progress on disorders afflicting them, perhaps even unique to them—for example, improvement of palliative procedures to reduce discomfort from decubitus ulcers occurring in elderly persons with senile dementia. Denying those in captive populations the chance to agree to be research subjects automatically assumes they should not or could not *ever* actually make an altruistic decision to contribute to socially useful knowledge, rather than for the hope of "mere" personal gain.

Our society has tended to deal with these problems in procedural ways. We allow surrogates to make most decisions about participation in scientific protocols involving those without capacity when there appears to be the prospect for benefit from being a subject in a "therapeutic" project or where the risk appears to be minimal. IRBs have particular obligations for oversight regarding research on vulnerable populations, including children and fetuses.[5,45] Generally speaking, our society has concluded that research involving these special populations becomes increasingly problematic to the extent that it can be expected neither to benefit directly the patient-subject nor shed light on the disorder(s) afflicting the particular patient-subject. When we anticipate the possibility of direct benefit, we need to take care not to exclude these individuals or groups simply because the problem of authorizing their participation is more complex than it is with competent, autonomous individuals.

Commercial Sponsorship

In the 1980s and 1990s we have witnessed a growing concern over researchers' conflicts of interest when involved in research sponsored by commercial sources, especially when the investigators have a direct financial (equity) interest in the outcomes of the research.[46-48] The public attention has focused on cases of alleged improper interpretation or reporting of research data based on economic considerations, such as the researchers' interest in assuring continued support for their investigations, or because an investigator or the scientist's institution stood to benefit from the demonstration that a particular product or technique has commercial value.[49-51]

We should note, however, that, in principle, the source of support for science has little to do with the value of the research. The latter depends on the adequacy of a project's design, the risks and benefits of conducting the research, and ultimately the integrity of the individuals and institutions implementing the research plan. Even publicly funded research has the potential to bring fame and fortune to the scientist and/or his or her institution, through such mechanisms as academic advancement, increases in referrals of patients, patenting and commercial development of products, or even copyrighting and sale of intellectual property.[52]

Hillman and colleagues have recommended a protocol for an economic analysis to avoid bias in the conduct and reporting of pharmaceutical company sponsored research.[20] This protocol involves: (1) research grants to universities, rather than contracts to investigators or institutions, with provisions allowing the researchers to publish their results whatever they may be; (2) research designs that are clinically relevant, not just designed to showcase the value of the sponsor's products; (3) provisions to allow researchers to extend the study beyond the company's design so that a more comprehensive picture of the product's worth can emerge; (4) care, through the use of conservative analytic assumptions and procedures, to protect against "the temptation to produce favorable findings"; (5) efforts by researchers to publish the "results regardless of their promotional value to the sponsoring company"; (6) avoidance of consulting relationships with the sponsor during the active research period; and (7) efforts to obtain adequate funding for "methodologically sound, clinically relevant results with enough statistical power to detect important differences among the alternatives compared" rather than having just enough data and analysis to meet marketing aims.[20]

Clinical Examples of Research Problems in Surgery

The above ethical concerns in surgical research and innovation are illustrated by developments in the surgical management of short bowel syndrome and hypoplastic left heart syndrome. The focus is primarily, though not exclusively, on the treatment of children, with which the authors are most familiar and which is not otherwise prominent in this volume. The lessons to be learned seem readily applicable to the entire world of surgery and the general ramifications will be highlighted following the narratives describing these surgical controversies.

Surgery for Short Bowel Syndrome

Short bowel syndrome (SBS) afflicts adults and children. Adult patients develop the problem after surgical and radiation treatment for cancer, after mesenteric vascular catastrophes, and from Crohn's disease and various other disorders.[53,54] SBS is more common in children and is associated with necrotizing enterocolitis, principally in premature infants, with congenital anomalies such as intestinal atresia or gastroschisis, and with midgut volvulus, as well as other problems.[53] The primary problem involves insufficient surface area to absorb the nutrients and fluids needed to sustain life, though a host of other physiologic disturbances make up the syndrome—for example, secretory losses of fluids and minerals, renal and gallbladder stone formation, and, in those receiving parenteral nutrition support, reversible or progressive toxicity to the liver.

In the mid-to-late 1990s, three quite distinct approaches to SBS have emerged: primary medical therapy; nontransplant surgical options; and bowel transplantation. For purposes of this chapter, it is easiest to focus the discussion on the treatment of children, in part because of the higher incidence of SBS in that population and in part because of a higher degree of uncertainty about the right or best thing to do. One fundamental question involves the ability of the small intestine to adapt (hypertrophy) sufficiently to permit avoidance of major surgery (i.e., surgery other than catheter insertion). Recently Kurkchubashche, Rowe, and Smith suggested the possibility of successful adaptation of the small bowel with a combination of enteral and parenteral support with a much lower limit of residual intestine, as little as 10 cm, than had been the previously "accepted" minimum of 30 or 40 cm.[55] Important questions remain about the optimal way to provide nutrition, the proportion of enteral versus parenteral feeding, type of enteral solutions, the importance of the ileocecal valve, the length of small bowel one needs to have in order to eventually achieve bowel "autonomy," and how long one can or should wait before proceeding to surgical interventions, as well as other related matters.

Nontransplant surgical options have included techniques to slow intestinal transit times and thereby increase the opportunity for absorption of nutrients and prevent diarrhea. Examples include creation of valves and reversing segments of intestine in the anti-peristaltic direction; techniques to increase the absorptive surface area, such as "patching," whereby new functional mucosa overgrows the interposed segments or longitudinal transection with sequential anastomosis to double a segment's length; and procedures to improve function, such as those that remove strictures or those that taper dilated, dysmotile segments.[56]

Finally, intestinal or multivisceral transplantation has become more and more common since the late 1980s following sporadic attempts earlier. After two reports of unsuccessful attempts with four children, two each in Pittsburgh and Chicago, Moore called for a clinical moratorium on further efforts until additional basic and animal research led to solid optimism that the results would improve, especially with respect to the avoidance of prolonged suffering on the part of the patients.[57] Moore attacked the approach of "desperate remedies" for desperately ill patients without substantial reason to believe that an operation had some reasonable likelihood of success beyond immediate survival of the procedure.[57]

Since that time, a number of centers in the United States and elsewhere have embarked on bowel transplant programs. A review of recent editorials,[58] a "clinical update,"[59] and abstracts from The Fourth International Symposium on Small

Bowel Transplantation (fall, 1995) demonstrates a wide diversity of views about the clinical benefits and utility of intestinal transplantation. At the very least, the following issues about the safety and effectiveness of transplantation remain unsettled: (1) the relative value of including organs other than the small bowel, especially the liver and colon, (2) the relative value of chimeric states, especially the contribution of inducing chimerism through simultaneous donor bone marrow infusions, (3) the optimal immunosuppressive regimen to prevent sepsis, rejection, and graft versus host disease, (4) the best methods to prevent post-transplant lymphoproliferative disorder (PTLD), (5) the best methods to treat PTLD, (6) strategies to prevent or treat cytomegalovirus-induced complications, (7) the acceptability of using living donors for intestinal segments, and (8) access to and socioeconomic justice involved in this high up-front and high long-term cost treatment.

From the above, it seems clear that even at this stage of fairly rapid evolution of the various treatments for SBS, only comparative clinical trials, preferably with random assignment of comparable patients, can begin to answer the many questions regarding the relative merits of the myriad interventions. As Moore cautioned, when the situation is desperate, "offering" unproven therapies as if they were validated clinical services—at great economic and psychosocial costs with considerable medical morbidity and personal suffering—risks considerable ethical hazard.[57] It seems ethically obligatory to attempt systematic evaluation of the relative benefits, risks, and costs of the different approaches used for SBS.

Hypoplastic Left Heart Syndrome (HLHS)

Until the 1980s, children born with HLHS, once diagnosed, were made as comfortable as possible and permitted to die without high-technology intervention. With the advent of competing treatments, namely the staged reconstructive treatment developed by Norwood and cardiac transplantation, new options were offered to parents of these infants. Now, some centers offer all three options (no surgery and death, palliative surgery, and transplantation), some centers offer one or another surgery but willingly or reluctantly refer patients for an alternative to the locally favored procedure, and some centers now apparently feel justified in at least *urging* all parents to accept surgical intervention, perhaps considering or threatening child protective service referrals for court-ordered treatment if the parents reject a surgical approach. Leaving aside the question of whether nonsurgery remains ethically acceptable, the obvious question is which surgery works best. There is no clear answer at present.

The Norwood reconstructions involve multiple stages ending in a modified Fontan procedure. This surgery necessarily leaves the patient with persistent cyanosis with the potential for lethal cardiac failure due to the inadequacy of the single ventricle to provide both pulmonary and systemic circulation. While Norwood's recent (since 1991) reports indicate a 19% mortality associated with the initial palliative surgery and 6% and 5% mortality respectively for the second and third stage,[60] others report less success—for instance, a first-stage operative mortality of 46% and overall actuarial survival *among stage-one survivors* at seven years varying between just under 80% to approximately 25%, depending on the original anatomy.[61] Those authors claim "overall results similar to those currently offered by cardiac transplantation" for the patient subgroup with a combination of mitral stenosis and aortic stenosis, who make up roughly 25% of the total initial presenting population.[61] A 1995 report from a multi-hospital consortium indicated a 53% Norwood stage-one operative mortality, compared to a 42% operative mortality for those infants undergoing heart transplantation (among those who survived to surgery).[62] According to the University Hospital Consortium report, "The higher initial costs of transplantation are offset by the need for 2 additional open-heart operations in infants managed by the Norwood technique. . . ."[62] Moreover, in discussing the fact that more than 15% of the patients were discharged after a decision by the parents and physicians to forgo surgical intervention, the Consortium report notes that with the Norwood approach "the initial operation is only a prelude to lifelong specialized cardiac care including frequent physician visits, daily medication, multiple cardiac catheterizations . . ." and, of course, two more major surgeries.[62]

One of us recently reviewed ethical issues associated with heart transplantation for HLHS and other aspects of heart, heart-lung, and lung transplantation in children.[63] As suggested above, a major obstacle involves the scarcity of donor organs, such that many infants die in ICUs of various complications while awaiting transplantation. If a donor heart becomes available, especially in the first month of life, some evidence suggests this population of children with HLHS will have an especially good prognosis. This notion is based on the apparent plasticity of the infant immune system, such that the donor heart is recognized as "self," and many early-transplanted children can be weaned from immunosuppression and thus not suffer from the hazards of infection and PTLD associated with anti-rejection treatment.[64] For those not so fortunate, additional hazards of the need for and complications of immunosuppression have been rapidly progressive coronary artery occlusion (especially associated with cyclosporin) and sudden death from arrhythmia as an apparent complication of rejection.

Again, it seems clear that these competing treatments offer a variety of clinical, psychosocial, and economic questions most directly, efficiently, and clearly addressed by a controlled clinical trial. Certainly no consensus exists among pediatricians, pediatric cardiologists, or pediatric cardiothoracic surgeons as to the preferred route, though surely individual families and physicians do and will continue to have strong feelings about one type of surgery versus another. In any case, taking Freedman's notion of "equipoise" in the medical community, the conditions seem right for a randomized trial of transplantation versus staged reconstruction for HLHS.[65]

Before leaving this part of the discussion, it should be said that the two situations, SBS and HLHS, pose somewhat different problems in the ethics of research. Though HLHS patients can be supported, using prostaglandins, without surgery for days or weeks, a definitive clinical decision must be made with some urgency. Moreover, the decision not to intervene has a clear result, namely death. Urgent circumstances in which the choice is innovation (with or without formal research) or certain death sometimes seems to permit less strict adherence to scientific method. But a view that death justifies any proposed "lifesaving" intervention frequently fails to account for the burdens associated with new measures that provide temporary but unsatisfactory prolongation of life. These burdens include the physical pain and suffering of the patient, economic costs of the intervention, psychological hardships for loved ones, and so forth. These more comprehensive considerations should be part of what is evaluated for any proposed surgical innovation, no matter the age or other specific characteristics of the likely patient population.

What can be learned from the evolution of competing treatments such as those for SBS and HLHS? In each case, innovation took place without much, if any, independent peer review. Independence is a key concept here. Intra-institutional consultation and scrutiny, even formal review of a research protocol by an IRB, can be problematic because of the interconnected web of relationships and interdependencies among colleagues.[13] Thus, surgeons should be willing to submit their ideas for innovation to inspection and critique by peers throughout their discipline. Moreover, once appropriately reviewed, innovators need to clearly disclose the nature of the "experiment" to potential patients or their surrogates. That is, the standards for informed consent under circumstances of innovation and research need to be substantively greater than disclosure requirements for customary care. Not only should patients and their loved ones know that the proposed intervention constitutes a departure from what has usually been done in similar circumstances, but the amount of experience and success or failure rates in carrying out the new technique should be discussed with the patients or guardians. The experiences with Norwood operations as well as cardiac and intestinal transplantation, as with most treatments, demonstrate a learning curve, often very steep in the initial stages of a program, with substantially increased risks. As noted above, the risks may well transcend that of death, which might have occurred in any case. The problem is that sometimes when life is extended, the quality of that life may be severely compromised by physical or emotional suffering. Patients or their surrogates deserve information relevant to the fact that innovation may well add to the patient's burden, rather than relieve it. Indeed, those engaged in innovation and research have a positive obligation to record and measure, insofar as possible, outcomes well beyond simple mortality and morbidity.

It seems reasonable then that after relevant scientific scrutiny, innovation enters a pilot phase aimed at identifying technical "bugs" to be ironed out and, most importantly, more clearly specifying the objectives and hypotheses to be addressed in a formal research protocol. That is, innovators should undertake a feasibility study to make sure that proper evaluative research can be carried out. During this phase it may become clear that the obstacles to progress loom larger than anticipated. Therefore, the innovators should have a well-defined plan to discontinue the pilot, pending analysis of the problems and rational proposals to take corrective action. Once the pilot is concluded, based on well-thought-out criteria for prematurely stopping or completing the feasibility study, surgeons should undertake an appropriately designed controlled clinical trial with sufficient patients (i.e., statistical power) to reach generalizable results about the efficacy of the new treatment.

Again, we believe that at each stage there should be broad and candid disclosure about the nature of what is being undertaken—that it is in fact innovation, a pilot study, or a formal research project, the amount of experience the involved surgeons have with each of the alternative treatments, and the success to date with procedures being used. Of course, IRB consent requirements mandate disclosure about the conditions, benefits, and risks involved in formal research. We believe that such information should be provided *regardless* of any institutional or federal regulations and that, in most cases, bureaucratic requirements governing informed consent represent only the minimum of what patients and families want to and deserve to know in order to make satisfying choices.

Just as research about the usefulness of new surgical approaches should attend to more than survival and assess the quality of life for survivors, investigations must now address how surgical alternatives save or use additional resources. In comparing available surgeries for HLHS, it helps to know that although initial costs for transplantation (for survivors) are higher than for palliative surgery, long term costs are likely to be lower with organ replacement. Similarly, in assessing endoscopic surgery, it has sometimes turned out that even with shorter hospitalizations, the additional operating room time and charges associated with amortizing the costs of new equipment, the overall impact is to minimize or offset hoped-for savings. Actually, the study of economic impact should look beyond direct costs of care and consider such factors as work time lost or gained, use of health care related services not typically covered by insurance, and so on. No doubt the move to managed care will provide incentives to pay increased attention to the economic consequences of our attempts to design "better" treatments.

Finally, just as independent intellectual scrutiny at the outset of innovation makes sense, the best research will include well-thought-out and peer-reviewed plans for periodic assessment of the results of clinical trials with lucid criteria for halting the study when the balance of harms or benefits weighs clearly for or against one treatment alternative. Confidence in such "stopping rules" may well be enhanced by the appointment of independent data safety and monitoring boards or committees. Such boards, made up of individuals without a direct stake in any particular conclusions that the study may reach, should have the authority to stop enrollment of new patients when the data suggest continuing the trial would unethically jeopardize those assigned to one or more arms of the trial.

Clinical Conclusions

We have identified several key ethical questions regarding innovation and research in surgery. Two sets of clinical issues seem especially problematic for surgeons. First, when should the innovating surgeon make his or her "deviations" from standard practice the object of systematic research? How much change should trigger scientific scrutiny? Second, when competing techniques intended to address essentially the same clinical problem emerge, how and when should the surgical community undertake comparative clinical trials? These problems seem particularly troubling to surgeons because of their understandable dedication to and pride in the personal craft of surgery.

On the question of when to subject innovative practice to rigorous inquiry, the biggest problem is the inherent bias of the innovator. Regardless of his or her clinical wisdom, experience, and judgment, the innovator is bound to be influenced by enthusiasm for the "better mousetrap." The potential for rewards—be they fame, fortune, or career advancement—cannot but help to affect his or her appraisal of the invention. So what to do? The best answer for now is perhaps more procedural than substantive. When the surgeon begins to wonder about the value of a new way of doing things or when the surgeon appreciates that others are asking evaluative questions, that is the time to begin systematic assessments. Like the old saw exhorting urban political loyalists to vote early and often, surgeons and others should take medical history seriously and ask questions soon after new practices surface and as frequently as necessary until satisfactory answers appear. We have suggested that innovative ideas be circulated and discussed by peers before implementation, that after such discourse innovators execute pilot studies designed to lead to larger and more thorough-going controlled clinical trials. The research queries should address whether the practice really works and with what rate and severity of complications, if it works better than what used to be done, and whether the cost—however measured—is justified, how commonly the procedure will be used and the impact of the resource use on the availability of other care and so on. These questions should help the surgeon or anyone seeking to evaluate the surgical innovation to know if the new approach can be said to offer an advance over no treatment or standard treatment.

Along this path from generation of new ideas, dissemination of plans for innovation, feasibility testing, and full-scale clinical investigation, patients/subjects and when appropriate their legal surrogates should be treated as partners in the attempt to improve surgical practice. The principal technique for ensuring this shared adventure should remain open, honest discussion of what is at stake (i.e., the risks and benefits of participation in the process). This undoubtedly requires a higher level of disclosure of the uncertainties about the outcomes than many would like. But, we need to remember that, legal requirements concerning informed consent aside, the patients ultimately bear the largest share of the burden of treatment and research. Those who desire to innovate, especially without undertaking formal research, should be prepared to demonstrate to colleagues and "consumers" that they have an adequate *prima facie* case to go ahead.

Clearly, we believe comparative clinical trials should play a larger role than has been customary in surgery and should occur prior to a technique's widespread diffusion through the surgical community. This is not to minimize the obstacles we have noted, including differences in skill among surgeons, different success rates according to experience with a procedure, and strong preferences for or against one approach. Various research strategies can lessen the logistic and moral concerns about surgical and patient preferences and allegiances. It seems important to restate the obvious: surgical practice is not fundamentally different from other types of medical care. The assessment of change and progress in surgery does not require an altogether different approach.

The principal goal of clinical research, of innovation, or of "mere" treatment is unitary: to accomplish benefit for patients. Assuming practitioners and investigators alike compassionately undertake to communicate fully what is and isn't known and what and how surgeons must all collaborate to learn what practice works best, then surgeons properly respect our patients/research subjects via the vehicle of informed consent. In the long run, diminishing the distinctions between scientific inquiry, innovative practice, and therapeutic intervention in ways that encourage critical appraisal of whatever surgeons do seems the wisest course.

References

1. Ernest M. Barsamian, "The Rise and Fall of Internal Mammary Artery Ligation in the Treatment of Angina Pectoris and the Lessons Learned," in *Costs, Risks and Benefits of Surgery*, John P. Bunker, Benjamin A. Barnes, Frederick Mosteller, eds. New York: Oxford University Press, 1977, pp. 212–220.
2. Henry K. Beecher, "Ethics and Clinical Research," *New England Journal of Medicine* 274 (1966): 1354–1360.
3. David J. Rothman, "Human Experimentation and the Origins of Bioethics in the United States," in *Social Science Perspectives on Medical Ethics*, George Weisz, ed., 1990, Philadelphia: University of Pennsylvania Press, 1990, pp. 185–200.
4. President's Commission for the Study of Ethical Problems in Medicine and Biomedical and Behavioral Research, *Protecting Human Subjects: The Adequacy and Uniformity of Federal Rules and their Implementation*. Washington, D.C.: U.S. Government Printing Office, 1981.

5. Department of Health and Human Services, "Children Involved as Subjects in Research; Additional Protection," *Federal Register* 48 (1983):9814–9820 (45 CFR 46.401–409).

6. National Commission for the Protection of Human Subjects of Biomedical and Behavioral Research, "The Belmont Report: Ethical Principles for the Protection of Human Subjects of Research." *OPRR Reports*, Washington, D.C.: U.S. Government Printing Office, 1979.

7. David J. Rothman, "Ethics and Human Experimentation: Henry Beecher Revisited," *New England Journal of Medicine* 317 (1987): 1195–1199.

8. Leslie Francis, "IRBs and Conflicts of Interest," in *Conflicts of Interest in Clinical Practice and Research*, Roy G. Spece, David S. Shimm, Allen E. Buchanan, eds. New York: Oxford University Press, 1996, pp. 418–436.

9. Bernard Barber, John J. Lally, Julia Loughlin Makarushka, et al., *Research on Human Subjects: Problems of Social Control in Medical Experimentation*. New York: Russell Sage Foundation, 1973.

10. Jerry Goldman and Martin D. Katz, "Inconsistency and Institutional Review Boards," *Journal of the American Medical Association* 248 (1982): 197–202.

11. Bradford H. Gray, "An Assessment of Institutional Review Committees in Human Experimentation," *Medical Care* XIII (1975): 318–328.

12. Murray Levine, "IRB Review as a 'Cooling Out' Device," *IRB: A Review of Human Subjects Research* 5 (1983): 8–9.

13. Peter C. Williams, "Why IRBs Falter in Reviewing Risks and Benefits," *IRB: A Review of Human Subjects Research* 6 (1984): 1–4.

14. Roy G. Spece and David S. Shimm, "An Introduction to Conflicts of Interest in Clinical Research," in *Conflicts of Interest in Clinical Practice and Research*, Roy G. Spece, David S. Shimm, Allen E. Buchanan, eds. New York: Oxford University Press, 1996, pp. 361–376.

15. John Lantos, "How Can We Distinguish Clinical Research from Innovative Therapy?" *American Journal of Pediatric Hematology/Oncology* 16 (1994): 72–75.

16. Charles W. Lidz, Alan Meisel, Eviatar Zerubavel, et al., *Informed Consent: A Study of Decisionmaking in Psychiatry*. New York: Guilford Press, 1984.

17. Renée C. Fox, *The Sociology of Medicine: a Participant Observer's View*. Englewood Cliffs, New Jersey: Prentice Hall, 1989.

18. Benjamin A. Barnes, "Discarded Operations: Surgical Innovation by Trial and Error," in *Costs, Risks and Benefits of Surgery*, John P. Bunker, Benjamin A. Barnes, Frederick Mosteller, eds. New York: Oxford University Press, 1977, pp. 109–123.

19. Lawrence I. Bonchek, "Are Randomized Trials Appropriate for Evaluating New Operations?" *New England Journal of Medicine* 301 (1977): 44–45.

20. Alan L. Hillman, John M. Eisenberg, Mark V. Pauly, et al., "Avoiding Bias in the Conduct and Reporting of Cost-Effectiveness Research Sponsored by Pharmaceutical Companies," *New England Journal of Medicine* 324 (1991): 1362–1365.

21. D. J. Roy, P. McL. Black, and B. McPeek, "Ethical Principles in Research," in *Principles and Practice of Research: Strategies for Surgical Investigators*, 2nd ed., Hans Troidl, Walter O. Spizer, Bucknam McPeek, et al., eds. New York: Springer-Verlag, 1991, pp. 91–103.

22. D. J. Benjamin, "The Efficacy of Surgical Treatment of Cancer," *Medical Hypotheses* 40 (1993): 129–138.

23. Stephen J. Haines, "Randomized Clinical Trials in the Evaluation of Surgical Innovation." *Journal of Neurosurgery* 51 (1979): 5–11.

24. S. Challah and N.B. Mays, "The Randomised Controlled Trial in the Evaluation of New Technology: A Case Study," *British Medical Journal* 292 (1986): 877–879.
25. John P. Gilbert, Bucknam McPeek, and Frederick Mosteller, "Statistics and Ethics in Surgery and Anesthesia," *Science* 198 (1977): 684–689.
26. Thomas C. Chalmers, "Randomization and Coronary Artery Surgery," *Annals of Thoracic Surgery* 14 (1972): 323–327.
27. Mike Gross, "Innovations in Surgery: A Proposal for Phased Clinical Trials," *Journal of Bone and Joint Surgery (Britain)* 75B (1993): 351–354.
28. Willem van der Linden, "Pitfalls in Randomized Surgical Trials," *Surgery* 87 (1980): 258–262.
29. Thorkild I.A. Sorensen, "Effects of Treatments in Clinical Trials: Surgery," *Journal of Surgical Oncology* Supplement 3 (1993): 186–188.
30. Michael J. Solomon, Andres Laxamana, Linda Devore, and Robin S. McLeod, "Randomized Controlled Trials in Surgery," *Surgery* 115 (1994): 707–712.
31. N. Kadar, "The Operative Laparoscopy Debate: Technology Assessment or Statistical Jezebel?" *Biomedicine & Pharmacotherapy* 47 (1993): 201–206.
32. Kenneth F. Schaffner, "Ethical Problems in Clinical Trials," *Journal of Medicine and Philosophy* 11 (1986): 297–315.
33. Leonard A. Cobb, George I. Thomas, David H. Dillard, et al., "An Evaluation of Internal-Mammary-Artery Ligation by a Double-Blind Technic," *New England Journal of Medicine* 260 (1959): 1115–1118
34. E. Grey Dimond, C. Frederick Kittle, and James E. Crockett, "Comparison of Internal Mammary Artery Ligation and Sham Operation for Angina Pectoris," *American Journal of Cardiology* 5 (1960): 483–486.
35. Henry K. Beecher, "Surgery as Placebo: A Quantitative Study of Bias," *Journal of the American Medical Association* 176 (1961): 1102–1107.
36. Gordon M. Stirrat, Stephen C. Farrow, John Farndon, et al., "The Challenge of Evaluating Surgical Procedures," *Annals of the Royal College of Surgeons of England* 74 (1992): 80–84.
37. B. McPeek, F. Mosteller, M. F. McKneally, et al., "Experimental Methods: Clinical Trials," in *Principles and Practice of Research: Strategies for Surgical Investigators*, 2nd ed. Hans Troidl, Walter O. Spizer, Bucknam McPeek, et al., eds. New York: Springer-Verlag, 1991, pp. 114–125.
38. Michael S. Kramer and Stanley H. Shapiro, "Scientific Challenges in the Application of Randomized Trials," *Journal of the American Medical Association* 252 (1984): 2739–2745.
39. Gordon H. Guyatt, Jana L. Keller, Roman Jaeschke, et al., "The n-of-1 Randomized Controlled Trial: Clinical Usefulness," *Annals of Internal Medicine* 112 (1990): 293–299.
40. Susan S. Ellenberg, "Randomized Designs in Comparative Clinical Trials," *New England Journal of Medicine* 310 (1984): 1404–1408.
41. Don Marquis, "An Argument that All Prerandomized Clinical Trials Are Unethical," *Journal of Medicine and Philosophy* 11 (1986): 367–383.
42. Robert H. Bartlett, Dietrich W. Roloff, Richard G. Cornell, et al., Extracorporeal Circulation in Neonatal Respiratory Failure: A Prospective Randomized Study," *Pediatrics* 76 (1985): 479–487.
43. John D. Lantos and Joel Frader, "Extracorporeal Membrane Oxygenation and the Ethics of Clinical Research in Pediatrics," *New England Journal of Medicine* 322 (1990): 409–413.

44. P. Pearl O'Rourke, Robert K. Crone, Joseph P. Vacanti, et al., "Extracorporeal Membrane Oxygenation and Conventional Medical Therapy in Neonates with Persistent Pulmonary Hypertension of the Newborn: A Prospective Randomized Study," *Pediatrics* 84 (1989): 957–963.

45. National Commission for the Protection of Human Subjects of Biomedical and Behavioral Research, "Report and Recommendation: Research Involving Children," *Federal Register* 43 (1978): 2084–2114.

46. American Federation for Clinical Research, "Guidelines for Avoiding Conflict of Interest," *Clinical Research* 38 (1990): 239–240.

47. Executive Council of the Association of American Medical Colleges, *Guidelines for Dealing with Faculty Conflicts of Commitment and Conflicts of Interest in Research*. Washington, D.C.: Association of American Medical Colleges, 1990.

48. David S. Shimm and Roy G. Spece, "Industry Reimbursement for Entering Patients into Clinical Trials: Legal and Ethical Issues," *Annals of Internal Medicine* 115 (1991): 148–151.

49. American Medical Association, Council on Scientific Affairs and Council on Ethical and Judicial Affairs, "Conflicts of Interest in Medical Center/Industry Research Relationships," *Journal of the American Medical Association* 263 (1990): 2790–2793.

50. Anonymous, "Pharmaceutical Funds for Clinical Research: A Mixed Blessing," *Lancet* 1 (1987): 257–258.

51. Paul Cotton, "Knee Implant Problem Has Orthopedic Surgeons Begging for Independent Data," *Journal of the American Medical Association* 263 (1990): 1889–1890.

52. Joel E. Frader, "Researcher Conflict of Interest," in *Handbook on Integrity in Biomedical Research*. Pittsburgh, Pa: University of Pittsburgh School of Medicine, 1992, pp. 21–23.

53. J. M. D. Nightingale and J. E. Lennard-Jones, "The Short Bowel Syndrome: What's New and Old?" *Digestive Diseases* 11 (1993): 12–31.

54. Jon S. Thompson, Alan N. Langnas, Lewis W. Pinch, et al., "Surgical Approach to Short- Bowel Syndrome: Experience in a Population of 160 Patients," *Annals of Surgery* 222 (1995): 600–607.

55. Arlet G. Kurkchubasche, Marc I. Rowe, and Samuel D. Smith, "Adaptation in Short-bowel Syndrome: Reassessing Old Limits," *Journal of Pediatric Surgery* 28 (1993): 1069–1071.

56. Jon S. Thompson, "Surgical Aspects of the Short-Bowel Syndrome," *American Journal of Surgery* 170 (1995): 532–536.

57. Francis D. Moore, "The Desperate Case: CARE (Costs, Applicability, Research, Ethics)," *Journal of the American Medical Association* 261 (1989): 1483–1484.

58. R. F. M. Wood and C. L. Ingham Clark, "Small Bowel Transplantation: Results Not Yet Too Hopeful," *British Medical Journal* 304 (1992): 1453–1454.

59. R. J. Ploeg and A. M. D'Alessandro, "Intestinal Transplantation: A Clinical Update," *Scandinavian Journal of Gastroenterology* 30, Supplement 212 (1995): 79–89.

60. William I. Norwood, Marshall L. Jacobs, and John D. Murphy, "Fontan Procedure for Hypoplastic Left Heart Syndrome," *Annals of Thoracic Surgery* 54 (1992): 1025–1030.

61. Joseph M. Forbess, Nancy Cook, Stephen J. Roth, et al., "Ten-Year Institutional Experience with Palliative Surgery for Hypoplastic Left Heart Syndrome: Risk Factors Related to Stage I Mortality," *Circulation* 92, Supplement II (1995): II 262–266.

62. Howard P. Gutgesell and Thomas A. Massaro, "Management of Hypoplastic Left

Heart Syndrome in a Consortium of University Hospitals," *American Journal of Cardiology* 76 (1995): 809–811.

63. Joel E. Frader, "Pediatric Heart, Heart-Lung, and Lung Transplantation: Ethics," *Progress in Pediatric Cardiology* 3 (1994): 20–25.

64. Leonard L. Bailey, Michael Wood, Anees Razzouk, et al., "Heart Transplantation During the First 12 Years of Life," *Archives of Surgery* 124 (1989): 1221–1226.

65. Benjamin Freedman, "Equipoise and the Ethics of Clinical Research," *New England Journal of Medicine* 317 (1987): 141–145.

13

Preventing and Managing Unwarranted Biases against Patients

LORETTA M. KOPELMAN
DONALD R. LANNIN
ARTHUR E. KOPELMAN

"The patient is a forty-five year old African-American male . . . a thirty-year-old Asian-American female . . . an eighty-year-old white male." Case reports begin in this familiar fashion because the patient's age, race, and gender may hold the key to his or her needs. The patient's mode of livelihood, living companions, sexual orientation, lifestyle or socioeconomic group may also be relevant factors in selecting medical care. Subspecialty clinics develop around such differences, such as gynecologic surgery for women or pediatric surgery for children's special problems and unique reactions. Studies also reveal group differences. For example, middle-aged caucasian men are more likely to have coronary artery disease than premenopausal white women. Age can also be predictive to such a degree that people over eighty or under two years of age might be excluded from consideration for some surgeries because they are unlikely to survive the procedure.

Race, age, gender, lifestyle choices, sexual orientation, work habits, socioeconomic background, or social background, then, can be legitimate factors in providing medical care generally, and surgical care in particular. Surgeons use this information to help identify patients' needs and interests. In contrast, such considerations would generally be regarded as unjustified in most social institutions. In law or education, for example, it would be unwarranted to decide how to treat people because of their race, religion, or gender.

On the other hand, concern has been expressed that clinicians may be unjustifiably biased by race, age, gender, lifestyle choices, sexual orientation, work habits, socioeconomic background, or social background in directing patients' care and treatments. Gornick[1] and her associates analyzed the 1993 Medicare data, the most recent available, correlating it with 1990 census data to compare the health care of 24.2 million caucasians and 2.1 million African-Americans. Despite similar insurance coverage they found that income, race, and gender affect how patients receive costly, scarce, or life-saving resources. For example, for patients with ischemic heart disease the black-white ratio for percutaneous transluminal coronary angioplasty was 0.46 and for coronary-artery bypass surgery 0.40. Adjustments for income slightly reduced these differences. African-American patients were also more likely to have procedures such as hysterectomies and amputation, suggesting that they are "at higher risk for procedures associated with less than optimal management of chronic diseases."[1] In an editorial published on this study, Geiger notes that well-designed studies controlled for such factors as age, disease severity, co-morbid conditions, and background incidence and prevalence rates support the disturbing conclusions that African Americans with comparable insurance are less likely to "receive renal transplants, receive hip or total knee replacements, and undergo gastrointestinal endoscopy, among other procedures, but are more likely to undergo hysterectomy and amputation."[2] He also points out the consistency of these findings with a growing body of evidence of unwarranted bias in medicine.

Other studies suggest disturbing patterns of unjustified bias by clinicians against specific groups of patients, including those who are female, poor, elderly, Latino, and African-American. One study from the University of California at Los Angeles Emergency Medical Center reported, "Hispanics with isolated long-bone fractures are twice as likely as non-Hispanic whites to receive no pain medication . . . No covariate measured in this study [such as the severity of the injury, the degree of pain, the accuracy of assessment that analgesics were given, or the ability to communicate] could account for this effect."[3] A follow-up study concluded, "Physician ability to assess pain severity does not differ for Hispanic and non-Hispanic white patients,"[4] supporting the view that the different use of pain medication might reflect bias.

Another study set out to "describe the process of care and clinical outcomes associated with acute myocardial infarction (AMI) in the Medicare population, and to examine differences in the process of care and outcome of care as a function of patient age, gender, and race."[5] The investigators concluded that the use of procedures varied by gender and race, but mostly by age. A follow-up study found, "[a]mong Medicare enrollees, whites are more likely than blacks to receive revascularization procedures after coronary angiography. Racial differences of similar magnitude occur in all types of hospitals."[6] Still another study of 12,402 patients with coronary diseases concluded: "Blacks with coronary disease were significantly less likely than whites to undergo coronary revascularization, particularly bypass surgery—a difference that could not be explained by the clinical features of their disease."[7] These investigators did not have information about patient preferences, however, and speculated that this group of patients might not want to accept the initial risks inherent in these procedures. The possibility of unwarranted bias on the part of physicians, they acknowledge, could not be dismissed either.

Three studies report that, among equally disabled men and women, women are less likely than men to have major procedures for diagnosis or therapy of coronary heart disease.[8-10] For example, Wenger and her colleagues found that women with cardiac disease were less likely to be treated aggressively and had higher mortality rates than men.[10] There is also a widespread perception that diseases affecting women are studied less, and that women and minorities tend to be unfairly excluded from clinical trials, thereby denying them important health opportunities.[11,12] The General Accounting office, at the request of Louise Slaughter[13] and other members of the U.S. Congress, studied the problem and concluded that women, African-Americans, and certain ethnic groups have been significantly underrepresented in studies and clinical trials, and this had caused bias in their diagnosis and treatment. Working groups at the National Institutes of Health,[14] the Institute of Medicine,[15] and the Council on Ethical and Judicial Affairs of the American Medical Association[16,17] reached similar judgments.

Unwarranted biases may harm patients, even if unintended, by distorting how doctors make diagnoses, frame issues, describe and compare options, consider prognosis, treat patients, assess outcomes, and form relationships. Unfortunately, despite increasing evidence of their existence among clinicians, little time is spent discussing the ethical hazards of unjustified biases against patients. After discussing the meaning of "unwarranted bias," we consider how it violates professional duties, values, and virtues and why surgeons need to work to prevent unwarranted biases against patients to fulfill their professional goals. Finally, we discuss several related strategies to prevent unwarranted bias.

Ethical Analysis of Unwarranted Bias

The first step in managing unwarranted bias is identifying it. The very concept of "unwarranted bias" carries a negative connotation, but "bias" has other uses that are not pejorative.[18,19] Some legitimate interests may be described as biases. A private foundation or public agency might have a legitimate bias toward aiding children, the poor, or elderly members of society. As we have seen, many times the patient's age, race, gender, lifestyle choice, or work habits is relevant— or a warranted bias—in considering medical or surgical care. Considering individual differences leads to good clinical judgments, but can also cause unwarranted bias. Our focus is on unwarranted biases, which include such notions as *prejudices, misconceptions*, and *unjustifiable self-interests*. Because the concept of bias is complex, we will begin by clarifying terms.

Types of Unwarranted Bias

Prejudice is a special form of unwarranted bias, having two components: faulty or unwarranted *beliefs*, such as overgeneralizations, and *attitudes* for or against certain persons or things based on those unsubstantiated or faulty beliefs.[20] For example, people would have a prejudice against surgeons or automobile mechanics if they distrusted them all based on an encounter with one of them. What is distinctive about prejudices is that the negative attitudes persist after the faulty beliefs and reasons allegedly supporting them are exposed. As Allport[20] has shown, prejudiced people resist having their rash reasoning exposed and shape "reasons" to accommodate their attitudes.

Misconceptions differ from prejudices. While both are based on faulty beliefs, we correct misconceptions when presented with appropriate evidence. The difference between misconceptions and prejudices then, concerns our willingness to change our beliefs and attitudes in light of new information. In 1992 there was a sharp exchange of letters in *The Lancet*,[21,22] in response to the views of Benson,[23] who held that men generally make better surgeons because women tend to panic, are too diffident, lack confidence, and respond poorly when sleep deprived. While Benson did not reply, it is important to ask, under what circumstances would someone with views such as Benson's be likely to alter those views? People who change their views appropriately as evidence changes correct misconceptions.

Unjustifiable self-interests are also unwarranted biases, but they need not be based on faulty beliefs. People may be aware that they are selfish, greedy, or operating from other unjustified interests. For example, some physicians and surgeons refuse to take care of HIV-infected patients because they want no association with them, and accept no risk, however low, of infection. They may have no misconceptions about the resulting burdens placed on others, but simply place their own interests ahead of other considerations. Unwarranted interests may sometimes lead to inappropriate neglect of patients or unfair imposition of risk on other surgeons. Such unjustified interests should not influence surgical judgment or practice.

Often there are difficult lines to draw between unjustified and legitimate interests. Clinicians are generally praised for helping their own patients and programs. Advocacy, however, can become unfair when it leads to the disregard of other patients' rights or welfare. Suppose, for example, that an organ transplantation program collects organs from a large region promising to distribute them fairly to all in that area. Despite such assurances, those who run the program devise strategies to ensure most organs go to their own patients. Such bias would violate the ground rules for acquisition of organs and thus jeopardize the program. To avoid this bias, national organizations prevent the retention of organs by the institution that procures them (see Chapter 6).

Self-interest can be a form of unwarranted bias that is particularly difficult to limit or manage. For example, suppose that smaller adults have greater morbidity and mortality following bypass surgery because of greater difficulties manipulating and repairing smaller blood vessels. Surgeons would be acting from unwarranted self-interest if they refused to do bypass surgery on smaller adults, mostly women, and were motivated by the inappropriate reason that such surgery would only contribute to the surgeon's higher mortality rates and thus to a worse postoperative profile for complications. Without being aware of crossing a boundary of unwarranted bias, such surgeons might even justify or rationalize such exclusions as being in the patients's best interest. This line may not be clear.

Sometimes it is apparent that clinicians refuse to treat patients for self-interested reasons such as risk of infection, economics, risky of litigation, complexity of illness, bothersome interactions, or discomfort to the physician. An orthopedic surgeon refused to treat an otherwise healthy gay man's fracture dislocation of the right ankle following an automobile accident, claiming that the patient should be transferred to a university medical center, an hour away, where physicians could both fix his ankle and evaluate his cough. The physicians at the receiving hospital did not challenge the thinly disguised excuse to avoid taking care of a patient who was gay.

The AMA Principles of Medical Ethics[16] affirm the traditional privilege of physicians to refuse to accept patients in non-emergencies. Principle VI states, "A physician shall, in the provision of appropriate patient care, except in emergencies, be free to choose whom to serve, with whom to associate, and the environment in which to provide medical services." The AMA clarifies that this is intended to help physicians avoid caring for patients outside their area of expertise or those who are threatening or troublesome. Do surgeons, therefore have the right to refuse patients who make them feel uncomfortable because of the clinicians' unwarranted biases? This tradition, however, does not give them the right or privilege of refusing to treat homosexuals, people with AIDS, people with contagious diseases, and so on. Such group exclusions would harm the profession by seeming to sanction prejudiced and self-interested behavior. It also would be likely to harm surgeons because their unjustified bias would not only go unchecked, but could change the character of the surgical profession in detrimental ways. Patients may be better off with surgeons who do not have unwarranted biases against them, but patients may have few options to leave a surgeon's care—for example, in public systems of medical care or managed care organizations with only limited numbers of surgeons on referral.

The Role of the Surgical Community

The medical community sets moral standards for physicians's conduct, including the tolerated limits of self-interested behavior.[16,24] Medicine is a profession because it promises or "professes" special duties, values, and virtues to patients. Among the most ancient and central are moral commitments to act so as to merit patients' trust and confidences. These include pledges to act compassionately, honestly, fairly, and as advocates of patients' best interests when they need medical attention. These commitments also include pledges to act without excessive self-interest and with a measure of humility. In short, these are promises to respect patients and act to enhance their well-being. Such duties, values, and virtues are central to the enterprise of medicine, transforming it from a business shaped by self-interest and market forces to a profession.[24,25] Accepting the benefits of being a member of the medical profession obligates clinicians to adhere to professional norms that limit individual self-interest. All physicians must strike some balance between self-interest and professional duties and professional associations help determine what constitutes unjustifiable practices. Pellegrino and Thomasma[24] argue that medicine, as other professions, has fuzzy boundaries about where to draw the line between acceptable and unacceptable behavior. Consequently, certain members of the profession push the limits of the sort of self-interested behavior that is tolerated. Often these gray zones are characterized by (1) the use of power and privilege for personal gain, (2) the wish to avoid risks or responsibilities in caring for those the profession should serve, and (3) rationalizations in terms of self-interest. Given these features, unjustified self-interest may be among the most difficult of the unwarranted biases to prevent or manage. For example, recent studies have shown that many physicians (57%) refuse to provide care for uninsured or Medicaid patients because they mistakenly believe that they are at increased risk of being sued.[26] If this misconception is exposed and they persist in their belief, it may really show self-interest or prejudice against the poor. This is one important test of unwarranted bias, revealing the link between ethical and factual issues.

Given our analysis of unwarranted biases, it should be clear why they are incompatible with the professional medical standards. Misconceptions and prejudices are, by definition, based on flawed reasoning, so they thwart commitments to ground judgments on the best available information. Moreover, these unwarranted biases presuppose attitudes founded on unsubstantiated or faulty beliefs, so they are generally unfair in assessing people and their needs. Doctors inclined to "see" certain groups as lazy, might "see" a genuine illness of a member of that group as malingering. Unwarranted biases can also thwart the equitable selection of research subjects or the just allocation of treatments and scarce resources for patients.

If patients sense unwarranted biases against them, they are unlikely to establish a good surgeon-patient relationship. People, especially those who have faced past discrimination, are sensitive to its possible existence. An African-American man was on hemodialysis for four years due to chronic renal failure related to uncontrolled hypertension. Because his living relatives were tissue-type incompatible and could not serve as living kidney donors, he was placed on a waiting list for a cadaveric transplant. After two years, he became convinced "the system" discriminated against him. While a variety of complex and interrelated factors might explain why fewer kidney transplants are done for African-American persons compared with other groups, this man's suspicions proposed only one answer.

Unwarranted bias is a potent form of disrespect that, even if unintended, undermines patients' trust in surgeons. Distrustful patients, for example, may withhold sensitive information, not cooperate in treatment plans, find another physician, or be more prone to sue. Furthermore, unwarranted biases undermine patients' trust not only in their surgeons, but in the medical profession and health care institutions. Exposing unwarranted biases helps clinicians practice in environments that make it possible for them to do what is right and be good. People have difficulty functioning at their best when they face unchecked prejudices from their peers, superiors, or institutions. Exposing unwarranted biases is also an important part of professional education, because they rest on flawed reasoning or unjustifiable attitudes. A central tenet of this chapter is that clinicians' unwarranted biases undercut important ethical commitments of the medical profession in general and surgery in particular. In what follows, we consider strategies to help deal with unwarranted biases in the clinical setting.

Clinical Topics

Surgeons, surgery residents, and medical students seem to find it easier than others to discuss some unwarranted biases than others. They readily discuss patients who object to being treated by certain groups. They will also discuss their negative reactions to patients who are self-destructive and irresponsible or abuse drugs or who are so-called "street people." They freely consider the challenge of how to respond respectfully and professionally, while finding strategies to cope with their attitudes. They become more cautious, however, in speaking about some of the unwarranted biases they perceive in their supervisors or peers. Surgeons, surgery residents, and students sometimes recognize unwarranted biases in remarks, jokes, or the allocation of goods and services, yet feel uncomfortable about speaking up. This not only harms patients but weakens the duties, values, and virtues central to the medical profession. In this section we propose several strategies to diagnose and treat unwarranted biases.

First, to foster an atmosphere of open discussion, we recommend more conferences be focused on controversial subjects generally. Because discussion about surgeons' unwarranted biases are among the most sensitive of issues, this strategy should help make free exchanges on controversial subjects more comfortable. For example, an area of current controversy in pediatric surgery concerns appropriate treatment of hypoplastic left heart syndrome (see Chapter 12). Is it most compassionate for these babies to get comfort care, transplantation, or palliative surgical treatment? Should doctors make recommendations to families about which of these three modes of care is best, or ask families to make the decisions? If physicians make recommendations, should they do so initially, or reluctantly at the conclusion of extensive counseling and educational sessions? Is surgical treatment of this condition a good use of resources? Expression of conflicting but reasoned views on such topics is not only an important part of surgeons' continuing education but also promotes an atmosphere of open discussion of ideas. Such exchanges could also be tied to questions about unwarranted bias by examining outcomes data about whether infants of certain gender or ethnic background are more likely to be treated in certain ways.

Second, we recommend the use of case conferences to discuss the line between warranted and unwarranted biases. Some years ago a 78-year-old woman came to her local physician with a two- to three-centimeter palpable mass in the upper right breast, which an aspiration biopsy showed was ductal carcinoma. She was on medication for hypertension, but otherwise in good health. She was referred to a surgeon who discussed the following options with her: mastectomy with or without reconstruction; breast preservation; axillary dissection; systemic adjuvant therapy; and lumpectomy with or without radiation. Her surgeon believed that different treatments were justified for older women and tailored his recommendations accordingly. As we noted earlier, sensitive physicians and surgeons may judge, even ahead of aggregate data, that persons from certain groups ought to be treated differently. Discussion of such a case with other surgeons, residents, and medical students serves many purposes, including consideration of whether a different recommendation based on age is warranted. Subsequent studies have vindicated that the best treatment for older women with breast cancer may be different from that for younger women. In some cases, therefore, different recommendations for identifiable groups, such as for elderly women, do not represent prejudice but sound clinical judgment. As an exercise, surgeons could even consider cases blinded by age, race, and gender to see what judgments are made in the absence of such information. This exercise would serve as an antidote to powerful and subtle forms of unwarranted bias, especially age-related bias.

Third, surgeons, as a part of their continuing education, should review the growing body of literature that shows unwarranted bias in the way medical care resources are distributed. This should sensitize surgeons to possible unwarranted bias and to how physicians may be perceived by certain communities. During this review, surgeons might usefully consider outcomes data from their own practices to determine if it reflects similar trends.

Fourth, health care institutions, such as hospitals and managed care organizations (MCOs), now routinely gather and analyze outcomes data. With some forethought they might study the allocation of medical resources in their centers based on age, race, gender, or other areas of potential bias. This would help them recognize possible unwarranted biases and thus take an important first step.

Fifth, one of the best ways to dispel unwarranted bias is to learn more about the group about which misconceptions exist, preferably from the people themselves. This promotion of diversity in the exchange of ideas and formation of policies can undercut a variety of mistaken beliefs and attitudes supporting unwarranted biases. Particular religious groups face discrimination in certain regions, for example, and some education of surgeons, surgery residents, and medical students about these religions may be very important to providing their patients with compassionate medical care. These discussions can sometimes be tied to specific cases, such as the treatment plans for someone with particular religious obligations.

Sixth, equitable institutional policies can help manage unwarranted biases. Health care organizations, including hospitals, nursing homes, and rehabilitation centers, have increasing responsibility for combating unfair biases, because these institutions increasingly make decisions affecting patients' access to health care. Because these organizations are hierarchical, they can be very effective in identifying and rooting out prejudices, special interests, and misconceptions. They also tend to be more carefully regulated and have more diversity than small or private agencies. On the other hand, organizations with systematic and unwarranted biases can create difficult environments for clinicians and patients. Reiser,[27] and Bulger and Cassel,[28] recommend that health-care institutions, including hospitals and MCOs, reflect on their ethical and social commitments to patients and staff. These institutions should critically examine the values and goals expressed in their codes of conduct and mission or vision statements to see if they are fairly serving the entire population's needs.

In addition, health care organizations must conform to social policies, regulations, and oversight agencies that enforce certain moral standards. These include federal regulations about research and patients' rights and powerful nongovernmental agencies such as The Joint Commission on the Accreditation of Healthcare Organizations (JCAHO). The JCAHO regulates and evaluates health care institutions' effectiveness in protecting the rights and well-being of all patients. It determines whether these health care organizations have adopted suitable policies and procedures regarding such matters as patient rights, confidentiality, sexual harassment, respect for cultural diversity, and conflict resolution.

Unjustified biases within institutions harm many people. For example, in their report "Gender Discrimination in the Medical Profession," the American Medical Association's Council of Ethical and Judicial Affairs concludes:

> In addition to the effects on women's careers, many deleterious effects on the medical profession result from the inequality between men's and women's professional status. Patient care may be compromised in an environment which does not respect the competence and talents of women. Undermining the professional capabilities of female surgeons and surgery residents damages the trust of patients in their surgeons, and an environment of harassment and hostility can distract attention and energy from the care of patients.[17]

This report also underscores the importance of addressing other unfair biases in medical schools and teaching hospitals.

Finally, we recommend that ethics and other humanities be taught as part of continuing education programs to help clinicians explore the difference between warranted and unwarranted biases in medical practice. A historical perspective about the abuses of subjects in the Tuskegee syphilis studies, for example, illuminates why many African-Americans still mistrust medical institutions and investigators.[29] Although this study ended in the early 1970s, understanding its impact on the African-American community helps clinicians understand suspicions of the medical establishment even decades later. Literature can also be used to help surgeons, surgery residents, and students understand and empathize with different groups or perspectives. Philosophy can provide both a theoretical basis for discussion about bias and resource allocation, consent, confidentiality, and so on, as well as how science that is mistakenly thought to be value-free can incorporate unjustified biases. For example, many medical studies report findings by race. Those with mixed racial backgrounds are often forced to state one particular race in such studies from a narrow range of choices that may not reflect biological categories. Self-selected racial classifications lack standardization and create hazards for interpretation. In addition, race is sometimes taken as a reliable surrogate for socioeconomic factors, when it is not. Studies based on such errors may "show" unreliable differences between people in such matters as access to and utilization of health care or morbidity and mortality.[30,31]

Clinical Conclusions

In surgery, as in other branches of medicine, clinicians must sometimes consider the patient's age, race, gender, lifestyle choices, sexual orientation, work habits, or socioeconomic background in providing medical care. Such factors may be salient to identifying the patient's needs and interests. Yet there is growing evidence that patients sometimes suffer from unwarranted clinician bias based on the misuse of these variables. With no clear demarcation between legitimate and unwarranted bias in medicine, we have argued that surgeons should pay more attention to the ethics of unwarranted biases against patients and within institutions.

Because there is no single way to expose and manage unwarranted medical biases, we have recommended several strategies to use in combination to combat prejudices, misconceptions, and unjustified self-interests. *First*, introduce humanities teaching to enhance understanding of the moral and social issues facing clinicians and to prevent unwarranted biases. *Second*, foster open discussions about controversial subjects in general to help create an environment where challenging and probing questions are more welcome. *Third*, use case conferences to discuss the line between warranted and unwarranted biases. *Fourth*, review and discuss the growing body of literature that shows unwarranted bias in the way medical care is distributed. *Fifth*, hospitals, MCOs, and other health care institutions should incorporate such factors as patients' age, race, gender, and so on in analyzing outcomes data. Identifying and recognizing unwarranted biases in one's own practice is an important first step toward eliminating it. *Sixth*, provide more education about the diverse groups in the patient population served, preferably from the members of those groups themselves. *Seventh*, review institutional policies and procedures. Prejudices and misconceptions are based on faulty beliefs or unwarranted attitudes, and as such threaten the scientific and moral foundations on which medicine in general and surgery, in particular, are based.

References

1. Marion E. Gornick, Paul W. Eggers, Thomas W. Reilly, et al., "Effects of Race and Income on Mortality and Use of Services Among Medicare Beneficiaries," *The New England Journal of Medicine* 335 (1996): 791–799.
2. H. Jack Geiger, "Race and Health Care—An American Dilemma?," *The New England Journal of Medicine* 335 (1996): 815–816.
3. Knox H. Todd, Nigel Samaroo, and Jerome R. Hoffman, "Ethnicity as a Risk Factor for Inadequate Emergency Department Analgesia," *Journal of the American Medical Association* 269 (1993): 1537–1539.
4. Knox H. Todd, Tony Lee, and Jerome R. Hoffman, "The Effect of Ethnicity on Physician Estimates of Pain Severity in Patients with Isolated Extremity Trauma," *Journal of the American Medical Association* 271 (1994): 925–928.
5. I. Steven Udvarhelyi, Constantine Gatsonis, Arnold M. Epstein, et al., "Acute Myocardial Infarction in the Medicare Population. Process of Care and Clinical Outcomes," *Journal of the American Medical Association* 268 (1992): 2530–2536.
6. John Z. Ayanian, I. Steven Udvarhelyi, Constantine A. Gatsonis, et al., "Racial Differences in the Use of Revascularization Procedures After Coronary Angiography," *Journal of the American Medical Association* 269 (1993): 2642–2646.

7. Eric D. Peterson, Linda K. Shaw, Elizabeth R. DeLong, et al., "Racial Variation in the Use of Coronary-Revascularization Procedures," *The New England Journal of Medicine* 336 (1994): 480–486.
8. John Z. Ayanian and Arnold M. Epstein, "Differences in the Use of Procedures Between Women and Men Hospitalized for Coronary Heart Disease," *New England Journal of Medicine* 325 (1991): 221–225.
9. Richard M. Steingart, Milton Packer, Peggy Hamm, et al., "Sex Differences in the Management of Coronary Artery Disease," *New England Journal of Medicine* 325 (1991): 226–230.
10. Nanette K. Wenger, Leon Speroff, and Barbara Packard, "Cardiovascular Health and Disease in Women," *New England Journal of Medicine* 329 (1993): 247–256.
11. Marcia M. Angell, "Caring for Women's Health—What Is the Problem?" *New England Journal of Medicine* 329 (1993): 271–272.
12. Ruth B. Merkatz, Robert Temple, Solomon Sobel, et al., and the working group on women in clinical trials, "Inclusion of Women in Clinical Trials—Policies for Population Subgroups," *New England Journal of Medicine* 329 (1993): 288–296.
13. Louise M. Slaughter, "Prepared Remarks of Congresswoman Louise M. Slaughter (D- NY) to the Office of Research on Women's Health Science Meeting," in *Recruitment and Retention of Women in Clinical Studies*. Office of the Director, National Institute of Health. Washington, DC: U.S. Department Health and Human Services Public Health Service, National Institute of Health, 1994, pp. vii–x. NIH Publication NO95–3756.
14. National Institutes of Health: Office of Research on Women's Health Office. *Recruitment and Retention of Women in Clinical Studies*. Washington, DC: U.S. Department Health and Human Services Public Health Service, 1995. National Institutes of Health Publication NO95-3756.
15. The Institute of Medicine: Committee on the Ethical and Legal Issues Relating to the Inclusion of Women and Clinical Trials. *Women and Health Research: Ethical and Legal Issues of Including Women in Clinical Studies*, Vol. 1, A.C. Mastroianni, R. Faden and D. Federman, eds. Washington, DC: Institute of Medicine, National Academy Press, 1994.
16. American Medical Association, Council on Ethical and Judicial Affairs, *Code of Medical Ethics: Current Opinions with Annotations*. 150th Anniversary Edition. Chicago, IL: American Medical Association, 1997.
17. American Medical Association, Council of Ethical and Judicial Affairs, "Gender Discrimination in the Medical Profession,"in *Code of Medical Ethics* IV:2 (1994): 127–139.
18. Eugene Garver, "Margins of Precision—Response to the Essay: Point of View Bias and Insight," *Journal of Thought* 23 (1988): 139–155.
19. Loretta M. Kopelman, "Case Method and Casuistry: The Problem of Bias," *Theoretical Medicine* 15 (1994): 22–37.
20. Gordon W. Allport, *The Nature of Prejudice*. Redding, MA: Addison-Wesley Publishing Company, 1976 (first published in 1954).
21. Judith A. Barden, "Surgical Career and Female Doctors," *Lancet* 340 (1992): 56.
22. Nish Chaturvedi and Allyson Pollock, "Surgical Careers and Female Doctors," *Lancet* 340 (1992): 56–57.
23. J. R. Benson, "Surgical Careers and Female Students," *Lancet* 339 (1992): 1361.
24. Edmund D. Pellegrino and David C. Thomasma, *The Virtues in Medical Practice*. New York: Oxford University Press, 1993.

25. Loretta M. Kopelman and M.G. Palumbo, "The U.S. Health Delivery System: Inefficient and Unfair to Children," *American Journal of Law and Medicine* 23 (1977): 319–337.

26. Miriam Komaromy, Nicole Jurie, and Andrew B. Bindman, "California Physicians' Willingness to Care for the Poor," *Western Journal of Medicine* 162 (1995): 127–32.

27. Stanley J. Reiser, "The Ethical Life of Health Care Organizations," *Hastings Center Report* 24 (1994): 28–35.

28. Roger J. Bulger and Christine K. Cassel, "Health Care Delivery: Health Care Institutions," in *Encyclopedia of Bioethics*, 2nd ed., Warren T. Reich, ed. New York: Macmillan, 1995, pp. 1046–1049.

29. Vanessa Northington Gamble, "A Legacy of Distrust: African Americans and Medical Research," *American Journal of Preventive Medicine* 9 (1993): 35–38.

30. Thomas A. LaVeist, "Beyond Dummy Variables and Sample Selection: What Health Services Researchers Ought to Know About Race as a Variable," *Health Services Research* 29 (1994): 1–16.

31. David R. Williams, "The Concept of Race in Health Services Research: 1966–1990," *Health Services Research* 29 (1994): 261–274.

14

Self-Regulation of Surgical Practice and Research

R. SCOTT JONES
JOHN C. FLETCHER

The ethical basis of self-regulation in the profession of medicine is our main subject, especially as understood in surgical practice and research. We must first persuade readers that self-regulation is ethically justified, because professions, as Buchanan[1] shows, "are social constructs, not facts of nature." Is it right and good that surgeons regulate and police themselves? Other sections of the chapter discuss self-regulation in the context of overlapping spheres of accountability and as applied to selected clinical topics.

Surgeons belong to the medical profession, which is supposed to be guided by its own ideal norms and values.[2] Buchanan[1] sets forth five elements of an "ideal" conception of profession: special knowledge of a practical sort; a commitment to preserve and enhance that knowledge; a commitment to excellence in the practice of the profession; an intrinsic and dominant commitment to serving others rather than personal gain; and effective self-regulation by the professional group. To be effective, practices of self-regulation should develop loyalty to these ideals and define standards of competence for members of the profession, means of developing loyalty to these standards, and sanctions (including expulsion from the profession) to ensure compliance with these standards.

Buchanan further identifies a "sociological" concept of a profession with three main elements: special status (public acknowledgement of worth, marks of prestige, etc.); special privileges, including financial (public subsidies for training and education and insulation from economic competition); and a large sphere of professional autonomy (substantial freedom from external regulation of the main activity). He points out that professions that embody these characteristics are "socially constructed inequalities" and may therefore be questioned and evaluated as to the actual good that they do for society. He argues persuasively that a simple argument from expertise is neither a necessary nor sufficient justification for such a favored position. Physicians and surgeons could be regulated externally. Why should society permit them such a large sphere of professional autonomy? Buchanan further notes that there is no necessary connection between the ideal elements and the favored economic position of medical professionals.

In this vein, social critics of medicine have challenged the integrity of self-regulation, as well as the authenticity of the claim that physicians and surgeons belong to a profession, especially if that claim is evaluated against the evidence of a service commitment. For example, Berlant[3] examined the progress of organized medicine in Great Britain and the United States in the light of Weber's theory of professionalization as a form of monopolization. In 1975, he concluded that self-regulation and medical ethics were mere artifacts of a powerful merchant guild's need to protect its social and economic status. In his view, self-regulation and medical ethics are the "emperor's clothes" or evidence of the fox guarding the henhouse. Is the practice of self-regulation ethically justified, or is it a device that simply serves the collective self-interest of surgeons and other physicians?

Buchanan's[1] more recent challenge is to the ethical justification of the profession of medicine as a "socially constructed inequality" deserving of high status and income. Buchanan argues that, if the performance of U.S. physicians is measured against the ideal norms of a profession and especially the norm of a service commitment, a reasonable person would see the "myth of professionalism" thoroughly exploded. His moral and political data include medicine's monopoly on licensure, opposition to periodic relicensing, anemic response to self-referral, and organized political opposition to health care reform. Using a "social bargain" approach to the question, he concludes that the costs to society of giving physicians high privileges of professionalism presently outweigh the benefits to society. He makes several suggestions to promote a fairer social bargain, including the improvement of self-regulation and external regulation to control conflicts of interest.

Ethical Analysis of Self-Regulation in Surgical Practice

Our response to Berlant is to acknowledge a solid core of truth in the history of organized medicine's collective behavior as a monopoly. The "medical ethics" of the nineteenth and early twentieth centuries was largely a body of guidance reflecting the interests of and ethical conflicts among the members of the profession as such. Our response to Buchanan is to affirm his trenchant criticism, especially of medicine's service commitment to society as a whole and to its neediest members. We welcome his appeal for more effective practices of self-regulation.

We note that profound changes in medicine's recent history are turning the profession toward more reciprocal relationships with other power centers in the society. Socioeconomic, legal, and ethical changes altered the profession's collective power and diversified its scope of ethical reflection.[4,5] Brieger[6] notes that medicine and surgery once had more positive power as well as negative power to prevent unwanted developments in the society. This power has been blunted by change, especially in the last four decades of the twentieth century. We submit that the impact of these changes coupled with more internal reforms in medicine can gradually make the profession of medicine more accountable to society's ethical traditions and laws and to patients and families.[5]

The profession's collective self-interest does influence self-regulation because the economics of practice depends on good standing and recognition of competence. However, self-interest is one force among many others. The interests of government, large and small employers, taxpayers, and third-party insurers today more successfully compete with the political and economic interests of physicians. Although surgeons are in a position to police themselves, other authorities now justifiably share this position. Accountable to one another, surgeons are also answerable to other weighty sources of evaluation and judgment. The central place of outcomes studies and other measures[7] in surgical practice today easily rebuts any claim to exclusive knowledge by surgeons. Exclusivity and secrecy may have marked self-regulation in the past, but such traits cannot survive in today's practice and research environments. These settings are both more open and more economically constrained by third parties.

As a result, self-regulation is now less a creature of a powerful medical monopoly than a complex ethical adaptation of an evolving profession's relationship to society, to government, to patients, and to economic conditions. Surgeons, like other American physicians, are ethically and economically adapting to a changed professional, legal, and economic environment. Furthermore, this process of social change is far from finished. In direct response to Buchanan's challenge, we offer the following ethical framework for self-regulation.

Ethical Framework of Self-Regulation

We view self-regulation in medicine in an ethical framework with three main features: (1) the goal of self-regulation is to inform and maintain professional integrity; (2) four duties of surgeons as physicians inform self-regulation in the service of this goal; and (3) self-regulation maintains professional integrity by methods of accountability that aim to identify causes of errors and ethical lapses and make individual surgeons and group practices answerable to the profession.

Rightly understood, the goal of self-regulation is to inform and maintain professional integrity in and among surgeons as they pursue the larger goals of medicine. Professional integrity encompasses the internal morality of medicine, rather than the whole of medical ethics. Professional integrity has two elements, an objective understanding of and a subjective loyalty to the duties, norms, and values that are internal to medicine as a profession. Professional integrity requires the subordination of personal and economic interests to these duties and the penumbra of norms, values, and virtues that must be learned to be consistently loyal from case to case. Some negative examples are cited below, but actual cases may have complex circumstances.

We follow closely an important discussion of professional integrity by Miller and Brody.[8] They identify four major duties of physicians:

1. To practice competently: A surgeon's primary duty is to practice competently in accord with the goals of medicine. Competence involves scientific, technical, and humanistic knowledge and skills. The humanistic skills include the ability to communicate openly and attentively with patients and family members.

2. To benefit patients and avoid disproportionate harm: The effectiveness of modern medicine, especially surgery, depends on invasive procedures. Patients surrender their bodily integrity and are vulnerable to physicians. Patients also expect some harms in the hope of cure, especially in the context of chemotherapy and surgery. The ethical maxim "Do no harm" is a fundamental ethical rule, applied in proportion to prospect of benefits. The art of clinical judgment builds on technical competence and balances harms to patients with anticipated benefits.

3. To avoid fraudulent misrepresentation of medical knowledge and skills: This duty restrains surgeons from unwarranted deviation from standard surgical practice, focusing on acts that pose as surgical practice but which conflict with the goals of medicine. Fraudulent misrepresentation is different from incompetence, although these may coincide in some cases. For example, a surgeon who performs phalloplasty[9] or breast enlargement for higher income may well be technically competent. But besides violating the rule against unjustified harm and risks, the science and art of medicine is misrepresented. These operations serve no goal of medicine. Also, these operations mislead the public to believe that surgery is proper in circumstances in which it is not.

4. Fidelity to the therapeutic relationship with patients: Fidelity is composed of two companion duties: to respect the trust that is a foundation of a therapeutic surgeon-patient relationship and non-abandonment of patients. Surgical patients are especially vulnerable to the surgeon's authority and power and are often in no position to judge the quality or the necessity of

surgery. Fidelity to patients protects vulnerable patients, and strong professional discipline is required for any surgeon who allows self-interest to overwhelm this duty.

In our framework of self-regulation, these duties have three functions: (1) to inform professional integrity, which is the goal of self-regulation, (2) to govern ethically appropriate means of medical practice, and (3) as resources to specify methods of accountability. This schema of ends, means, and duties requires more explanation and justification.

The Goals of Medicine, Spheres of Accountability, and Self-Regulation

Medicine is a goal-oriented profession. Kass[10] argues that medicine has one overriding and absolute end: healing. His claim is overstated because it is clearly problematic to fit other valid goals of medicine (e.g., prevention and research) under healing. Actual experience recommends viewing medicine as having multiple, complex, and sometimes competing goals: to save life and cure disease; to relieve pain, suffering, and disability; to rehabilitate and restore function; to prevent disease; to improve the quality of living and dying; and to seek new knowledge.

To be ethically praiseworthy, surgeons' conduct must first be an ethically acceptable means toward one or more of these goals. Surgery for phalloplasty or breast enlargement, mentioned above, clearly fails this basic test. Prescribing anabolic steroids for athletes or physician involvement in capital punishment also serve no ethically acceptable goals of medicine.

The profession must be guided by an internal morality as its members pursue the complex goals of medicine. To know and be loyal to the claims of these ethical obligations is to have professional integrity. Physicians are never more ethically authentic than when they reject personal or economic advantage in favor of the claims of their professional duties.

Good medical education and professional socialization provide a practical understanding of the facets of professional integrity. Good clinical supervision of medical students and resident physicians tests their loyalty and personal commitment to medicine's internal norms and values.

Surgeons, as members of the medical profession, strive to meet medicine's goals from within three overlapping spheres of accountability. They are accountable to one another, to patients, and to society for their knowledge of and loyalty to the ethical obligations that inform professional integrity and for their fitness and failures in progress toward the goals of medicine. Each sphere influences and enriches the other two. An account of the integrity of a whole professional life would be inclusive of decisions and actions in these three spheres.

It is important to note, however, that professional integrity does not encompass the entire scope of medical ethics but only that which is internal to medicine. For example, issues of allocation of resources, fair access to basic health care, and considerations that flow from respect for the autonomy of patients belong to larger bodies of social and ethical guidance.

Social ethics makes strong claims on the profession, as well as on other sectors of society,[11,12] for fairness in allocation of resources and access to preventive and primary health care. There is a historic unmet need in the United States for a national health policy to remedy problems of access to primary and preventive care and fairly to ration expensive resources. The results of this unmet need are a threat to professional integrity and the ethical obligation to benefit patients and avoid disproportionate harm. Neglect of national health policy fuels a marketplace revolution in managed health care that, in some forms, undermines the duties of professional integrity by economic incentives to do less for patients, to corporatize medicine,[4] and to weaken teaching and research.[13] Also, the lack of national allocation strategies creates a vacuum in which an individual's claims that there is a positive right to exotic but futile treatments are upheld by courts' interpretation of existing law. The Baby K case is a good example. Federal courts ordered "emergency treatment" for apnea consequent to anencephaly,[14] treatment that conscientious physicians saw as a violation of their professional integrity (see Chapter 9). Would a national allocation policy reflective of the values and preferences of the majority permit treatment in such circumstances?

Surgeons are clearly accountable to one another for their mistakes. Surgical errors and mistakes are a rich arena in which to examine the interface between the duty of fidelity and the claims of larger ethical and legal traditions of informed consent and disclosure. The duty of fidelity in therapeutic relationships requires surgeons to explain both their clinical reasoning on the patient's behalf and their mistakes that impact on the patient's course. The imperatives of informed consent and disclosure are operational throughout the history of a surgical case, not only at the beginning. Brody's[15] discussion of a "transparency standard" that ought to govern the informed consent process can also guide the degree of a surgeon's accountability to patients and families. Discussion of mistakes in mortality and morbidity conferences is incomplete without an account of disclosure to patients or surrogates of how the surgeon disclosed the error to the patient or surrogate and how this information was received and understood. The culture of such conferences needs changing in this regard.

Professional Autonomy and the Obligation of Surgeons to Regulate Themselves

Surgeons pursue the goals of medicine mainly by a combination of intellectual and manual skills. The primary duty of surgeons, as we noted above, is to practice competently. In training and beyond, surgeons must earn and maintain the professional autonomy to decide to operate or to recommend other means of therapy. Professional autonomy is not absolute but contingent on practices of peer review and self-criticism for continuing improvement of intellectual and manual skills. Professional autonomy is also balanced by the autonomous choices of patients, or their surrogates or guardians, to consent to or refuse treatments. Society itself interacts with professional autonomy, in that surgeons are regulated by federal and state laws for licensing, reimbursement from Medicaid and Medicare programs, and so on. Some states require continuing education of all physicians.

Professional accountability for surgeons focuses largely on the operation, which is the defining characteristic of surgical practice, in contrast to medical practice. An operation always poses some risk of disability, suffering, and death in addition to the disease and its natural history. Some operations are called major, some are called minor, but no surgical operation is inconsequential. The surgeon must be professionally autonomous to establish a diagnosis with reasonable certainty, to decide which operation is best, to evaluate the risks and benefits of the proposed operation, to evaluate the fitness of the patient to recover from surgery, and to assess risks and benefits for the short and long terms. Knowing when to avoid or defer an operation often becomes an important part of surgical practice. The success of a surgical operation depends on the surgeon's knowledge, judgment, diagnostic accuracy, and surgical technical skills.

Historical Roots and Development of Self-Regulation. The history of regulation of surgeons dates from antiquity. In ancient Babylon, laws were provided by the king. Law specified compensation for surgical care and also exacted punishments for surgeons whose practice resulted in adverse outcomes. For example, if a patient died following an operation, according to The Code of Hammurabi, one of the surgeon's hands would be cut off. In the Middle Ages, self-regulation was in evidence in guilds that established standards of practice. The guilds evolved into surgical societies throughout Europe—for example, The Royal College of Surgeons of England. The Royal College represented a collaboration between the crown and the profession to establish standards and foster quality care. In the United States the American College of Surgeons was founded in 1913 to foster the ethical practice of surgery based on the scientific method.[16]

Ethical Justification for Self-Regulation. Why is it justified for surgeons and other physicians to regulate themselves? Can regulation be better done by others? We find three sources of the ethical justification of self-regulation. The first source is in actual performance, Are surgeons regulating themselves well enough to merit the trust of the public? How have surgeons performed in this regard? We give some answers under clinical topics below. By historical comparison with the situation as viewed by Berlant until the early 1970's,[3] surgeons and other physicians are now required to reciprocate in many forms of accountability to the profession and to other sources of authority. Surgeons work in increasingly open environments focused on quantitative and qualitative outcomes. Since a surgical operation is an open and definable event, the responsibility of the surgeon in the totality of this event is so clear and precise there is usually no difficulty in linking outcomes of all types with the surgeon.

The second source of ethical justification arises from the fiduciary nature of medicine, in which ethical obligations transcend economic issues. Internalized by individual surgeons, this fiduciary sense shapes and defines the ethical sense of being a professional, over against the stereotype of a surgeon shaped by the marketplace and the merchant guild. There is no empirical way to measure the strength of the fiduciary sense, but we submit that surgeons are much more aware of ethical and legal expectations than in previous generations. Bosk's field study of the moral and social context of surgery was a sign of change and more openness to external evaluation, beginning in the mid-1970s.[17]

The third source of ethical justification for self-regulation arises from combining two reality factors: the vulnerability of patients and the expertise of surgeons. These two factors prompt the conclusion that no others are better situated to protect patients or to identify, prevent, and regulate the causes of harm and danger. Due to the biological, technical, and ethical complexity of surgical operations and to the high personal stakes of all involved, especially the patient, the issue of monitoring or quality control becomes a vital component of surgical care. Who is responsible for ensuring the quality of surgical practice? All of the givers of care bear responsibility but surgeons individually and corporately bear the greatest portion of that responsibility to the patient, to society, and to the medical profession. The concept of "captain of the ship" has its greatest validity as a description of where the brunt of responsibility in doing surgery falls (see Chapter 16).

The obligation of self-regulation stems from necessary experience. Surgeons have the knowledge and experience to analyze surgical outcomes effectively and accurately. No other group can regulate surgical practice truthfully and effectively. Lawyers, ethicists, or administrators cannot police surgeons, even if they desired to do so, although lawyers, ethicists, and administrators can contribute to the climate of self-regulation by their observations and criticisms of the profession.

Clinical Topics

The Impaired Surgeon

The duties to practice competently, to benefit patients, and to avoid disproportionate harm bear strongly on the topic of the impaired surgeon. The added vulnerability of patients in this context calls for utmost vigilance. The term "impaired physician" implies a victim of alcohol or drug abuse, but surgeons can also be impaired by mental or physical disease and injury. There has long been a consensus on the duty of the profession to confront, seek treatment, and restore impaired physicians to practice if possible. Discussing a 1971 Texas statute on the "sick" physician, the AMA Council on Mental Health said:

> The sick doctor statute defines the inability of a physician to practice medicine with reasonable skill and safety to his patients, because of one or more enumerated illnesses. It eliminates the need to allege or prove that a physician's clinical judgment was actually impaired or that he actually injured a patient. The defined inability can be the result of organic illness, mental or emotional disorders, deterioration through the aging process, or loss of motor skill. Further the inability can arise from excessive use or abuse of narcotics, drugs and chemicals, alcohol, or similar types of material.[18]

Springer[19] discusses the legal aspects for the medical staff and hospital in handling impaired physician cases. Who has the obligation to solve or initiate the solution to the problem? In the case of substance abuse, mental disease, emotional or character disorders, and the impairments of age, the responsible individuals depend on the specific work environment. No surgeon works alone. In an academic or teaching institution, professional hierarchies exist and a person (department head, division chief, etc.) is charged with such responsibilities. In private or community hospitals, members of the medical staff bear general responsibility for recognizing and dealing with impaired colleagues. Hospitals also have staff organizations to deal with issues of its members' competence. In group practices, the members of the group are responsible to detect and deal with impaired colleagues. Also the problem should be referred to the hospital medical staff, the state or country medical society, and finally to the state licensing body. Most states, according to Springer,[19] have reporting statutes requiring that suspicion be reported to the licensing body or the state medical society's impaired physician program. Following due process and a hearing, the licensing body may suspend the license and institute probation. In many cases, however, spouse, family, and close friends can aid the impaired surgeon to seek treatment. The license can be reinstated when he or she can demonstrate renewed competence to practice.

The Surgeon Who Should Retire

Federal law prohibits discriminatory hiring or firing because of age. Increasing age limits the effectiveness of surgeons because of loss of stamina, mental acuity, and cognitive skills. Unfortunately, these disabilities occur insidiously and their age of onset is highly variable. When a surgeon should retire becomes a matter of personal choice and of leadership by others (e.g., partners, department chairman, dean, hospital director). Interestingly, data from the American College of Surgeons show the average retirement age for general surgeons in the United States is 62.5 years. The decision of when a surgeon should retire is made difficult by the absence of legal definition and arbitrary retirement criteria such as age. Practically, retirement is dictated by the individual's choice, by gentle persuasion of professional leaders (e.g., department chairman) or by documentation of impaired competence. Clinical outcome data could be used to decide retirement. It is possible that elderly surgeons could properly delay retirement by performing simple procedures that are less taxing of skill, judgment, and stamina. The incompetent but unimpaired young surgeon must be identified by peer review, or outcome measures. The incompetent surgeon must have clinical privileges restricted or withdrawn. There have been instances in which surgeons have been asked to take remedial training. The profession has not organized remedial programs in a systematic manner.

Peer Review

The ethical basis of peer review is grounded in the first three duties of physicians. Peer review involves various methods of accountability. For surgeons, these methods focus mainly on the deaths and complications that accompany their operations. The preponderance of postoperative deaths and complications are due to the patient's prior condition. However, the error rate in hospitals and in surgery is high. A study of randomly selected medical records found that nearly 4% of 30,121 patients in 51 acute care hospitals in New York State were iatrogenically injured in one year, and nearly 14% of these injuries were fatal.[20] Close to half (48%) of the adverse events found in the entire study were linked to an operation. Technical error in performance of operations caused the majority of surgery-related adverse events, and negligence, defined as occurring when "the degree of error exceeds an accepted norm," accounted for 17% of these events. The study identified types of errors as (1) performance (technical error), (2) prevention (errors of omission), (3) diagnostic (failure to use indicated tests), (4) drug treatment (error in dose or method of use), and (5) system (defective equipment, supplies, inadequate training, etc.)

Our views draw on Leake's[21] lucid discussion of error in medicine and preventive strategies. He makes a telling criticism of the socialization process in medicine and its ideal of "error-free practice." Infallibility is unrealistic and promotes secrecy about mistakes. Leake notes that "all humans err frequently. Systems that rely on error-free performance are doomed to fail." Much earlier, McIntyre and Popper[22] pointed to negative consequences of the need to be infallible: intellectual dishonesty and covering up mistakes. Preventive approaches using techniques adapted from Total Quality Management, discussed below, are indicated. Honesty and forgiveness of error reduce its incidence. In this context, fallibility is not a source of shame but a resource for improvement. Patients also need information about their vulnerability in the hospital setting.

For reasons of professional integrity, especially in terms of fidelity to patients, we strongly advocate open disclosure by physicians to patients or their surrogates of the cause of injuries attributable to technical error or medical management. The case for disclosure assumes that the adverse event causes measurable disability or negatively affects the patient's course of illness or recovery. The therapeutic relationship with patients is grounded in fidelity and trust. Adverse events of consequence must be disclosed to patients to sustain trust. Disclosure also exposes and educates about fallibility and vulnerability. In our view, if errors have no negative impacts, disclosure is optional. One can be so compulsive about disclosure of inconsequential errors as to encourage mistrust.

The most egregious failures in surgery are not heeding the patient's signs and symptoms, or failure to see and evaluate the patient personally and regularly. These are "normative errors," as defined by Bosk as occurring ". . . when a surgeon has, in the eyes of others, failed to discharge his role obligations conscientiously."[17] A normative error occurs whenever a surgeon allows personal interests to supersede the primacy of the surgeon-patient relationship and the surgeon's total responsibility for a given patient. Such errors include failure to stay abreast of a patient's condition, being absent at an important time or event in a patient's illness, or placing personal convenience or negotiable family obligations above responsibilities to patients. In our framework of professional integrity the surgeon has duties not to abuse the trust of the physician-patient relationship and not to abandon patients. Our list also includes failure to improve in interpersonal relations, failure to work effectively with colleagues, nurses, and other technicians, or dishonesty in any task related to surgery and patient care. The remedies for such serious errors occur in sincere acceptance of responsibility and distinct changes in self-awareness and behavior. Failure to accept responsibility and improve in these matters should be cause for reprimand or dismissal.

Quality, effectiveness, and cost of health care depend on systems and on individuals, in this case, surgeons. Systems and surgeons can be monitored and reviewed by statistical methods. Peer review involves evaluation of surgeons by other doctors, usually other surgeons. Peer review may involve one or more of such approaches as retrospective medical record review, direct observation of performance, pre-admission certification, and intersurgeon comparison.[23]

The Morbidity and Mortality Conference is a traditional method of peer review in surgery. Conducted properly, it provides an excellent opportunity for professional self-regulation. To be effective, all surgical deaths and complications must be on the agenda and discussed forthrightly. All participants should be able to ask questions. Ideally, the discussion should be closed by the surgeon who was responsible for the particular case. Such conferences require probing honesty and sensitivity to emotionally charged statements. The conference is an effective and important teaching vehicle for practicing surgeons and trainees. By its mere existence, the conference heightens surgeons', surgery residents', and students' awareness. They realize in advance that if there is an adverse outcome, they will have to explain to their peers what they did and why. It should be possible to study whether and how an effective weekly conference improves quality of care in a hospital.

The weaknesses of weekly conferences are their nonquantitative process and exclusive focus on individuals and their acts rather than on root causes. Cases are discussed but information tends not to be recorded, analyzed, tabulated, or evaluated in any other way. Conferences tend also to be anecdotal experiences and do not relate frequencies of complications to any standards or benchmarks. As a result, even though detailed minutes are recorded, no meaningful quantitative memory of the events remains. These drawbacks suggest that the contribution of total quality management and continuous quality improvement is important.

Another *structured* means of self-regulation and quality control is an effectively operating Tissue Committee. The systematic correlation of pathologic findings with the operation and its outcome provide an effective mechanism for self-regulation and quality control. Peer review in surgery also occurs in informal consultation and discussion of cases with colleagues.

Total Quality Management and Continuous Quality Improvement

Total quality management (TQM) and continuous quality improvement (CQI) refer to concepts and processes developed by Deming. Deming was educated as a mathematician and a physicist but subsequently studied statistics. He ultimately developed statistical methods to apply to quality control. In the 1980s, American industry began to employ his techniques and many large corporations presently adhere to TQM and CQI. In the late 1980s, he suggested that his methods should be applied to American health care and since 1988 many hospitals and practice organizations have implemented these techniques.[7,24]

The cornerstone of Deming's concept is the application of statistical theory, methods, and control processes to the improvement of quality. Deming developed methods for observing variance in many parameters of industrial production. He found that by observing variance and reasons for it that reduction of variance enhanced performance quality.

TQM and CQI as applied to the hospital surgical service or to a department of surgery will provide statistical control of 85% of the important variability in quality of surgical services. The use of protocols, guidelines, and critical pathways with prospectively established control levels of variability will establish, maintain, and improve the quality of the service and the care provided to patients. Furthermore, as an added feature, the improved quality of the care will reduce the cost of the care. However, 15% of the quality improvement process is dependent on the behavior of individuals, so that the practice of individual surgeons must undergo scrutiny as well.[23]

To show how peer review could be improved by objectivity, Scher and Scott-Conner[25] conducted a study of 1,500 consecutive abdominal operations performed by general surgeons working at three hospitals in a single community. They developed an outcome profile for each surgeon that was compared statistically to the cumulative profile of the surgical community. They adjusted for variations in physiological status of the patients and the clinical circumstances. They were able to identify outlying performers whose results were significantly different from the rest of the surgical community and could not be explained on the basis of case mix or complexity of procedures. It is therefore possible to develop valid statistical comparisons of individual surgeons' outcomes profiles with colleagues and the prospect of using this methodology may be preferable to the usual retrospective review of deaths and complications. One disadvantage is the time and effort to accumulate and analyze the data. Hospitals must be committed to this process and provide the resources. Accordingly, the University Hospital Consortium is developing methodologies to monitor the outcomes of individual practitioners and their participating hospitals. Statistical methods will allow comparison of an individual with other surgeons in the same hospital or with the entire group and also allow for observation of interhospital variability.

Credentialing for New Procedures

We should initially consider the meanings of the terms certification, credentials, competence, and clinical privileges. Most surgical education and formal training is documented by issuing certificates to those who have successfully completed such training. An individual surgeon's credentials consist of an enumeration of educational or training experiences as well as previous professional performance and work history. Most surgeons therefore possess credentials consisting of a medical school diploma, a residency training certificate, and a specialty board certificate. While credentials are important, indeed essential, they do not always assure clinical competence. Competence refers to an acceptable level of skill to provide comprehensive patient care and, in the case of surgery, to perform technical procedures of specific types.[26]

Although boards can issue certificates, oversight for competence becomes the responsibility of medical staffs and ultimately a matter of peer assessment.[23] Hospitals and clinics grant clinical privileges. Clinical privileges ideally should be awarded on the basis of credentials as well as assessments of clinical competence.[27] Some hospitals grant privileges provisionally for a period of observation until full privileges can be earned.

Technical components of medicine and surgery continue to change rapidly. New procedures are introduced as others become obsolete. Technical change requires that surgeons continue to upgrade their knowledge and skills to remain competent. For example, in 1989, DuBois and others[28] showed that cholecystectomy could be performed laparoscopically and that the laparoscopic technique had many advantages. Very few surgeons who performed cholecystectomy had knowledge or skill in laparoscopy. A great conflict ensued, because there were limited resources at the time for all surgeons in the United States to learn laparoscopic techniques. The new procedure was quickly adopted by residency training programs. However, those trainees would not be available to practice for several years, assuring a short supply of trained surgeons for this procedure. Consequently, training programs developed throughout the country to teach practicing surgeons the techniques of laparoscopy and how to perform laparoscopic cholecystectomy. These courses included didactic material and hands-on use of the instruments in an animal laboratory. Many hospitals also required a period of proctoring by an individual familiar with the procedure.

The surgical profession must take the lead in providing advice and educational opportunities for surgeons to learn new procedures. The introduction of laparoscopic cholecystectomy caught academic institutions and surgical organizations unprepared. The lessons learned prepared U.S. surgeons to address the introduction of endovascular techniques, ultrasound, and mammographically directed core needle biopsy into surgical practice. The development of advanced laparoscopic techniques and technology and the development of robotics will provide additional challenges for the near future.

Whether technology will permit a surgeon to operate on a patient at a remote site remains to be seen. The ethical conflicts for the physician-patient relationship, preservation of trust, and physicians' professional and legal accountability may present more daunting challenges than the technological.

Self-Regulation in Surgical Research

Professional Integrity: Honesty and Fairness in Research

Surgical research is a branch of the larger community of science.[29] The values, norms, and practices of biomedical research are informed by that community's systematic ethical reflection in reciprocity with broader ethical and legal traditions[30] (see Chapter 12). However, wherever surgical research is done by physicians, especially involving their patients, the sources for professional integrity are also informative and morally binding. Whenever physicians engage in research, they stand within dual sources of ethical guidance. As scientists, surgeons share in a tradition of self-regulation to monitor and maintain ethical integrity of the conduct of research and publication of findings. As physicians, a commitment to submit all aspects of medical practice to tests of evidence is the ideal pathway to avoid fraudulent misrepresentation of medical knowledge and skills. As in the practice of surgery, self-regulation in research is justified because researchers are best situated and competent to detect misconduct in research. Researchers are the best "whistle-blowers," that is, one who alleges ethical violations in research to his or her employer, to a governmental body, to a professional society, or to the general public.[31]

The tradition of self-regulation in research is grounded in two ethical principles that inform the ends and means of seeking new knowledge. Truthfulness is required in collecting, managing, and reporting research data. If parts of the scientific record are untrustworthy, many errors will ensue and eventually persons and society itself will be harmed. The second principle is fairness in dealings with colleagues, trainees, and the peer review process of science and the institutions that support research. These two principles guided the reflections and recommendations of the Commission on Research Integrity,[32] created by Congress in 1993.

Challenges to Self-Regulation in Research

Self-regulation in research has been sharply criticized and partly reformed in the United States for two main reasons. The first was strong evidence that "whistle-blowers" suffered harm or ruin to their professional careers.[32,33] A second was the lack of an impartial institutional process to investigate allegations of scientific misconduct. Prior to the 1980s, the authority figure in charge of the laboratory was generally the judge and jury. Biased and personalistized motives intruded. Levine recalled that "most scientists thought that anyone who faked data had to be crazy."[30] If the authority figure had a strong investment in the career of an offender, impartiality suffered, as Braunwald[34] acknowledges in his reflections on a famous case. The better alternative today is inquiry by a non-involved peer group[35] with the prerogative of enlisting its own consultants.

Local self-regulation by peers in science is now coupled with federal oversight[36] and a bureaucracy to oversee local investigations. Congress and federal agencies have reformed the tradition of self-regulation into a quasi-legal process. Universities receiving federal funds are required to have procedures for internal investigations that must be reported to an oversight agency in the Public Health Service, the Office of Research Integrity (ORI). The accused have the right of legal counsel during formal hearings, should an investigation reach that stage. The ORI has authority to conduct its own investigations. The severity of the violation determines a variety of outcomes; for example, reprimand, suspension from scientific activities and grant applications for a period, loss of employment, or in the worst case, prosecution under federal fraud statutes. Surgical researchers should be thoroughly familiar with the policy and practices of their institution in this regard.

Reforming self-regulation is controversial in the scientific community.[37] The incidence of actual misconduct, as opposed to reported cases, is hard to ascertain. Scientists debate the severity of the problem and disagree on definitions of scientific misconduct. This debate should not detract from the richness of the topic of research integrity.

What topics and ethical concepts should senior investigators cover with trainees in surgical research? An adequate course[38] will cover at least these topics: types of research misconduct; data management; publication practices and authorship; conflicting loyalties to science and industry; ethical issues in clinical and epidemiological research; rules of confidentiality governing peer review of privileged information; and the process for reporting allegations of misconduct. Ethical concepts include the veracity and public trust on which science depends, practices of voluntary informed consent or "waived consent" under specific conditions in human investigations, and methods of risk/benefit analysis.

Have surgical researchers maintained research integrity? ORI investigations are made public. Only one U.S. surgeon, Dr. Anand Tewari,[39] has been found to have violated research integrity by fabricating ophthalmologic examination results and falsifying test results in clinical research. He was disqualified from applying for federal research grants or contracts and from participation in peer review activities for a period of five years. A Canadian surgeon, Dr. Roger Poisson,[40] intentionally falsified patient records and reports over several years to make subjects eligible for inclusion in the NIH-supported National Surgical Adjuvant Breast and Bowel Project. This controversy had large repercussions in the National Institutes of Health and in Congress.[41]

How Can Research Misconduct Be Prevented?

There is evidence that the pressure to publish, associated with one's status in science as well as promotion and advancement in academic medicine, is a strong influence on research fraud. In several scandals in the 1980s, the violators worked in laboratories whose chiefs had prolific publications but low participation on many papers co-authored with junior faculty members. Woolf[42] documents this source of pressure. Pollock and others[43] conducted a study of NIH T32 surgical investigators with a control group. The questionnaire included a section on expectations of productivity. Both groups of trainees felt unhealthy pressure to publish research findings rapidly as well as to secure funding early in their careers. However, a majority in both groups did not understand the level of research productivity expected of them by authorities.

The pressure to publish will continue but must be countered by professional norms. The crux of the issue is never the number of publications but whether the individual's research is at a stage of fruition when publication is timely and appropriate. Caution in regard to the scientific maturity and integrity of the research project is the greatest protection against a rush to publication that may induce ethically unacceptable ways to speed the process. Discussion of the options with a senior researcher not directly involved in the project and with the mentor can prevent mistakes. Promotion committees can strengthen these precautions by reassuring candidates that the quality of their research rather than the quantity is the basis for judgment and make this policy actual practice. Rhetoric without action in this area will breed a cynicism corrosive of professional integrity. The committee can also limit the number of articles for submission to a specific number, as do many institutions today, but not all.

Ethical conflicts about authorship can be prevented. Writing and revising a scientific paper should actively involve each author. Each should be prepared to defend her or his specific contribution to the research and to the publication. Each should be generally familiar with the contributions of co-authors. The laboratory chief should have the opportunity to review each manuscript prior to initial submission and may wish to examine the data base from which conclusions are drawn, regardless of who is to be listed as senior author. A significant safeguard is to decide place of authorship prior to writing the article and to follow guidelines for ranking authors.

We commend these authorship guidelines:[44]

1. To be listed as first author of an original scientific article, the investigator must (a) have adapted a general hypothesis (his or her own or the senior author's) in a detailed, systematic fashion, down to the actual details of Methods and Materials, (b) have participated in a major way in the analysis and interpretation of data, and (c) have written the paper. It is desirable, but not obligatory, that the first author have also participated substantially in the performance of the research and the data collection.

2. To be listed as a co-author, an investigator must be recognized as an individual who made significant contributions to the planning and execution of the research, the methods and procedures, the collection and analysis of data, and so forth.

3. To be listed last as a senior author, a scientist must (a) have either formulated the original general hypotheses or have provided significant intellectual resources for the work, (b) have provided constructive criticism of the paper during and/or after its composition, (c) accept overall responsibility for all the findings of the final version of the paper and for the order of authorship, and (d) have provided the laboratory space and/or the finances for the experiment.

Responsibilities of the Senior Investigator. The senior or principal investigator has primary responsibility for the design and conduct of a research project and the competence to carry it out or to supervise those who will do so. In this role, she or he has five major duties prior to the beginning of the research itself. The first duty is to ascertain that all other investigators are sufficiently competent to carry out their roles in the study. Additional training of junior investigators may be necessary in the prelude period to the actual study. The codes of Nuremberg and Helsinki[45] stress the issue of competence; however, the senior investigator is the arbiter of this question. The second duty is to ascertain the soundness of the scientific design of the study to answer the study's questions. If the design is flawed, subjects will be taking risks for unjustifiable reasons. The third duty is to lead in creating a written protocol that justifies and explains the research plan along with a thorough risk-benefit assessment of the subjects' participation. The writing of the protocol is an exacting scientific and ethical task. Randomization must be ethically justified in each instance. Seeking opinion or review from peers in and outside the institution is an important standard. The fourth duty is to interact and cooperate with the Institutional Review Board's (IRB) ethical and legal duty to assess the risks to subjects and their rights and welfare. The final duty is to act as the responsible party for the quality of informed consent of prospective subjects. The Nuremberg Code stipulates that the determination of the quality of consent rests with "each individual who initiates, directs, or engages in the experiment" and cannot be delegated to others. This imperative translates into a duty of the senior investigator, who might delegate the task of obtaining consent to another qualified colleague, but who cannot escape the ethical responsibility for its quality. In practical terms, the senior investigator is required to train and monitor any others who conduct the consent process. The senior investigator and the IRB may collaborate on accountability methods in some instances. For example, we favor the use of qualified consent auditors to ascertain the integrity of consent or substituted judgment of legally authorized representatives or surrogates in studies that involve cognitively impaired subjects.

Testing Medical Devices. A medical device is a diagnostic or therapeutic article that does not achieve any of its principal intended purposes through chemical action within or on the body. Such devices include diagnostic test kits, imaging equipment, electrodes, pacemakers, arterial grafts, intraocular lenses, orthopedic pins, artificial joints, or other orthopedic equipment.[46]

The 1976 Medical Device Amendments give the Food and Drug Administration (FDA) authority to assure safety and effectiveness in devices intended for human use before they are placed on the market. Surgical researchers and IRB members should be thoroughly familiar with the terms of art regarding medical devices. An ethical and regulatory distinction is made between a "significant" and "nonsignificant" risk device. *Significant* means one that presents a potential for serious risk to the health, safety, or welfare of a subject and is intended as an implant, is used in supporting or sustaining human life, and/or is of substantial importance in diagnosis, curing, mitigating, or preventing impairment of human health.[47] Insignificant risk devices, such nonsterile tongue depressors and cotton swabs, are exempt from FDA clearance. Others, such as surgical staples, require clearance through determining that they are substantially equivalent to predecessor devices.

The manufacturer and the IRB must decide whether the device to be tested is a significant or insignificant risk device. Testing of an insignificant risk device can proceed without FDA knowledge. A significant risk device requires an Investigational Device Exemption (IDE) from the FDA to test it. Disagreements about risk levels appear to be frequent in testing medical devices. Sherertz and Streed[48] give an account of a confusing and stressful experience in a trial of three urinary catheters in which there was disagreement between the sponsor and the FDA about the risk involved. Representatives of the FDA[49] comment and advise about medical device testing in this context. In 1994, the Office of Inspector General found serious problems in clinical testing in four investigational devices, including two used in surgery.[50]

The conduct of ethically acceptable research and development of medical devices is a complex confluence of business ethics and research ethics. Samuel[51] describes ten stages of the development of a medical device, but surgeons will typically be mainly involved at the stage of clinical trials for FDA approval.

Use of Animals

The use of animals in research, including surgical research, has for centuries been a subject of ethical debate. Researchers need to know this history and the arguments on various sides of the debate.[52] Bulger[53] gives the scientist's perspective, based largely on the benefits for human beings, society, and animals that come from research. The clinical benefits of animal research are especially clear in surgery, for example, in cardiovascular surgery and transplantation.[54]

Singer,[55] Regan,[56] and Rollin[57] are contemporary philosophers who have mounted a sustained and effective critique of the use and abuses of animals in research. Their arguments were informed by an imperative to reduce suffering, a theory of animal rights, and the view that most animals have a biologically determined nature that is entitled to respect. Other philosophers,[58] legal scholars,[59] and veterinarians[60] take a critical but more moderate position, that supports an ethically justified use of animals in the goals of medicine. In this view, animals are not understood to be equal to human beings in terms of rights but have shared interests that must be taken seriously from a moral point of view. Because animals have a capacity to suffer pain and loss of natural habitat, it is in their interest to avoid or minimize pain and suffering and cruel forms of confinement and abuse during periods of experimentation. This position places the burden of proof on researchers for the uses they propose to make of animals. It is also the position that is currently supported by federal law and regulation. Since 1985, federal law[59] has required that experiments involving virtually all species of animals receive prior approval by institutional animal care and use committees, which have functions and goals similar to those of institutional review boards. The most important ethical issues addressed in this context are the necessity for the proposed research, its nature, duration, effects, and management of pain. The senior investigator should take the lead in the assessment of these matters and see to it that regulations regarding the use of animal subjects are followed.

Clinical Conclusions

This chapter has reviewed why and how the tradition of self-regulation is ethically justified in the practice of surgery and in surgical research. In concluding, we begin with two particular areas of clinical practice that have a strong impact on this tradition: managed care and peer review. We also make concluding comments on issues in surgical innovation and institutional practices of protecting whistle-blowers and investigations of allegations of research misconduct.

Spiraling costs have led to marketplace regulation of medical and surgical practice in the form of managed care.[13] Although managed care may reduce costs and increase efficiency of health care, it can create at least three serious ethical conflicts. The first is that particular clinical judgments can be compromised or set aside by techniques and practices of utilization review. Our discussion of professional integrity and patient-centered accountability is ethically relevant to this conflict. Surgeons should be advocates for their patients in every model of health care reimbursement. Use of the appeals process and unrelenting commitment to the patient's best interest is the best interim strategy in such conflicts.

The second conflict is that some managed care organizations seeking profit enroll the healthiest patients and exclude the most vulnerable. The claims of social justice on the profession of medicine require reforms of access that will not be resolved by managed care. All physicians have an interest in extending the benefits of contemporary medicine to the greatest number.

A third serious issue for surgical research is managed care's lack of contribution to new knowledge. Managed care benefits from society's investment in clinical research but tends to provide little funding for new knowledge and technology. Collective action by organized medicine and state and federal legislatures will be necessary to go to the root causes of these problems.

Traditional forms of peer review like the Mortality and Morbidity Conference will continue, but the tradition can be enriched by the techniques of TQM and

CQI as applied to surgical services and its component parts and processes. A quantitative profile of individual surgeons, prospectively collected and contemporaneously analyzed, will allow optimal monitoring and improvement in the quality of surgical care.

The evolution of laparoscopic cholecystectomy revealed the need for standards and guidelines.[26] The American College of Surgeons developed guidelines[61] on introducing new technologies and the evaluation of credentials in this context. The statement stressed that any new technology should proceed through a series of steps to ensure safety, appropriateness, and cost effectiveness. These points were made: (1) new technology must be accompanied by scientific assessment of safety, general efficacy, and need; (2) diffusion into clinical practice requires appropriate education of surgeons and evaluation of their use of new technology and in-depth knowledge of the relevant disease and its management gained through formal training and clinical experience as a prerequisite; acquisition of new technical skills and the development of appropriate support facilities must follow and must be subject to initial assessment and periodic monitoring of outcome; and (3) widespread application of new technologies must be continuously assessed and compared with alternative therapies to ensure appropriateness and cost-effectiveness through outcome studies.

To evaluate credentials of individuals for the purpose of awarding surgical privileges in new technologies, the guidelines are (1) the surgeon must be a member in good standing of the department or service from which the privileges are to be recommended; (2) a defined educational program in the technology, including didactic and practical elements must be completed and documented either as a post-residency course of instruction or as a component of an approved residency program; (3) the surgeon must be qualified, experienced, and knowledgeable in the management of the diseases for which the technology is applied; (4) the qualifications of the surgeon to apply the new technology must be assessed by a surgeon who is qualified and experienced in the technology and should result in a written recommendation to the department or service head; in the case of a resident trained in the technology during residency, recommendation by the program director is acceptable; and (5) maintenance of skills should be documented through periodic outcome of assessments and evaluation in association with the regular renewal of surgical privileges.

The Commission on Research Integrity[32] made several important recommendations for new federal regulations to protect whistle-blowers. Institutions need not wait for final regulations to make improvements. The better to protect whistle-blowers, institutions should anticipate these measures: (1) defining retaliation by an individual or institution against a whistle-blower as "prohibited obstruction of investigations of research misconduct" and investigating accordingly; (2) defining the whistle-blower's obligation to respect institutional rules of confidentiality; (3) providing whistle-blowers with an opportunity to defend themselves in a proceeding where they can present witnesses and confront those they charge with retaliation against them; (4) responding to allegations in a timely way; and (5) crediting promptly those whose allegations are substantiated and being prepared to reprimand those who make allegations in bad faith.

In terms of institutional policy for the process of inquiry and investigation into scientific misconduct, the Commission stressed the value of (1) mediation by an ombudsman from inside or outside the institution who is independent of the dispute, (2) institutional procedures that are accessible from multiple entry points, (3) oversight by individuals or by committees whose members are free from bias and conflict of interest—for example, *at least one person who is not from the institution in which the allegation arose should be included in the investigation phase*, (4) the independence of the investigation, (5) oversight by bodies that are separated in their investigatory and adjudicatory functions, (6) balancing advocacy, (7) capacity to prevent retaliation against participants, and (8) openness, wherever possible. Our impression from the available literature on the subject[62,63] and the Commission's proceedings[32] is that there is wide variation among institutions as to the quality and impartiality of practices.

References

1. Allan E. Buchanan, "Is There a Medical Profession in the House?" in *Conflicts of Interest in Clinical Practice and Research*, Roy G. Speece, Jr., David S. Shimm, and Allen E. Buchanan, eds. New York: Oxford University Press, 1996, pp. 105–136.
2. David T. Ozar, "Profession and Professional Ethics," in *Encyclopedia of Bioethics*, 2nd ed., Warren T. Reich, ed. New York: Macmillan, 1995, pp. 2103–2111.
3. Jeffrey L. Berlant, *Profession and Monopoly: A Study of Medicine in the United States and Great Britain*. Berkeley, CA: University of California Press, 1975.
4. Paul Starr, *The Social Transformation of American Medicine*. New York: Basic Books, 1982.
5. David Rothman, *Strangers at the Bedside*. New York: Free Press, 1992.
6. Gert H. Brieger, "Medicine as a Profession," in *Encyclopedia of Bioethics*, 2nd ed., Warren T. Reich, ed. New York: Macmillan, 1995, pp. 1688–1695.
7. David Blumenthal and Ann C. Sheck, *Improving Clinical Practice. Total Quality Management and the Physician*. San Francisco, CA: Jossey-Bass, 1995.
8. Franklin G. Miller and Howard Brody, "Professional Integrity and Physician-Assisted Death," *Hastings Center Report* 25 (1995): 8–17.
9. Lisa Bannon, "Growth Industry. How a Risky Surgery Became a Profit-Center for Some L.A. Doctors," *Wall Street Journal*, June 6, 1996: A1.
10. Leon R. Kass, *Toward a More Natural Science*. New York: Free Press, 1985.
11. Tom L. Beauchamp and James F. Childress, *Principles of Biomedical Ethics*, 4th ed. New York, Oxford University Press, 1994.
12. President's Commission for the Study of Ethical Problems in Biomedical and Behavioral Research, *Securing Access to Health Care*. Washington, D.C.: U.S. Government Printing Office, 1985.

13. James C. Thompson, "Seed Corn. Impact of Managed Care on Medical Education and Research," *Annals of Surgery* 223 (1996): 453–463.
14. George J. Annas, "Asking the Courts to Set the Standard of Emergency Care—The Case of Baby K," *New England Journal of Medicine* 330 (1994): 1542–1545.
15. Howard Brody, *The Healer's Power*. New Haven, CT: Yale University Press, 1992.
16. Gert H. Brieger, "The Development of Surgery," in *Textbook of Surgery*, 15th ed., David C. Sabiston, Jr. and H. Kim Lyerly, eds. Philadelphia, PA: W.B. Saunders Company, 1994, pp. 1–15.
17. Charles L. Bosk, *Forgive and Remember*. Chicago, IL: University of Chicago Press, 1979.
18. Council on Mental Health, "The Sick Physician," *Journal of the American Medical Association* 223 (1973): 684–687.
19. Eric W. Springer, "Peer Review/Hospital Privileges/Credentialing," *Legal Medicine* (1994): 57–81.
20. Lucian L. Leake, Troyen A. Brennan, Nan M. Laird, et al., "The Nature of Adverse Events in Hospitalized Patients: Results of the Harvard Medical Practice Study," *New England Journal of Medicine* 324 (1991): 377–384.
21. Lucian L. Leake, "Error in Medicine," *Journal of the American Medical Association* 272 (1994): 1851–1857.
22. Neil McIntyre and Karl Popper. "The Critical Attitude in Medicine: The Need for a New Ethics," *British Medical Journal* 287 (1983): 1919–1923.
23. Douglas S. Wakefield and Charles W. Helms, "The Role of Peer Review in a Health Care Organization Driven by TQM/CQI," *Journal on Quality Improvement*, 21 (1995): 227–231.
24. Louis E. Teichholz. "Quality, Deming's Principles and Physicians," *The Mount Sinai Journal of Medicine*, 60 (1993): 350–358.
25. Kenneth S. Scher and Carol E.H. Scott-Conner, "Making Peer Review Statistically Accountable," *The American Journal of Surgery* 17(1996): 441–444.
26. Thomas L. Dent, "Training, Credentialling, and Granting of Clinical Privileges for Laparoscopic General Surgery," *The American Journal of Surgery* 161 (1991): 399–403.
27. Frank C. Wilson, "Credentialing in Medicine," *Annals of Thoracic Surgery* 55 (1993): 1345–1348.
28. F. Dubois, P. Icard, G. Berthelot, and H. Levard, "Coelioscopic Cholecystectomy. Preliminary Report of 36 Cases," *Annals of Surgery* 211 (1990): 60–62.
29. R. T. Mathie and K. M. Taylor, *Principles of Surgical Research*, 2nd ed. Oxford, England: Butterworth-Heinemann, Ltd., 1995.
30. Robert J. Levine. *Ethics and Regulation of Clinical Research*, 2nd ed. New Haven, CT: Yale University Press, 1988, p. 32.
31. President's Commission for the Study of Ethical Problems in Medicine and Biomedical and Behavioral Research, *Whistleblowing in Biomedical Research*. Washington, D.C.: U.S. Government Printing Office, 1992.
32. U.S. Department of Health and Human Services, *Integrity and Misconduct in Research*, Report of the Commission on Research Integrity. Washington, D.C.: U.S. Government Printing Office, 1996.
33. James S. Lubalin, Mary-Anne E. Ardini, and Jennifer L. Matheson, "Consequences of Whistleblowing for the Whistleblower in Misconduct in Science Cases: Final Report," Unpublished. Submitted to ORI by Research Triangle Institute, Contract No. 282-92-0045, October 2, 1995.

34. Eugene Braunwald, "Cardiology: The John Darsee Experience," in *Research Fraud in the Behavioral and Biomedical Sciences*, David J. Miller and Michel Hersen, eds. New York: John Wiley and Sons, 1992, pp. 55–79.

35. Kenneth F. Schaffner, "Ethics and the Nature of Empirical Science," in *Research Fraud in the Behavioral and Biomedical Sciences*, David J. Miller and Michel Hersen, eds. New York: John Wiley and Sons, 1992, pp. 17–33.

36. U.S. Department of Health and Human Services, Public Health Service, "Responsibilities of Awardee and Applicant Institutions for Dealing with and Reporting Possible Misconduct in Science," *Federal Register* 54(151): 32446–32451 (August 8, 1989).

37. Jocelyn Kaiser, "Scientific Misconduct. HHS is Still Looking for a Definition," *Science* 272 (1996): 1735.

38. Robin L. Penslar, *Research Ethics: Cases and Materials*. Bloomington, IN: University of Indiana Press, 1995.

39. Public Health Service, Office of Research Integrity, *Annual Report*, April, 1994. Washington, D.C.: U.S. Government Printing Office: 1995.

40. Public Health Service, Office of Research Integrity, *Annual Report*, September, 1994.

41. Mackenzie Carpenter and Steve Twedt, "Anatomy of a Scandal," *Pittsburgh Post-Gazette* (Dec. 26, 1994): 4–10.

42. Patricia K. Woolf, "Pressure to Publish and Fraud in Science," *Annals of Internal Medicine* 104 (1986): 254–256.

43. Raphael E. Pollack, Steven A. Curley, and Eva Lotzova, "Ethics of Research Training for NIH T32 Surgical Investigators," *Journal of Surgical Research* 58 (1995): 247–251.

44. University of Virginia School of Medicine, *Research Ethics: Guidelines for the Faculty*, August 9, 1994. (unpublished document)

45. "Nuremberg Code," "Declaration of Helsinki," in *Encyclopedia of Bioethics*, 2nd ed., Warren T. Reich, ed. New York: Macmillan, 1995, pp. 2763–2767.

46. Office of Protection from Research Risks, *Protecting Human Research Subjects. Institutional Review Board Guidebook*. Bethesda, MD: National Institutes of Health, 1993, pp. 5–17.

47. U.S. Department of Health and Human Services, Food and Drug Administration, *Investigational Device Exemptions Manual*. Washington, DC: U.S. Government Printing Office, 1992, p. 32. FDA-92-4159.

48. Robert J. Sherertz and Stephen A. Streed, "Medical Devices. Significant vs Insignificant Risk," *Journal of the American Medical Association* 272 (1994): 955–956.

49. Joanne R. Less, Susan Alpert, and Stuart Nightingale, "Institutional Review Boards and Medical Devices," *Journal of the American Medical Association* 272 (1994): 968–969.

50. U.S. Department of Health and Human Services, Office of Inspector General, "Investigational Devices: Four Case Studies," April 1995, OEI-05-94-00100.

51. Frank E. Samuel, Jr., "The Perspective of the Medical Device Industry," in *New Medical Devices*, National Academy of Engineering and Institute of Medicine. Washington, DC: National Academy Press, 1988, pp. 145–150.

52. Tom L. Beauchamp, "Problems in Justifying Research on Animals," in National Institutes of Health, *National Symposium on Imperatives in Research Animal Use: Scientific Needs and Animal Welfare*. Bethesda, MD: NIH Publication No. 85-2746, 1984, pp. 79–94.

53. Ruth Ellen Bulger, "Use of Animals in Experimental Research: A Scientist's Perspective," *Anatomical Record* 219 (1987): 215–220.
54. Lawrence H. Cohn, "Contribution of Animal Research to Progress in Cardiovascular Surgery," in National Institutes of Health, *National Symposium on Imperatives in Research Animal Use: Scientific Needs and Animal Welfare*. Bethesda, MD: NIH Publication No. 85-2746, 1984, pp. 27–38.
55. Peter Singer, *Animal Liberation*. New York: Avon Books, 1975.
56. Tom Regan, *The Case for Animal Rights*. Berkeley. CA: University of California Press, 1983.
57. Bernard E. Rollin, *Animal Rights and Human Morality*. Buffalo, NY: Prometheus Books, 1981.
58. Arthur L. Caplan, "Beastly Conduct: Ethical Issues in Animal Experimentation," *Annals of the New York Academy of Science* 406 (1983): 159–169.
59. Rebecca Dresser, "Assessing Harm and Justification in Animal Research: Federal Policy Opens the Laboratory Door," *Rutgers Law Review* 43 (1988): 723–795.
60. Michael A. Fox, *The Case for Animal Experimentation: An Evolutionary and Ethical Perspective*. Berkeley, CA: University of California Press, 1986.
61. American College of Surgeons, "Statement on Emerging Surgical Technologies and the Evaluation of Credentials," *Bulletin of the American College of Surgeons* 79 (1994): 40–41.
62. Institute of Medicine Committee on the Responsible Conduct of Research, *The Responsible Conduct of Research in the Health Sciences: Report of a Study*. Washington, D.C.: Institute of Medicine, National Academy Press, 1989.
63. National Academy of Sciences Panel on Scientific Responsibility and the Conduct of Research, *Responsible Science: Ensuring the Integrity of the Research Process*, Vol. 1. Washington, D.C.: National Academy Press, 1992.

15

Surgery and Other Medical Specialties

NANCY S. JECKER
MARGARET D. ALLEN

The Tangled Web of Referral Practice

The ethics of relationships among surgeons and other medical specialists is fraught with potential ethical conflicts. As referral specialists, surgeons sometimes find themselves at the center of a tangled web of relationships, composed of multiple medical specialists with overlapping and competing authority, responsibility, and interests. Potential for ethical chaos within these relationships is hardly new; it is apparent both in traditional, fee-for-service and newer, managed care settings (see Chapters 17, 18, and 19). In this chapter, we identify and address ethical issues that arise in relationships among surgeons and medical specialists, particularly referring physicians.

Typically, the referral process functions remarkably well and ethical conflict is avoided. Colleagues properly work up and refer patients, obtain the patient's consent to perform surgery, and at the appropriate juncture the surgeon returns the patient's care to the referring physician. Occasionally, these stable referral patterns become disrupted and conflicts arise. For example, a surgeon functioning within a multispecialty team may disagree with a referring physician regarding a patient's diagnosis and whether or not surgery is medically indicated for the patient's—now corrected—diagnosis. Surgeons working as part of multispecialty teams must tread carefully to maintain collegial relationships. Institutional policies and practices, such as third-party payers, can enhance or frustrate such relationships through rules governing, for example, which health professionals and institutions are authorized to provide the patient's care preoperatively, perioperatively, postoperatively, and long term. Public policies, such as prospective payment for hospitalized Medicare beneficiaries, also affect relationships among surgeons and other medical specialists.

The policies and practices of private payers and managed care organizations (MCOs) exert direct and indirect influences on the relationships among surgeons, referring physicians, and other specialists. Indeed, a major business strategy of MCOs is to manage referral patterns carefully and to control the utilization of expensive resources, such as surgical procedures, especially those that entail hospital admission. For hospitals to survive current market changes, hospital managers and administrators must encourage and discourage various referral patterns in an effort to segment the market to obtain the hospital's economic advantage.

Ethical Analysis

Our ethical critique of the relationships among surgeons and other medical specialists begins by describing the terrain of potential conflicts. We present three typical case scenarios to illustrate the sort of conflicts that can and do arise. General lessons drawn from these illustrations set the stage for presenting an ethical framework to manage conflicts among surgeons and other physicians.

Mapping the Terrain of Potential Ethical Conflicts

The first of our three cases concerns a patient with end-stage heart failure who required a heart transplant. His insurance was through an MCO that covers heart transplants at a local tertiary care center through a "center of excellence" contract. The patient was referred for evaluation to the tertiary care transplant cardiology team, which also runs the tertiary care end-stage heart failure clinic. He was accepted on the heart transplant waiting list, with an estimated wait of several months to a year for an organ to become available. The first ethical problem to arise involved pre-transplant patient management. The tertiary care transplant cardiologists reviewed the patient's medication regimen and determined that his condition was critical, and that his symptoms, quality of life, and perhaps his life expectancy (i.e., chance of dying while on the waiting list) could be improved by admitting him to the hospital, instituting invasive monitoring in the cardiac care unit, and putting him on a different medical regimen. Without adjustment of pulmonary arterial pressures and some determination of the reversibility of pulmonary hypertension the patient could not be transplanted.

The patient's MCO informed the tertiary care team that the patient's care could be handled by the MCO's cardiologist. The referring physician at the MCO agreed to consider the recommendation of the tertiary care transplant cardiologist regarding a new medical regimen for the patient. Nonetheless, the tertiary care transplant cardiologist was concerned that management of the patient by a primary care physician or cardiologist who was not well versed in transplantation might not be as aggressive as that offered by the transplant specialists. Such secondary sequelae of heart failure as pulmonary hypertension might go unrecognized without periodic monitoring. Other potential risks included renal failure or other secondary organ failure, which would preclude a transplant altogether. The tertiary care transplant cardiologist worried that even if the managed care cardiologist recognized potential problems, pressure from the managed care group to control costs might discourage physicians from hospitalizing the patient or instituting early invasive monitoring.

A second ethical problem arose once the patient's medical condition deteriorated. The patient, after waiting for six months for a donated heart, developed worsening heart failure. At this point, both the MCO cardiologist and the transplant cardiologists agreed that the patient should be admitted to an intensive care unit and intravenous inotropic medications instituted. Yet they disagreed about whether the patient should be hospitalized at the MCO contract hospital or at the transplant center. The transplant surgeon believed that, although hospitalization at the transplant center might be a greater cost to the insurer, it would improve the patient's chances of receiving an organ. Should an organ be offered on short notice, a patient in the transplant center could take advantage of this, whereas there might not be time for an ambulance transfer or airlift from the managed care intensive care unit to the tertiary care transplant center. As the patient becomes more critically ill, the risk of destabilization during the transport by ambulance or airlift would become a significant risk. If the patient's condition were to become more critical, his access to specialized care available at the transplant center would also become essential, to prevent him from reaching a point where the transplant itself would become too great a risk and the possibility of transplant might be permanently lost. For example, if this patient were cared for at a transplant center and his condition acutely deteriorated before transplant he could be placed on a life-saving left ventricular assist device, a device unavailable at the managed care hospital.

A third ethical problem concerned responsibility for the patient's long-term care postoperatively. The patient eventually received a heart transplant and was cared for post-transplant by the transplant team at the transplant center. Once discharged, he visited the transplant center twice weekly to be treated for several episodes of rejection and to modify immunosuppressive drugs. Finally, several months after the transplant, the patient's condition stabilized. The MCO stipulated that all further care was now to be provided by the managed care team.

The transplant cardiologist considered whether or not the patient's care should return to the referring cardiologist or primary care physician at the managed care institution; the transplant team was concerned that neither of these physicians had experience prescribing, modifying, or monitoring immunosuppressive drugs. A solution was agreed upon whereby the tertiary care group advised the managed care group on immunosuppression and other transplant-specific issues.

The question of post-transplant management was further complicated by the requirement that all U.S. transplant centers report early and late transplant survival rates to UNOS, the United Network of Organ Sharing, which contracts with the federal government to run the national organ procurement and transplantation network and to keep a national database on all transplanted patients. UNOS publishes a center-specific report, available to the general public, that delineates the early and long-term transplant survival results for every program in the United States for every organ. The government, therefore, holds the transplant team, and not the MCO, responsible for the long-term survival results, which, in turn, are dependent on careful adjustment of immunosuppression medications and detection and treatment of post-transplant complications. These statistics are used not only by patients in helping them choose a transplant center, but also by insurance companies and managed care groups in looking for "centers of excellence" to perform transplant services, as well as in negotiating competitive contracts for other tertiary services, such as end-stage organ failure.

A fourth ethical concern arose when a serious post-transplant complication developed. Two years following the heart transplant, the patient was diagnosed with post-transplant lymphoproliferative disease. This is an unusual form of lymphoma, often Epstein-Barr virus–related, which is unique to transplant recipients. Once diagnosed, the question arose as to who should prescribe the chemotherapy and modulation of the immunosuppressive regimen for this patient. Frequently, this type of lymphoma can be eradicated by careful withdrawal of immunosuppression; however such an approach carries a risk of fatal donor organ rejection under accompanying immunosuppression withdrawal. The MCO argued that having already funded the transplant, such complications could be treated by its oncologists. The transplant team felt strongly that oncologists at the transplant center should manage the patient's care because they were the only oncologists in the region with experience caring for patients with this unusual condition. The transplant team, in addition to feeling personal concern for the patient whom they had transplanted, were concerned about their published survival results and how a potentially preventable late death might affect the viability and public image of their program.

The patient himself wished to receive treatment from subspecialists at the transplant center experienced with his type of disease, and he identified with them as the group of physicians who had treated his previous life-threatening illness. The MCO physician was clearly caught between his role as patient-advocate, favoring referral for tertiary care to the transplant team that he himself had now been involved with for two years in joint management of this patient, and loyalty to his employer, the MCO. An administrative disagreement ensued among the managed care administrators on the one hand, and the patient, managed care physicians, and transplant team, on the other hand, with the latter group *all* favoring referral for tertiary care to the transplant center. The MCO administration was persuaded that, in this unusual situation, a referral to the transplant center was in the patient's best interests. The decision was made to respect the patient's preference and, despite the extra costs involved, the patient was treated by the transplant center oncologists. He recovered from his lymphoma. This case and other similar cases resulted in the transplant team and managed care group working together to develop a policy for transplant patient care that carefully defines the responsibilities of each group.

The next two cases illustrate the complex association between referral patterns, patient care decisions, and shifting responsibilities among medical colleagues. In the second case, a patient was told by her primary care physician that she required heart valve replacement. The primary care physician referred the patient to a well-respected community cardiologist for evaluation. The cardiologist performed two diagnostic tests, an echocardiogram and a cardiac catheterization with left ventriculogram, a dye-based estimation of the amount of valvular leak. Although these tests provided somewhat conflicting results, the cardiologist's opinion was that the patient would be best served by valve replacement at this time. He informed the patient that he would schedule surgery at the tertiary care hospital with a surgeon well-experienced in valvular techniques. The cardiologist called the tertiary care cardiothoracic surgical service, scheduled the patient's surgery with one of the surgeons, arranged for the patient's hospital admission the night before surgery, and forwarded diagnostic test results to the surgeon.

Upon reviewing the diagnostic information and talking with the patient the night before surgery, the surgeon suspected that one of the diagnostic tests, the echocardiogram, had overestimated the extent of valve leakage; the surgeon surmised that in this case, the ventriculogram, which showed only a mild degree of leak, provided a more accurate indication of the patient's status. A tertiary care cardiologist specializing in echocardiography confirmed the surgeon's suspicion and pointed out that echocardiography equipment available at the community hospital did not have the resolution power of the new state-of-the-art equipment at the tertiary care center. A repeat echocardiogram was done at the tertiary care center and read by the tertiary care center cardiologist ; it confirmed a lack of severe valvular regurgitation. The surgical operation was canceled and the surgeon advised the patient that it might be possible to continue for several more years with aggressive medical therapy before the valve replacement became necessary.

The cardiac surgeon wondered how best to communicate his opinion to the referring community cardiologist and to the patient in a manner that would avoid undercutting the authority and competence of the referring cardiologist in the eyes of the patient. The surgeon considered the possibility that the referring cardiologist might reject his recommendation to defer surgery and felt he could not perform the surgery "on demand." The referring cardiologist would also have the option of asking another cardiac surgeon to perform the operation. The surgeon considered that another cardiac surgeon, especially in fee-for-service private practice, might feel more obliged to the cardiologist for the referral than he did, and might operate in deference to the referring cardiologist.

The patient was returned to the care of the referring cardiologist with discussion of the new echocardiographic findings. The cardiac surgeon, the tertiary care echocardiologist, and referring cardiologist all agreed that results from the tertiary care center's more sophisticated echocardiogram equipment warranted changing the patient care plan. All agreed that it was in the patient's best interest to postpone surgery. All advised careful follow-up on a yearly basis by echocardiography.

One year later the patient made a direct self-referral to the tertiary care cardiac surgeon and an appointment for an echocardiogram at the tertiary care center, rather than rescheduling an appointment with her local cardiologist. Arranging follow-up care at the tertiary care center seemed the logical course to the patient, who wished to avoid repeating the experience of having multiple echocardiograms. However, the patient's approach bypassed the referring cardiologist (who did not have privileges at the tertiary care center); moreover, bypassing the cardiologist was inappropriate as the tertiary care cardiac surgeon lacked the training required to evaluate the echocardiogram and to follow the patient medically. The cardiac surgeon recognized that the patient would need follow-up by a cardiologist. The surgeon felt a responsibility to supporting the delicate balance of relationships among the patient, tertiary care cardiologist and referring cardiologist, which were of importance for the patient's long-term care. The surgeon called the patient and told her she should be seen by her referring cardiologist, although the echocardiogram could be done at the tertiary care center.

In our third and final case, a patient was referred by his private cardiologist to the tertiary care transplant team for a heart transplant. The diagnosis was cardiac decompensation secondary to unrecognized aortic valve disease. An appointment was made for the patient with the tertiary care transplant cardiologists, who also run the tertiary care center's heart failure clinic. Upon reviewing the cardiac catheterization data provided by the referring private cardiologist, the transplant cardiologist determined that the patient might be better served by conventional aortic valve replacement. Although the valve replacement operation carried a higher risk in the short run, the patient's ventricle might return to normal function over a year or so following valve replacement, thus precluding, or at least deferring, the need for a heart transplant with its accompanying risks of long-term complications. Because valve replacement surgery was a high-risk operation for this patient, the transplant cardiologist called the transplant surgeon for consultation. The transplant surgeon, who had also performed routine cardiac surgery, agreed that valve replacement could be done, but only if the patient's heart failure was meticulously managed preoperatively to improve the patient's ventricular function as much as possible prior to surgery, thereby minimizing the risk of mortality from the valve replacement operation. The patient, who was told previously by his private physician that he was dying of heart failure with no recourse except a transplant, was taken aback to learn that there was a possibility he might have full recovery with conventional therapy and that his own cardiologist had not explored this option further.

Because both the transplant cardiologist and the transplant surgeon care for nontransplant patients, they were both essentially referring the patient to their own services. Because the operation advised by the surgeon was one that nontransplant cardiac surgeons could perform, there were obviously many surgeons to whom the patient could have been sent. The surgeon wondered if the referring cardiologist had the impression that the surgeon was being self-serving by advising surgery. Should the cardiac surgeon and transplant cardiologist function merely as technicians, performing whichever procedures the referring physician deemed best, in this instance a transplant? Or should each determine independently what they judged to be in the best interest of the patient, possibly coming up with an opinion that differed from that of the referring cardiologist, and then persuade the referring cardiologist and patient to do what they considered in the patient's interest? They worried about the possible effects that a disagreement with the referring cardiologist might have on future patients' care and future referrals to the transplant center. Would the referring cardiologist send his patients to other centers in the future, to avoid what may seem to be an embarrassment? Would the referring physician be slower to refer patients for transplant in the future and possibly advise high-risk conventional surgery instead of transplant to future patients for whom recovery potential might be less and for whom surgery might be unwise or inappropriate? Would further decisions be made without consulting the transplant team? Further delays in referral for transplantation could potentially also result in patients' being referred at too late a stage in their disease processes for safe transplant operations to occur, thereby precluding transplant options for some patients. On the other hand, for the transplant team to be uncompromising about the care of an individual patient might also have adverse future consequences for their program in general, potentially jeopardizing the welfare of future patients.

The patient eventually decided to proceed with high-risk valve replacement and was advised to undergo intensive heart failure management for one to two months prior to surgery. As it turned out in this situation, the referring cardiologist was happy to find that in the opinion of the tertiary team, the patient could be treated by conventional means. The next question that arose was who should manage the heart failure—the referring cardiologist or the heart failure specialists at the tertiary care center? Before this question could be settled among the physicians, the patient's daughter stepped in and stipulated that her father's care was to be given by the tertiary care cardiologists, as it was the tertiary care center's cardiologists who had recommended the present course of treatment in the first place. On further work-up the tertiary care cardiologists learned that the patient had a history of alcohol abuse that he had been unwilling to confide to his private cardiologist, perhaps in an effort to put his best foot forward when seeing the private physician. This finding provided another, potentially reversible, cause of poor ventricular function, namely, alcoholic cardiomyopathy. The tertiary care cardiologists persuaded the patient that abstaining from alcohol was essential and, with a combination of a more aggressive medical regimen and abstinence, his ventricular function improved to a point where he was at significantly less risk of mortality from valve replacement surgery.

The operation was performed and the patient had a good recovery. Another ethical dilemma arose concerning the responsibility for long-term follow-up care postoperatively. Patients undergoing routine cardiac surgery are usually returned at hospital discharge to the care of their referring cardiologists after one post-surgical checkup. Yet this patient still had heart failure; to achieve the best chance of full ventricular recovery following surgery the patient might need a full year of medical management by a specialist in the field. Thus, in the surgeon's view, the patient's interests would best be served by follow-up care given by the heart failure specialists at the tertiary care center

In light of these considerations, it was unclear to the tertiary care cardiac surgeon whether or not he had a responsibility to return the patient to the referring cardiologist, although he wanted to exercise care in maintaining the relationship between himself and the referring cardiologist. Although there was no monetary gain to the cardiac surgeon, advising the patient to stay within the tertiary care system might be perceived by others as self-serving. The cardiac surgeon was uncertain what his responsibility was to the referring cardiologist, from whom he would like to receive future referrals.

The surgeon decided to advise the patient to stay with the heart failure cardiologists for a year, or until his ventricular function had improved significantly, even at the risk of losing future referrals for both transplant and non-transplant cardiac surgery. Although the patient's daughter agreed, the patient decided to return to the care of his private cardiologist, citing convenience of location and a long-standing relationship with the referring cardiologist as major factors.

An Ethical Framework for Managing Conflicts among Surgeons and Professional Colleagues

In any relationship among medical and surgical colleagues, conflicts may arise about patient management. In the second and third cases discussed above, surgeons arrived at diagnostic judgments or treatment recommendations that differed from the referring physician's. In all three cases, tensions developed over who should provide care and where care should be delivered. In each case, the surgeon felt an obligation to the referring physician and expressed concern about undercutting the patient's trust in the referring physician. At the same time, the surgeons recognized as a primary obligation the duty to promote their patients' welfare.

In addressing situations where conflict exists among professional colleagues, it is worth remembering that medicine's success has brought with it the development of new diagnostic and treatment modalities, so that in many cases there is no single best treatment for the patient.[1,2] As pointed out in Chapter 2, when alternative medically acceptable treatments exist, it should be the competent patient, rather than the surgeon or referring physician, who exercises the final authority to decide among treatment options.[3,4] Often reasonable, nonsurgical alternatives exist—for example, in the care of acute, but not yet emergent, patients (see Chapter 7). Examples include the alternatives of surgery versus "watchful waiting" for benign prostatic hypertrophy (see Chapter 8), and lumpectomy versus mastectomy for breast cancer. In these kinds of cases, the referring physician and consulting surgeon should provide information and recommendations to the patient, acknowledging openly where differences exist and discussing them to the patient's satisfaction.

In other situations, the surgeon may believe there is a single best medical treatment and that the treatment the referring physician has recommended would result in the patient receiving substandard care. In most instances, disagreements of this kind prove to be only temporary, reflecting the fact that the surgeon has information that the referring physician does not. Thus, in the second case, the cardiac surgeon had information from repeating the echocardiogram using state-of-the-art equipment and from consulting with the tertiary care echocardiologist, information that was not initially available to the referring physician. Once apprised of this information, the referring cardiologist agreed with the cardiac surgeon's recommendation to change the treatment plan.

In other clinical situations, however, the surgeon and referring physician may look at the same factual data and the referring physician may recommend a course of care that the surgeon believes is medically unacceptable. In these instances, the surgeon may suspect (as in the first case) that the referring physician lacks the specialized knowledge and experience pertinent to the patient's condition, or that the physician is acting under financial or other constraints that limit the physician's ability to provide optimal patient care. In such a situation, the surgeon's ethical obligation to the patient is paramount.[5,6] A "collusion of anonymity" can occur when this obligation is not met because neither referring physician nor surgeon assume ultimate responsibility for promoting the patient's best interest.[7]

To avoid abdicating responsibility in the face of conflict, both the referring physician and surgeon should address conflicts of medical opinion openly, seeking an outside opinion where appropriate. In addition, each should (1) maintain high standards of competence in order to promote the patient's interests; (2) avoid harming the patients by referring patients elsewhere when medical judgments or procedures fall outside his or her competencies; and (3) support the patient's right to make important health care decisions by communicating information necessary for the patient's informed choice. So, for example, if appropriate post- or presurgical care cannot be provided by the referring physician (as in the first case) it is unethical for the surgeon to turn over care to the referring physician. Expressing this point, the American College of Surgeons has stated that "Post-operative care will be rendered by the operating surgeon unless it is delegated to another physician who is well qualified to continue this essential aspect of total surgical care."[8]

In many respects the current U.S. reimbursement system exacerbates conflicts between referring physicians and consultants. Thus, Medicare does not reimburse generalists who provide concurrent care with a specialist when both physicians are treating the same patient for the same diagnosis. Some MCOs do not reimburse specialists who provide primary care services because such services can be provided by primary care physicians at a lower cost. These reimbursement policies can conflict with optimal patient care and frustrate efforts by surgeons and medical colleagues to work cooperatively in promoting patients' interests. They also can encourage a "pieces and parts" approach to patient care by discouraging surgeons and other specialists from caring for the whole person.[9]

In negotiating and attempting to forestall ethical conflicts, both surgeons and their medical colleagues should avoid exercising undesirable forms of dominance over each other. Thus, the surgeon should seek to avoid any general tendency "to dictate therapeutic action or to take over the action entirely, withholding responsibility, credit, and learning from the primary physician."[10] Likewise, the surgeon's medical colleague should avoid approaching the surgeon as a mere technician, rather than a colleague of equal stature.[10] As health system reform increases the primary physician's authority and control of health care resources, it will become even more important that primary care physicians avoid abuses of newfound power and authority,[11,12]

Summary

Each of the three cases discussed above highlights ethical aspects of relationships among surgeons and other medical specialists. The first case brings to the fore ethical concerns regarding balancing the third-party payer's interest in providing competent care at the lowest possible cost against the surgical specialist's concern to provide adequate care to the patient. Clinical decisions about who should provide patient care and where patients should receive medical services reflect a balancing of these considerations. In addition, institutional policies can facilitate or inhibit communication and referral processes among health professionals. National policies assigning responsibility for patient outcomes exclusively to the surgical team, while ignoring the role of other providers in producing these outcomes, can create misleading appraisals of the quality of care surgeons provide.

The second and third cases underscore the problems that can ensue when surgeons and referring physicians reach different conclusions about a patient's diagnosis or plan of care. Disagreements sometimes reflect a discrepancy in information or clinical experience (as in the second case); in other instances they reflect a lack of consensus within the broader medical and surgical communities. Both kinds of situations pose ethical quandaries for surgeons related to communication, decision-making authority, and patient advocacy. Thus, surgeons in cases two and three felt obligated to advocate for their patients' interests by questioning the referring physicians' judgment. Each may also have believed that the referring physician was obligated to promote the patient's interest and so should openly invite the surgeon's opinion concerning the patient's best interests. At the same time, the referring physicians in these cases may have assumed that the surgeons would not "take over" the management of their patients.

Finally, the fact that the patient in the third case was willing to disclose a previously undisclosed history of alcohol abuse to the tertiary care physician, but not to his private cardiologist, suggests a reason why patients should have a role in choosing their physicians and surgeons: namely, patients know best whom they can trust and with whom they feel comfortable. This, in turn, can affect patients' compliance with medical advice, disclosure of pertinent medical information, and willingness to initiate follow-up care should problems arise.

Clinical Topics

We turn now to the relationships among surgeons and other medical specialists, referring physicians in particular. In the course of this discussion, we further develop the general ethical framework suggested above to guide the appropriate management of surgeons' relationships and potential conflicts with other physicians.

Financial Constraints on Patient Advocacy

The surgeon's primary ethical obligation is to advocate for patients' best interests. Reflecting this stance, the ethical principles upon which the American

College of Surgeons was founded include a pledge to "place the welfare and the rights of my patient above all else."[8] However, as U.S. health care delivery systems move increasingly toward MCOs that provide both the financing and delivery of health care under a single corporate structure, there has been growing concern among surgeons and other physicians about the restrictions that financial constraints place on patient advocacy.[13, 14, 15] Among the strategies managed care organizations use to control costs are reducing "unnecessary" services, including excessive diagnostic testing, extended hospital stays, specialist referrals, and unnecessary surgery. Surgeons increasingly find their relationships with referring physicians mediated by MCOs and other third-party payers that impose quality assurance and utilization management requirements.

In response to these requirements, some surgeons express concern that the quality of surgical services, as well as pre- and postoperative care, may be compromised in the desire to rein in health care costs. Thus many of the ethical issues that arise in the three cases described above relate to economic constraints placed on patient care.

The American College of Surgeons recently issued recommendations that address the ethics and economics of managed care. These recommendations emphasize that "[t]he surgeon must be the patient advocate so that all patients will be ensured access to high-quality [care] and the appropriate range of surgical care, regardless of disincentives, financial or otherwise, employed by the managed care organization."[16] Among the College's other recommendations are that managed care organizations document the quality of surgical care, including documenting that "[r]eferrals to surgeons are timely and appropriate, regardless of financial incentives"; "[s]urgical response is timely and appropriate, regardless of financial incentives"; and "[s]atisfaction is measured and used in assessing and improving performance of the system . . . [including] surveys of the patient, referring physician, and surgeon."[16] Certainly, to the extent that managed care plans develop valid and reliable quality measures, all patients will benefit from having more rigorous and systematic mechanisms available to evaluate the competence of health plans and physicians.[17] Yet critics of managed care express concern that the factors selected to measure the quality of patient care are often misleading, driven by financial incentives to cut costs rather than by incentives to enhance the quality of patient care. For example, regarding low mortality and short hospital stays as a mark of quality can potentially reduce health care costs by encouraging surgeons to avoid operating on more costly, high-risk patients (as occurred in the third case).

The ethical issues that are perhaps most poignant for surgeons who function in managed care environments concern limits on referrals received from primary care physicians, the appropriateness of providing presurgical management and postsurgical follow-up versus returning the patient to the referring physician for these services, and recommendations to pursue more costly surgical treatment versus less costly medical therapy.

Although MCOs typically assume that referrals to specialists will result in more costly services and a greater volume of services, this is not always true. Thus, in the second case it was the cardiothoracic surgeon who advised against valve replacement and recommended less expensive medical therapy, whereas the referring cardiologist directed the patient to the more expensive surgical treatment. This example illustrates that high quality patient care and cost control are not always antagonistic goals in surgical practice. Surgical specialists can benefit individual patients by bringing to bear their greater knowledge and experience; these benefits, in turn, may provide patients the most cost-beneficial care over the long run. Similarly, although surgical management of pre- and postoperative care is typically perceived as more expensive, it can potentially reduce health care expenditures by providing timely identification and response to medical problems.

In situations where specialty care is expected to increase the overall health care expenditures for a particular patient, a potential conflict exists between the surgeon's goal of providing the best possible care to the patient and the health plan's goal of providing competent care at the lowest possible cost.[18,19] At a policy level, it is widely (but not unanimously[20,21]) held that controlling health care costs and providing optimal delivery of health care requires the overall number of primary care physicians to make up roughly half or more of all physicians.[22,23] Yet even if such a policy goal could be achieved, individual surgeons and other medical specialists would still face conflicts about promoting patients' best interests versus abiding by health care plans' goals of reducing health care costs. Several resolutions to this conflict are possible.[24] First, it might be argued that the surgeon's primary ethical responsibility is to advocate on behalf of the individual patient's best interests, and that the goal of cost containment prevents the surgeon from fulfilling this responsibility. Expressing this view, Angell has argued that "as individual physicians, we must do the very best we can for each patient. The patient rightly expects his physician to act single-mindedly in his best interests. If very expensive care is indicated, then the physician should do his utmost to obtain it for the patient."[25] Voicing a similar view, Levinsky maintains that the doctor cannot serve two masters: the patient and the society.[26] According to Levinsky, "physicians are required to do everything that they believe may benefit each patient without regard to costs or other societal considerations."[26]

The problem with this approach is that it conceives of patient advocacy as an absolute or unlimited obligation. Although patient advocacy is a central and important goal for surgeons, it does not automatically trump all other ethical considerations. Especially in the transplantation field, the surgeon assumes another ethical responsibility, namely, to make the best use of limited, donated organs, in order to benefit potential recipients (see Chapter 6). If one patient's risk of mortality becomes too great, the surgeon is obligated to consider that the risk of losing an organ could be reduced by providing it to another patient with a greater likelihood of survival. Thus, in the context of transplantation, the good of the larger group of patients is sometimes served by not transplanting a particular patient with little hope of success, even though, as individual patient advocates, transplant surgeons may feel inclined to provide a small, but realistic, chance for survival to the patient who is a poor transplant candidate.

Outside the transplant setting, the tension between the good of individual patients and other ethical goals is apparent in a variety of ways. Imagine a surgeon who promised to provide a patient with the best possible medical care regardless of the costs, and regardless of what was necessary to obtain it. If, in pursuit of this promise, the surgeon lied on insurance forms to obtain payment for an experimental therapy that may help the patient, the surgeon's action would correctly be subject to stringent ethical criticism. Generally speaking, surgeons are not ethically justified in advocating for patients by finding ways to bypass the system's rules while still appearing to honor them and thereby securing resources that were not, technically at least, intended for this patient.[27] Thus, figuring out what one ought, as a matter of ethical obligation, to do is not simply a matter of getting clear about what a specific relationship requires. Relationships have moral preconditions: certain commitments cannot be ethically made. They also have moral side constraints: under certain circumstances, even legitimate commitments cannot be ethically met.[28]

If the duty of patient advocacy is not unconditional, then the surgeon must determine the conditions under which patient advocacy can, with ethical justification, be limited. Clearly, the surgeon should not simply accept, at face value, whatever restrictions on patient advocacy a health plan imposes, especially constraints driven solely by cost reduction strategies. In many circumstances reimbursement incentives are not an ethically acceptable justification for limiting patient care. Although surgeons cannot always provide their patients with the best possible care, they are obligated to ensure that the care their patients receive meets professional standards and represents sound medical practice.

To this end, private-pay surgeons who participate in managed care plans should review the requirements of individual health plans before agreeing to participate, and refuse to enter into arrangements with health care plans that restrict or discourage provision of medically necessary services.[29] Emphasizing this obligation, the American Medical Association has directed physicians to refuse to participate in any health plan that "encourages or requires care at or below minimum professional standards."[29] In addition, because the surgeon stands in a fiduciary relationship with the patient, the surgeon should challenge restrictions that are at odds with the patient's best interests. Recognizing this fiduciary responsibility, some courts have held physicians legally liable for withholding care against their best medical judgment in order to comply with the rules of the reimbursement system.[30] Finally, to maintain trust in the surgeon-patient relationship, the surgeon should disclose to the patient financial and resource constraints that adversely affect the quality of care the patient receives. For example, in the three cases described above, restrictions on the location of care, the provider of care, and the surgeon's ability to consult with surgical specialists should be disclosed to the patient if the surgeon perceives that such restrictions are likely to result in substandard care.[31]

Shared Responsibility for Patient Management

None of the surgeons in the three cases discussed above stood in a simple dyadic relationship with the patient. Instead, surgeons in each case stood in relationships with physicians in other medical specialties, including primary care physicians, community-based, tertiary care-based and managed care-based cardiologists, cardiac surgeons, members of the tertiary care cardiothoracic surgical service, and oncologists. These cases demonstrate the importance not only of sustaining a positive relationship with individual patients, but also of consulting with and maintaining collegial relationships with others involved in patient care in an ethically responsible fashion (see also Chapter 16). In the context of caring for patients, there are several distinct relationships in which surgeons may stand with other physicians.

General Referral. First, the surgeon may stand in the relationship of consultant to a referring physician. In any kind of reimbursement setting, there are clearly factors that are not medical, technical, or related to the patient that potentially influence clinical decision making. Thus, concern for personal income, status in the local professional community, and generation of reciprocal referrals can affect the selection of surgeons or consultants.[32] Professional groups recommend minimizing the influence of nonmedical factors. Thus, the American College of Physicians ethics manual cites only two ethically acceptable motivations for patient referral: when assistance is required in the care of the patient, and when consultation is requested by the patient or surrogate.[33]

The College goes on to identify general ethical guidelines that govern the relationship between the referring physician and the physician to whom a referral is made. First, the level of consultation should be established at the outset, for example, a one-time visit, continuing cooperative care, or total transfer of care to the consultant. At the same time, patients (or patient representatives) are ethically and legally entitled to decide from whom they will seek care. Thus, a patient may make a decision to change physicians without obtaining the approval of the referring physician. The referring physician is then obligated to facilitate this decision—for example, by transferring the patient's medical records.

Second, the physician to whom a referral is made should communicate directly with the referring physician about recommendations. In making major decisions or requesting additional consultants, the physician receiving a referral is usually expected to obtain concurrence from the referring physician. Yet even when these ethical guidelines are followed, other conflicts may arise. For example, in the third case the referring physician had agreed with the consultant's recommendation for valve replacement surgery, yet a conflict later arose when the patient bypassed the referring cardiologist in attempting to schedule an appointment for follow-up care directly with the consultant.

Third, in interactions with the patient or members of the health care team, the consultant should try to avoid undercutting "the authority and dignity of the referring physician in this process."[33] This was a central concern in both the second and third cases. In the second case, the surgical specialist advised the patient to return to her referring cardiologist, although the tertiary care cardiologist was also competent to provide follow-up care. In the third case, when the surgeon initially disagreed with the referring physician's recommendation for transplantation, the surgeon had a responsibility to communicate this disagreement in a respectful and direct manner to the referring physician. The surgeon should avoid communicating to patients in a manner that wrongly suggests the referring physician is incompetent or negligent, especially in areas of medical controversy.

Finally, the consultant's primary responsibility is the patient's welfare. Therefore, when disagreements of the sort described in the second and third cases arise, consulting surgeons should not defer to referring physicians against their own best judgment. For example, if the referring physician in the second case continued to insist on valve replacement surgery, even after obtaining the results of the more accurate echocardiogram and the expert opinions of the cardiac surgeon and echocardiologist, the surgeon should not perform the surgery merely to satisfy the referring physician's wishes. Instead, the surgeon's ultimate responsibility is to the patient's welfare. As the American College of Surgeons makes clear, "the performance of unnecessary surgery is an extremely serious violation of ethical principles for which disciplinary action is indicated."[8] Although in the final analysis the patient (or the patient's representative) has the legal and ethical authority to decide which recommendations to accept, the referring physician influences the patient's decision by directing the patient to surgeons, or other consultants who provide the information on which the patient will ultimately base any decision.

Directed Referral. A second kind of relationship in which the surgeon stands with medical colleagues is a subset of the first. In directed referral, explicit financial constraints limit the avenue of referral. Directed referral characterizes many kinds of managed care arrangements, including health maintenance organizations and preferred provider organizations. As suggested already, the form of reimbursement a physician receives appears to influence the coordination of care between the surgeon and referring physician. When use of consultative services was compared among three groups of physicians practicing in the same hospital but reimbursed for their services in different ways, it was found that physicians in prepaid insurance plans used consultative services the least; unaffiliated, fee-for-service physicians ordered an intermediate number of consultations; and physicians in a large multispecialty fee-for-service group practice made the most referrals of all three groups.[34] In a different study, general internists reported that communication and coordination between primary care and specialist physicians were impaired when multiple health insurance plans with restricted panels of participating physicians were implemented in a community.[35] Despite clear differences in referral patterns, generalizations about MCOs should be made cautiously, in light of the variety of different types of MCOs and their rapidly changing structures.[36]

The finding that physicians within fee-for-service settings make the greatest number of referrals hardly demonstrates that referral practices in such settings are uninfluenced by financial considerations. Although fee-for-service settings are less likely than MCO's to discourage limiting medically appropriate referrals, they are more likely to encourage excessive referrals. Thus, the financial incentives that characterize some fee-for-service settings encourage physicians to make more, not less, referrals and to make referrals within the group, not outside it, in order to maximize profits shared by group members (see Chapters 18 and 19). Incentives to refer patients to colleagues within a multispecialty group can take various forms. According the AMA Council on Ethical and Judicial Affairs, the overt practice of fee splitting, defined as the payment by or to a physician solely for the referral of a patient, is unethical. The AMA holds that "[a] physician may not accept payment of any kind, in any form, from any source . . . for prescribing or referring a patient to said source,"[37] because doing so violates the requirement to deal fairly and honestly with colleagues and patients. Yet even without engaging in explicit fee splitting, physicians belonging to the same multispecialty fee-for-service group may stand to gain financially by referring patients within the group. Thus, referral decisions are potentially based on the group's financial interest, rather than being based exclusively on the patient's need for a referral, or on the skill and quality of the physician to whom a patient is referred. Self-policing remains the primary method to prevent excess referrals within fee-for-service settings. Although since 1992 federal law has prohibited physicians from referring Medicare patients to outside facilities in which the physician has a financial stake,[38] no federal law prevents the analogous practice of within-group referral where physicians have a financial stake in the group's profits.

As discussed above, the surgeon is obligated to ensure that the patient receives competent care. Surgeons should not feel comfortable in directed referral arrangements unless these arrangements are consistent with providing sound patient care. Against this view it is sometimes held that patients "choose" to participate in health plans or "choose" the physician groups in which they receive care, and therefore choose the financial conflicts of interest associated with each. Yet this argument is often unpersuasive. First, many patients have no real choice among different health plans because their employer provides only one plan option. Second, when they do have choices among plans, patients may not consider or understand fully the consequences of restricted choice until these impact directly upon their care. Health care plans reinforce patients' ignorance of plans' limits by advertising to potential consumers in a manner that emphasizes what the plan offers, not what it excludes or restricts.[39] Finally, patients may be unaware of physicians' financial conflicts of interest, or, when such conflicts are fully disclosed, patients may feel awkward asking for other referrals and thereby 'buying from the competition' rather than patronizing specialists within the physician's own group.[40]

To address the ethical conflicts surgeons and other providers in directed referral face, Cain and Jonsen propose a four-step decision process for managing patient care.[39] This process calls for addressing four distinct questions:

1. What is the best medical care for this particular patient, in light of this patient's specific medical condition, including the best medical personnel to deliver this care and the site with the best experience with this problem?
2. What are the financial constraints on this choice, for the physician, for the local group, and for the patient?
3. What are the social constraints on this choice, such as censure by group practice, clinic, hospital, or health maintenance organization?
4. What are you going to suggest to the patient?

According to this model, whenever answers to (4) and (1) differ, the surgeon should discuss with the patient the constraints on care that account for this difference. In support of this approach, Cain and Jonsen argue that when departures from ideal advocacy occur, the physician owes the patient a certain level of disclosure of the motives and supporting reasons that entered into the decision. This accountability is necessary to maintain the values of honesty and integrity in the surgeon-patient relationship.

Clinical Conclusions

Although the doctor-patient relationship is often pictured as a simple dyadic relationship, this picture does not accurately portray the surgeon's experience.

Medical care has become increasingly specialized, with the number of consulting physicians for each patient now higher than ever before.[10] Contemporary surgeons care for patients in tandem with many other medical specialists. At every stage of patient care, the surgeon consults with other health professionals: before seeing the patient for the first time, a contact is made between the surgeon and referring physician; after seeing the patient, the surgeon may consult with other specialists and with the referring physician; if surgery is performed, the surgeon may manage the patient's pre- and postoperative care together with other medical specialists. Especially when patients present with complex medical problems, their postoperative care, classically in the domain of the surgeon, is now commonly shared with other medical specialists. In light of these shared responsibilities for patient management, surgeons must not only establish and maintain positive relationships with patients, they must also form and nurture positive relationships with professional colleagues. Relationships with both patients and colleagues present ethical challenges when the financial incentives of health plans constrain patient advocacy by discouraging medically appropriate care or by encouraging excessive consultations and services. Financial incentives may disrupt patient care when referral or directed referral situations leads to questions about who should provide care and where care should be delivered; and when differences of opinion arise between surgeons and medical colleagues. In these situations, both surgeons and their medical colleagues are responsible to advocate for patients to receive competent care; avoid harming patients by providing services that fall outside their competencies; and provide patients with information necessary to make informed choices about treatment, including nonsurgical options.

Although all medical providers stand in a special, fiduciary relationship with their patients, in certain respects the surgeon's relationship with the patient is unique. Unlike his or her medical colleagues, the surgeon's relationship with the patient has special features—most prominently, the

> . . . actual physical interaction, including the act of making an intentional, permanent 'wound,' in which the therapy produces measurable pathophysiologic change and mixes with the disease process. . . . [This feature of the surgeon-patient relationship] creates unique bonds. Even though the acts may be skilled and ritualized, the fact remains that you have cut open the body, removed or rearranged organs, and left your mark. This extraordinary contact cannot but influence how you feel about the patient and how he or she feels about you.[41]

Especially in dramatic life-saving surgical situations, patient and surgeon develop a unique bond. The surgeon's challenge is to maintain this special and distinctive relationship with the patient while also maintaining positive relationships with other providers involved in the patient's care.

References

1. Robert M. Veatch, "Contemporary Bioethics and the Demise of Modern Medicine," in *Prescriptions: The Dissemination of Medical Authority*, Gayle L. Ormiston and Raphael Sassower, eds. New York: Greenwood Press, 1990, pp. 23–40.
2. John E. Wennberg, Jean L. Freeman, Roxanne M. Shelton, et al., "Hospital Use and Mortality Among Medicare Beneficiaries in Boston and New Haven," *New England Journal of Medicine* 321 (1989): 1168–1173.
3. Dan W. Brock, "The Ethical Responsibilities of Surgeons in Conflicts with Patients or their Surrogates About Treatment," *Rhode Island Medical Journal* 74 (1991): 227–232.
4. Dan C. English, "Surgeon's Role in Ethical Decisions," *American Surgeon* 51 (1985): 423–425.
5. Frank A. Chervenak and Laurence B. McCullough, "The Importance of Ethics to the Practice of Obstetric Ultrasound," *Annals of Medicine* 25 (1993): 271–273.
6. Michael D. Wertheimer, Sandra L. Bertman, H. Brownell Wheeler, et al., "Ethics and Communication in the Surgeon-Patient Relationship," *Journal of Medical Education* 60 (1985): 804–806.
7. Robert Rakel, *Essentials of Family Practice*. Philadelphia: W. B. Saunders, 1993.
8. American College of Surgeons, *Statement on Principles*. American College of Surgeons, 1993.
9. William H. Bruening, Jerald L. Andrew, Denise M. Smith, "Concurrent Care: An Ethical Issue for Family Physicians," *Journal of Family Practice* 36 (1993): 606–608.
10. Linda L. Emanuel, "The Consultant and the Patient-Physician Relationship," *Archives of Internal Medicine* 154 (1994): 1785–1790.
11. Kathleen E. Ellsbury, "Can the Family Physician Avoid Conflict of Interest in the Gatekeeper Role?: An Affirmative View," *Journal of Family Practice* 28 (1989): 698–701.
12. G. Gayle Stephens, "An Opposing View," *Journal of Family Practice* 28 (1989): 701–704.
13. Nancy S. Jecker, "Business Ethics and the Ethics of Managed Care," *Trends in Health Care, Law, and Ethics* 10 (1995): 53–55.
14. Nancy S. Jecker, "Managed Competition and Managed Care: What are the Ethical Issues?" in *Geriatric Clinics of North America*, Gregory A. Sachs and Christine K. Cassel, eds. Philadelphia: W.B. Saunders Co., 1994, pp. 527–540.
15. Nancy S. Jecker and Albert R. Jonsen, "Managed Care: A House of Mirrors," *Journal of Clinical Ethics* (in press).
16. American College of Surgeons, "Statement of Recommendations to Ensure Quality of Surgical Services in Managed Care Environments," *American College of Surgeons Bulletin* 79 (1994): 30–31.
17. Ezekiel J. Emanuel and Nancy Neveloff Dubler, "Preserving the Physician-Patient Relationship in the Era of Managed Care," *Journal of the American Medical Association* 273 (1995): 323–329.
18. Jack M. Colwill, "Where Have All the Primary Care Applicants Gone?" *New England Journal of Medicine* 326 (1992): 387–393.
19. Judith P. Swazey and Paul S. Russell, "Surgery," in *Encyclopedia of Bioethics*, 2nd ed., Warren T. Reich, ed. New York: Macmillan, 1995, pp. 2450–2455.

20. Richard A. Cooper, "Seeking a Balanced Physician Workforce for the 21st Century," *Journal of the American Medical Association* 272 (1994): 680–687.

21. David A. Kindig, James M. Cultice, and Fitzhugh Mullan, "The Elusive Generalist Physician," *Journal of the American Medical Association* 270 (1993): 1069–1073.

22. Council on Graduate Medical Education, *Third Report: Improving Access to Health Care Through Physician Workforce Reform: Directions for the 21st Century*. Rockville, MD: Health Resources and Services Administration, October, 1992.

23. Peter Franks, Carolyn M. Clancy, Paul A. Nutting, "Gatekeeping Revisited—Protecting Patients From Overtreatment," *New England Journal of Medicine* 327 (1992): 422–429.

24. Nancy S. Jecker, "Integrating Medical Ethics with Normative Theory: Patient Advocacy and Social Responsibility," *Theoretical Medicine* 11 (1990): 125–139.

25. Marcia Angell, "Cost Containment and the Physician," *New England Journal of Medicine* 254 (1985): 1203–1207.

26. Norman G. Levinsky, "The Doctor's Master," *New England Journal of Medicine* 311 (1984): 1573–1575.

27. Haavi Morreim, "Gaming the System," *Archives of Internal Medicine* 151 (1991): 443–447.

28. Nancy S. Jecker, "Impartiality and Special Relations," in *Kindred Matters*, Diana T. Meyers, Kenneth Kipnis, and Cornelius F. Murphy, eds. Ithaca, New York: Cornell University Press, 1993, pp. 74–92.

29. American Medical Association, Council on Ethical and Judicial Affairs, "Ethical Issues in Managed Care," *Journal of the American Medical Association* 273 (1995): 330–335.

30. *Wickline V. State of California*. 228 *California Reporter* 661, 1986.

31. Bernard Lo, "Incentives for Physicians to Decrease Services," in Bernard Lo, *Resolving Ethical Dilemmas*. Williams and Wilkins, 1995, pp. 293–300.

32. William A. Schaffer and Frank C. Holloman, "Consultation and Referral Between Physicians in New Medical Practice Environments," *Annals of Internal Medicine* 103 (1995): 600–605.

33. American College of Physicians, Ad Hoc Committee on Medical Ethics, "American College of Physicians Ethics Manual, Part I: History of Medical Ethics, the Physician and the Patient, The Physician's Relationships to Other Physicians, the Physician and Society," *Annals of Internal Medicine* 111 (1989): 245–252.

34. Roice D. Luke and Michael A. Thomson, "Utilization of Within-Hospital Services," *Medical Care* 18 (1980): 219–227.

35. Zese C. Roulidis and Kevin S. Schulman, "Physician Communication in Managed Care Organizations: Opinions of Primary Care Physicians," *Journal of Family Practice* 39 (1994): 446–451.

36. Robert H Miller and Harold S. Luft, "Managed Care Plan Performance Since 1980: A Literature Analysis," *Journal of the American Medical Association* 271 (1994): 1512–1519.

37. American Medical Association, *Code of Medical Ethics: Current Opinions with Annotations*. Chicago: American Medical Association, 1994.

38. John K. Iglehart, "Congress Moves to Regulate Self-Referral and Physicians' Ownership of Clinical Laboratories," *New England Journal of Medicine* 322 (1990): 1682–1687.

39. Joanna Cain and Albert R. Jonsen, "Specialists and Generalists in Obstetrics and Gynecology: Conflicts of Interest in Referral an Ethical Alternative," *Women's Health Institute* 2 (1992): 137–145.
40. Haavi Morreim, "Conflicts of Interest: Profits and Problems in Physician Referral," *Journal of the American Medical Association* 262 (1989): 390–396.
41. Michael A. Parmer, "Ethics of a Professional Surgeon," *Bulletin of the American College of Surgeons* 67 (1982): 2–5.

16

Obligations of Surgeons to Non-Physician Team Members and Trainees

RUTH PURTILO
BYERS W. SHAW
ROBERT ARNOLD

A *New Yorker* cartoon depicts several surgeons and other members of the operating team hovering over a shrouded clump amidst a clutter of lights, machines, and other paraphernalia of the operating suite. The perplexed chief surgeon says, to the nurse "I give up—where's the patient?" A Gary Larson cartoon shows a body part flying through the air from the direction of a patient's open incision. A member of the surgical team, agape with astonishment, shouts, "Watch where that thing lands . . . we may need it later!" A popular film, "The Doctor," opens with an operating team scene: the ruptured aorta having been repaired successfully, Dr. McKee leads the team across the suite in a dance to the radio's blaring, "Let's Get Drunk and Screw!" Only Nancy, the chief nurse, and the object of surgeon McKee's constant needling and harassment, is not amused.

Such stereotypes of the surgeon's role on the team are further fed today by popular television serials such as "E.R.," in which the "real action" of medicine often is portrayed as beginning only when the surgeon (or an inexperienced student or resident posing as a surgeon) arrives on the scene wielding a scalpel and creating an *ad hoc* surgical team by barking orders to everyone in sight. Although it is not the purpose of this chapter to explore why surgeons are the brunt of so much stereotyping, some of the recurring themes are instructive for our examination of the obligations of surgeons to team members. Our focus is on the relevant ethical obligations of surgeons toward non-physician surgical team members, obligations designed to assure that the surgical team can successfully meet its peculiar professional goal: *to ensure and foster competent, humane surgical practices that are directed to the optimum care of the surgical patient in the surgical suite and surrounding setting, and foster an environment of respect for all team members.* Other teams, which often include some members of the surgical team, will address larger clinical and social issues of this patient's care, as well as serve as a steward of public resources.[1] The surgeon, for instance, will assuredly be a member of another, multi-physician team directed to the perisurgical care of the patient and family. Therefore this chapter focuses on one small window of the complex and interrelated web of teams that, in fact, constitute the total clinical management of a patient's medical experience.[2] The chapter is divided into three sections: the surgeon's obligations to other professionals on the team (nurses, physician assistants, bioengineers, etc.); obligations to trainees (residents, students); and some comments on the collective nature of team decisions and the team members' obligation of mutual respect.

Two comments at the outset, elaborated later in the chapter, will help to orient the reader. First, an interdisciplinary health care team (IHCT), composed of physician and non-physician members, raises some ethical issues that are different from those that emerge on all-physician teams.[3] Second, a "team" composed of a surgeon or surgeons and trainees has important and different goals than those of an IHCT, so that the surgeon's obligation to trainees will differ in some significant ways from his or her obligations to IHCT members. Some ethical issues arise simply by virtue of these diverse goals, because trainees also serve as contributing members of IHCTs. A brief introduction to team organization of health care generally will be helpful for this later discussion.

Ethical Analysis: Ethical Foundations of Team Care

In the history of medicine, surgical teams were one of the first examples of team-organized intervention.[4] The surgeon always has needed the assistance of others, whether it be to hold down a hapless patient facing surgery without the benefit of anesthetic, or, in more recent times, to administer the anesthetic, hold a retractor, or supply instruments. It was only during and following World War II that team-organized care became more widespread as a focus of reorganization of health care services generally.

Not surprisingly, the ethical obligation to protect and promote the interests of patients created the primary motive for team-organized health care. Sociologists Brown,[5] and Nagi[6] studied this movement and concluded that the rapid increase in physician specialization during the 1940s and 1950s necessitated bringing together several physicians into "teams" in order to provide a comprehensive diagnostic and treatment regime for the patient. But there were other forces at work as well. During World War II, health professionals in the war effort worked shoulder to shoulder in a more equal and independent mode than they had experienced in civilian life. This raised health care professionals' awareness of how working together as an integrated team fostered comprehensiveness and continuity of care. Besides, the non-physician members enjoyed their new autonomy and strived to maintain this new work structure, having enjoyed the physicians' recognition of and respect for their contributions. A review of the nursing literature, for example, supports that this became a turning point in the further professionalization of nursing, as nurses became more cognizant of their own contributions and need for autonomy in their unique areas of practice.[7]

At the same time, Americans were moving to the cities. Urbanization supported the development of large centralized sites where patients could come for all of their health care needs. In the 1940s and 1950s (the original "shopping mall era") hospital administrators, too, supported the idea, concluding that it was more cost-efficient to gather the experts under one roof than send them out to patients.[1]

In short, professionals' commitment to patient needs during a period of medical specialization, the desire for more equality and autonomy by some health care providers, urbanization, and the value of institutional efficiency were some of the critical factors contributing to the team-oriented approach that today is taken for granted.

Team Rules and Ethical Obligations

The health care team phenomenon drew on sports and military team metaphors.[8] Such teams are a social entity studied by sociologists, philosophers, game theorists and others because *teams* and *teamwork* have parameters and functions that distinguish them from loosely knit or other more formally organized groups. *Teams* involve social contracts, the rules of which are constructed to meet a common goal of society or of the team members themselves. There is an assumption that the team structure is necessary and that the goal cannot be achieved any other way. Members volunteer or are chosen/drafted explicitly because of their utility in helping to meet this goal. Any personal recognition or blame is measured solely on the basis of that utility. *Teamwork* is the work directed toward meeting the goal, however that work activity is organized.[9] Surgical teamwork is easy to observe because, for the most part, it is conducted in close proximity over an identified period of time, with well-defined roles for each member. This fact holds even in an era of outpatient surgery, while traditional teamwork of other teams in health care is becoming more diffuse. Some key descriptors of a "good team" (which society has accepted as normative for judging how a team *should* work) are the following:

1. Each member agrees and personally is held accountable for meeting the team's goals and knowing and following its rules.
2. However, a team victory or loss is a collective affair, not an individual one.
3. A potential conflict is built into this description by virtue of the fact that there is also a *captain* of the team.
4. The captain's role is to "call the shots," therefore, loyalty to the captain has moral standing. It is a team "betrayal" to go against the "captain's orders."
5. Expertise is the major qualifying factor for captain and other team membership. A well working team depends on the special, often unique, skill of each individual, each doing his or her prescribed part and—only in well-planned and agreed-upon situations—assuming other roles.
6. Team secrets should not be shared with "outsiders."[2]

Embedded in this team ideal are many ways of thinking and acting that are totally compatible with the *traditional* medical ethic. In both instances moral obligations and rights are believed to be ascertained from an examination of the nature of the relationship and the role or roles assumed by the parties involved.[10] Philosophers call these *special* or *role* obligations in contrast to obligations that might arise simply by virtue of our being human.[11] For example, the duty to foster the well-being of another person is not an obligation of citizens in general. At the same time, there is a professional obligation to foster the well-being of the patient, derived from an understanding of what the physician-patient relationship is designed to accomplish.[12]

The surgeon and other team members generally can take guidance from this basic framework regarding their moral obligations (and rights) by examining how each arises and why, the behaviors that demonstrate an obligation is being met, and what should be done when they are not being met. In recent times there has been support for a more democratic conception of the health care team because of the greater level of expertise of many different professional groups in our technologically driven approach to health care. As the chapter unfolds, some areas where this conception may better serve the goals of the surgical team are considered.

The Surgeon's Ethical Obligations to Nonmedical Professional Team Members

The surgeon is the captain of the surgical team. (Obviously more than one surgeon may be on a team and other physicians also may be—i.e., anesthesiologists. Obligations of surgeons among these team members are covered in Chapter 15, therefore we are simplifying this discussion by suggesting that there is one surgeon in charge of the IHCT.) However, as the above section explains, the captain's authority and accountability, privileges and responsibility do not arise by virtue of innate characteristics but, rather, are determined by his or her special role on this type of team. The assumption is that the captain has the learned skills that enable her or him to be the key expert for the task to be accomplished. Another part of the equation is that the captain in this type of structure is not necessarily free to choose *who* will be on the team. The individuals on the team may be there solely by virtue of the role they play and not because the captain (or other team members) judged them competent for the task or that personally they would be compatible or a good fit. A surgeon colleague committed to providing outstanding leadership among her team members, and who had agreed to review this chapter, complained after one exasperating afternoon in the surgical suite:

> I find myself so frustrated over the years by the incompetence of the people assigned to work with me that the ideals of team work you espouse come up as a ludicrous dream. I have developed highly effective techniques that would allow me to do a procedure with three members of environmental services as long as they, unlike many surgical scrubs sent in, would pay attention to what I say.

A key question in this chapter, then, is "Under these stressful conditions, and in contrast to other team members, what is the captain nonetheless morally obligated to do?" The answer, elaborated throughout this section, is (1) to assure team behaviors and attitudes that will protect and promote the surgical well-being of patients and (2) to maintain an environment of competence, mutual respect, and enablement among team members. While related, the first has priority over the second. If the two goals come into conflict, the captain is held accountable for assuring that smooth teamwork never be bought at the price of a compromised quality of patient care.[13]

Obligation of Due Care

Due care, a legal notion, prescribes that appropriate diligence be exercised to bar the deliberate or negligent imposition of unreasonable risks to patients.[14] This includes maintaining high standards of competence and compassion towards patients.[15] As team captain, the surgeon is assumed to recognize when quality surgical care is being delivered. From this position the obligation arises to try to assure a high standard. For instance, an experienced surgeon should be aware when the error rate is likely to be highest in a procedure. One time is during a delicate moment in a tricky procedure. As an experienced pilot once said to one of the authors, "When I'm a passenger I want the pilot to have white knuckles when he's taking that baby up and when he's putting her down. Most of the rest of the time the pilot can relax a little." Some would suggest that risk is highest when the procedure is the most familiar, mundane, or boring, so that everyone's attention is only half directed to the task.

How can the surgeon dispense an obligation to ensure due care? First it helps to be cognizant that even a highly qualified team member may have bad days. Good communication with the team on an ongoing basis improves team morale. It also helps head off the likelihood that the surgeon will be "out of the loop" when a problem is brewing. For example, an otherwise competent team member trying to work under fear, severe stress, illness or other compromising factors will have an increased likelihood of making an error.[16] Moreover, the practice of an informal team meeting prior to an intervention (particularly if untoward side effects might ensue, or if the procedure is new or extremely complicated) encourages discussion of potential challenges and earmarks areas of team weakness before elbow-deep in the procedure. Whether from a motive of deep moral commitment to high standards or a desire to prevent difficulty with the law, it then behooves the surgeon to be vigilant throughout the procedure, take seriously the concerns of other team members, and act swiftly to correct the situation if a member of the team seems unable to meet the requirements of the task. All of these activities can help to maintain a high level of team functioning that assures due care.

Confronting the Etiology of a Problem on the Team

According to the team metaphor, the team captain is assumed to know best how to maintain the goals of good teamwork in this setting. Therefore, the obligation of due care extends to the surgeon's responsibility to locate the etiology of a problem related to a breakdown in the provision of quality care. Sometimes the focus of the problem lies in how the team has been structured. There are increased data to show that problems in quality assurance arise less from individual incompetence than from failing to recognize that errors are inevitable and safeguards must be built into the system.[17] The surgeon must be decisive and bring experience to bear when unforeseen events occur, such as bleeding problems. Part of the captain's role in promoting high quality team functioning is to honor a positive obligation to promote systems of quality teamwork rather than assume that the team is guaranteed to succeed when a group of competent individuals have been assigned to the team. At the same time, it falls to the surgeon personally to confront emerging patterns of incompetence that appear to be developing in a team member. Whether the incompetence is caused by impairment, lack of skills, ill intent, or sloppiness, the surgeon cannot absent himself or herself from moral and legal responsibility for harm that ensues during surgical intervention. This being the case, the surgeon is faced with confronting the errant team member in the name of maintaining an acceptable quality of care. Sometimes other team members already will have noticed and can be of assistance. For instance, a recent case discussed in the popular press involved an anesthesiologist. Team members had noticed his habit of falling asleep during surgical procedures. Several members of the team, including the surgeon, tried to intervene by urging the anesthesiologist to get up and walk around, have a cup of coffee or otherwise find a way to stay awake! By the time a patient had died during surgery all of the team members were aware of the problem and active in trying to correct it. A preventive ethics approach in this case emphasizes the need for rapid, early corrective action (i.e., getting another anesthesiologist) to prevent incompetence from harming a patient.

Other times non-physician team members will engage in a legacy of silence and protectiveness. (This legacy is well documented in the situation where health professionals resort to this "team ideal" in order to protect incompetent or impaired members of their profession at the price of compromised quality of care to patients.) The perceived power differential between surgeon and non-physician team members may exacerbate silence.[18] Beyond that the team assumption that team secrets should not be exposed may subtly be at work. While the surgeon as leader of the team should strive to maintain high standards of care *and* keep harmony on the team, the first goal should be primary.[19]

The only effective corrective to a legacy of silence and protectiveness is for the surgeon to exercise a parallel obligation to promote an ethos of the team in which the surgeon is equally open to the possibility that he or she could become a problem and be open to and expect constructive criticism from teammates, especially from non-physician members. Some readers may find that ideal naive, devoid of any possibility given the stereotypical personality of surgeons. We believe that the stereotype of surgeons as egotistical, omniscient, and controlling czars of the OR may correctly capture the personality profile of some individuals in that role but is greatly overrated. Most surgeons accept that effective leadership means being open to well-founded criticism from one's colleagues and setting an example of how to receive criticism in a thoughtful and disciplined fashion. In the end, whether from the ethical motive to promote high quality care or the prudential posture of saving oneself from the ravages of legal entanglements, the surgeon's acceptance of an obligation to expect and respond professionally to colleagues' legitimate criticisms will yield more positive results regarding team goals than older models of one-sided authority and responsibility.

Reporting Incompetent Behavior

Sometimes the difficulty can be addressed informally and corrected. The tension heightens when the surgeon believes it necessary to report the incompetence. Doing so does not mean that the surgeon has the power or responsibility to determine punishment; her or his job solely is to determine and provide data supporting that there is possible incompetence and ask for a fuller investigation. Obviously, in-house mechanisms are a useful first step in the process. When matters proceed beyond that step, new challenges arise. In many states the disciplinary committee of the state licensing board mandates reporting incompetence, impairment, or unethical behavioral only of persons in the same profession. Lingering doubt about the evidence, questions about the surgeon's ability to be fully aware of the parameters of competence in another's field of expertise, a desire not to spend time or money pursuing the issue, or the wish not to harm a well-liked team member are just some reasons the surgeon may be reticent to take the next step. Obviously a judgment has to be made at this juncture.

Once reported, the persons involved must honor due process. Due process involves *notification* and *hearing*. Due process requires that the person with the alleged difficulty had been given enough information to conform to the standard that apparently was broken. Notification means that the person should be given exact notice of the law or standard allegedly violated, and the evidence supporting the alleged violation. Confidentiality, as well as a presumption of innocence, also must be strictly maintained. After initial examination by the disciplinary group, the person has a right to a hearing if the matter has not been dropped. Fortunately not all reports of incompetence require this level of adjudication in order to be corrected.

Particularly in cases of impairment, most states have developed mechanisms to assist persons in rehabilitation, which usually is a mandatory condition for reinstatement to practice.[20] Because states vary in their procedures and mechanisms, it is a good idea to become familiar with them before a crisis.

The "Enabling" Ethical Obligations: Protecting the Integrity of the Professional Enterprise

The enabling objectives are effective *means* of assuring high-quality patient care. We address two major such objectives under the topics of obligations to (1) prevent and correct disparagement and harassment and (2) encourage truthful disclosure. Other enabling obligations include those that promote high levels of performance such as lifelong learning and self-education, or maintaining adequate equipment. We do not address them here separately because they are implied in the other obligations we address in this chapter. Although some authors place some or all of these obligations in the softer category of practice *ideals*, increasingly in the medical ethics and medicolegal literature they are treated as essential constituents of total quality management in team-organized health care and therefore have the moral stringency of obligations.

The Obligation to Prevent and Correct Disparagement

High stress in the surgical suite sometimes results in permission among team members to engage in disparaging comments or behaviors toward a patient or a "bottom rung" team member. While a certain amount of levity in the environment is needed to serve as an effective tension-reduction mechanism, overall the atmosphere and discussion must never slip into an arena that degrades the level of professionalism appropriate for this setting. One surgeon who reviewed an early draft of this chapter correctly captured the essence of this section in observing:

> It took me awhile to figure out the goal of this part of the paper. In the end, I think I discovered that it was to suggest to surgeons and others how their bad behavior isn't tolerated—or shouldn't be tolerated—anymore. I say that because much of what happens in the real world is based on personalities and not on these ideals you portray. Surgeons traditionally have huge egos, some are just plain assholes and believe they should be able to get away with anything they say or do as long as the procedure is a success.

His comment conveys that, yes, some expressions of a basically unpalatable personality should not be permitted because of the ethical foundations of the medical profession and society's understanding of what is entailed in showing respect for the dignity of other humans.

The surgeon, as captain, has the power to influence the behavior of everyone and therefore sets the tone in the surgical suite.[21] Women are at special risk because much of the tradition of teamwork is based on male models, and women are usually in the less powerful positions on the surgical team than men.[22] Because a patient's, nurse's, or surgical technician's interests never are served by being the brunt of a belittling or disdainful comment, the surgeon has an ethical obligation to provide strong leadership in enabling stress reduction and community-building behaviors that avoid and discourage disparagement of non-physician team members or patients.

Does this type of mistreatment affect the team's quality of care? We found no published studies in this area, but common sense leads one to suspect that the surgeon's attitudes toward the patient will influence the other members' judgment about what this patient "deserves." Furthermore, when a team member is him- or herself the brunt of disparagement, experts in this area tell us that there will certainly be less motivation to exert the exactitude, readiness, and overall excellence required for effective teamwork. Everyone wants to feel that he or she belongs and is important. In fact, common responses to ego blows in the workplace are retaliation, passive-aggressive activity, and other obstructive behaviors that can diminish effective teamwork.[17] In the absence of a strong and single-minded commitment to a "high road" approach to stress reduction and community building, the surgeon's obligation to enable total quality management is at risk of becoming thwarted.[23]

Harassment is a more serious form of disparagement or belittlement and obviously has no place on any health professions team. Harassment may include verbal slurs, lack of opportunity based on one's individual characteristics, malicious gossip about one, belittling comments, and the necessity of working in an environment that one experiences as "unsafe" or "hostile" because of the above behaviors or prevailing attitudes in that setting. Protections from harassment based on gender, race, sexual orientation, and religious affiliation have been evolving through the United States courts. A recent report of the AMA Council on Ethical and Judicial Affairs created guidelines to redress discrimination based on gender, including sexual harassment.[24]

The surgeon, again acting as the team captain, is required to know what constitutes harassment and try to prevent all displays of harassment. If and when it does occur on the team, the surgeon's ethical and legal obligation is to assure that damage is corrected and the harasser is disciplined. The surgeon also must help assure that due process is supported should the victim choose to pursue legal recourse.

The Obligation to Support Truthful Disclosure

Truthful disclosure to patients usually poses no challenge when things are going well and the news is good news. However, the crunch comes when the team is confronted with, say, an injury that occurs during a surgical procedure. Sometimes the injury is a random unavoidable event that occurs due to the slings and arrows of fate that fly to remind each of us of our mortality. There are nonblameworthy but avoidable injuries. Finally, there are blameworthy injuries (mistakes) that do not reflect on the physician's underlying ability. Of course, the distinctions seldom present themselves with the clarity one would like. It is not easy for anyone to recognize one's own failures, or those of other team members. Worse, sometimes what ought to be considered failures to honor the patient's well-being are simply considered routine practice or at least the prerogative of the surgeon to decide. But even with these complications taken into account, the basic obligation to enable good patient care through such discernment is required of the surgeon because we believe that there may be some comfort to the patient and family simply to be able to "understand" what happened.

What and to whom should this information be disclosed? Who should decide? In this case, the surgeon is morally obligated to provide leadership on the team in assuring that the course of action chosen is indeed in the best interests of the patient and, secondarily, will protect the effectiveness of teamwork.

Today the assumption by some ethicists and others is that a patient's interests generally are best served by the patient having all the facts. This rests on the notion of patient self-determination and the belief that respect for the patient must be consistent with enabling patients to make informed decisions about what is best for them. A more considered goal, and one to which we subscribe, was presented in Chapter 2 of this book. In that chapter the surgeon's obligation is portrayed as being determined by a reasonable person standard, which obligates the surgeon to relate clinically significant information to the patient. For example, suppose an event occurs during surgery that is not due to negligence but that is clinically significant; this event is addressed and reversed and has no clinically significant postoperative effects on the patient. That is, neither the event nor its immediate consequences affect the surgeon's plan for effective postoperative management of the patient. These sorts of events happen to every surgical team over the course of time but they aren't matters of negligence. Rather, they are the risks of surgery that have been corrected intraoperatively. In that case, they have no postoperative clinical significance. In contrast, there are some incidents that do have postoperative significance. For example, a patient undergoing a colostomy procedure has an episode of marked hypotension and bradycardia from anesthesia which is managed intraoperatively but which may be a risk factor on the follow-up operation to reconnect the colon. Because anesthesia with the same material may be a risk factor for the second surgery, the event's occurrence, management, and outcome would have to be discussed with the patient after recovery and as part of the decision making for the follow-up surgery.

Any departure from the practice of relating clinically relevant information to the patient or family places the burden of proof for this omission back on to the surgeon's shoulders.[25] Self- protection, protection of another member of the team or even the assumption that there was "no harm done" do not constitute sufficient reasons for nondisclosure of such information. From a pragmatic standpoint, nondisclosure also does not serve the team well in the long-term. For example, one or more members may experience deep discomfort with the nondisclosure and feel alienated from promoting patient welfare. Their perception that deception is tolerated to protect the surgeon or other team member will be interpreted as being inconsistent with their ethical responsibilities to the patient.[26] The troubled team member may begin to harbor resentment against the team leader (i.e., the surgeon), who is viewed as being the locus of control of the information flow. An important part of the psychology of this situation is that the person who decides to "break with the team" will have an easier time if he or she decides a great wrong has been perpetrated. To blow the whistle is never easy, and once the decision is made to do so, irrevocable damage probably will be done to the team.[27] In short, if there are compelling reasons for not disclosing clinically significant information to the patient and/or family, the surgeon should discuss this prospectively with all team members, and an understanding should be reached about the justification and desirability of choosing a course of medical paternalism in this situation.

The Special Case of Informed Consent

Informed consent includes an important information disclosure component. Chapter 2 details obligations of surgeons to patients in this process. But do surgeons have any special obligations to non-physician team members regarding this type of information disclosure? The point of reference for answering this question is again to assess what the surgeon should do in order to help assure quality patient management while, if possible, maintaining the smooth functioning of the team.

The process outlined in Chapter 2 assumes that the surgeon is personally on hand and is the sole agent in securing informed consent. However fitting as an ideal, this, as everyone knows, is not always the practice. The authors mention the anesthesiologist, but not highlighted are the numerous times in which nurses or other team members assume a primary role in the sequential process of preparing a patient for surgery and obtaining consent for the intervention or some aspect of it. It follows that the surgeon is obligated to obtain all relevant feedback regarding the team's efforts in regard to gaining informed consent prior to proceeding with the surgery. Simply knowing that a patient "consented" does not give the surgeon the prerogative to proceed without making sure that the patient has all the information he needs or desires about the process. In short, the obligation extends beyond "informing the patient" to also following up diligently with team members, reassuring all parties involved that they have been heard.[28]

Ethical Obligations toward Trainees

Because virtually all surgery is conducted in a team setting, training in surgery is, at its essence, training for leadership on the surgical team. The goal is for the trainee to be able to assume the surgeon's obligations to assure the provision of due care for each and every patient and enable that end in the ways outlined in the first part of this chapter.

The Obligation to Educate Future Surgeons

Not all surgeons are involved in educating future professionals. However, the profession as a whole has an obligation to perpetuate itself so that future health care needs that can be met by surgical intervention are addressed. Those not directly involved in meeting this obligation have a duty to support the efforts of those members who do assume such a responsibility.

The educator's task is to share knowledge and skills and then provide appropriate supervision to the trainee consistent with the level of expertise he or she brings to the situation.[29] The further along the trainee is, the more experience, authority, and responsibility he or she assumes. The surgeon educator has an obligation to monitor the appropriate type and level of contribution. Completion of the course of residency study signals that this person now has baseline expertise adequate for full specialty status. Along the way trainees should gain skills that allow them to become contributing members of the surgical team, bound by the rules and ethics of that team.

It goes well beyond the purpose of this chapter to examine the details of an adequate course of education for trainees in surgical settings. Generally speaking, a surgeon's training should be based on

1. A thorough understanding of the basic competencies required in this specialty or subspecialty area at the given level of undergraduate or graduate training;
2. Attention to opportunities for exposure and practice that will assist the trainee in mastering those competencies;
3. Vigilant supervision appropriate to the duty of due care;
4. Availability for questions and assistance; and
5. Fair but rigorous evaluation of performance.[30]

Attention to the individual strengths and idiosyncrasies of trainees is necessary in order to tailor their experiences to assure successful completion of the program and foster career satisfaction.[31]

In most academic settings too little time is devoted to teaching trainees the attributes and skills required for effective team leadership. A recent, otherwise thoughtful, piece entitled "Priorities in General Surgical Training" makes no mention of the surgical trainee's need to learn effective team leadership in order to apply his or her surgical technique, surgical judgment, or "book knowledge."[30] The old ideal of the apprentice who learns by observing a good role model still applies but does not fully prepare the next generation of surgeons for the challenges of providing due care in an evolving, team-intensive health care context.

Training in communication skills is necessary because good communication is an important factor in patient satisfaction and a skill required for leadership on the team. One recent study showed that patient satisfaction with students' provision of care correlated with the time students spent with them and whether they answered patients' questions.[32] Because trainees in both undergraduate and graduate medical education do spend time with patients, this is a golden opportunity for surgeon educators to help refine trainees' communication skills early in their training. However, trainees should no more be expected automatically to know how to talk to patients skillfully than they should know how to perform surgery. To become effective communicators they will require formal training in communication. A variety of programs designed to accomplish these goals has been developed.

The Obligation to Avoid and Prevent Mistreatment of Trainees

The obligation to avoid disparagement or harassment toward trainees is as binding in the trainee-surgeon relationship as in the surgical team setting. Trainees in medicine at all levels report mistreatment and abuse on a regular basis, a problem that is beginning to be addressed through studies and the promulgation of policies.[33-35] Of course, the dynamics they describe are not unique to the medical profession. As one article summarizes,

> The evidence in these studies suggests that abuse and mistreatment of all kinds comes from a variety of sources, including attending physicians, resident physicians, nurses, medical students and patients. The prevailing trend, as might be expected, is that a majority of perceived abuse suffered by an individual comes from those with greater rather than less authority.[36]

The studies cited here document high levels of perceived mistreatment and abuse. For instance, in a single school survey of third-year medical students, 84% said that they had experienced a little bit of humiliation, 24% reported threats of physical harm, 49% said that the assignment of tasks often seemed to be for punishment rather than for education, 49% were given a threat of having a grade lowered for something they did other than academic work, and 47% said that others had taken credit for work the student had done.[34]

One hopes that this report is extreme in its prevalence. However, the scope of mistreatment and abuse may not be. Strategies must be developed to prevent sexual or other harassment, discrimination, or other kinds of mistreatment at the institutional level.[37] At the same time, the surgeon educator has an obligation personally to avoid any form of mistreatment.

The Obligation to Nurture Trainees

The drafters of the Hippocratic oath showed wisdom in devoting attention to the well-being of colleagues and their offspring. In today's health care environment this mandate translates to mean that the physician must be attentive to the well-being of peers as well as the next generation of physicians, namely trainees. Therefore the obligation to avoid and prevent mistreatment has a positive corollary in the obligation to nurture trainees.

Nurturance is not limited to creating an environment for trainees that is conducive to inquiry, enables safe practice under supervision, and provides a sense of security while learning. Although those conditions are important aspects of an optimal learning environment, the obligation to nurture goes beyond that, requiring that the surgeon-educator provide encouragement, positive feedback, and support.[10] Such activities instill a sense of professional confidence in the trainee. Nurturance also requires showing a personal interest in events affecting the trainee's daily work, thereby showing the trainee that sympathy or even empathy toward colleagues is appropriate and an expected part of professional conduct.

The obligation to nurture is grounded partially in the commonsense understanding that willingness to offer support promotes trainees' ability to identify positively with the profession. One study showed that non-physician team members experienced more job satisfaction when they felt their supervisors were receptive to their problems.[38] It is reasonable to assume that attention and respect from someone with higher power and authority than the trainee (i.e., the surgeon-educator) will lead the trainee to respond similarly.

The obligation to nurture cannot be fulfilled if daily practices do not honor its importance. Traditional residency and other training often appears to be based more on models of fraternity hazing than nurturance. Long hours without sleep have been the norm for residents and only in recent years has this been addressed as a problem that can affect the competence and psychological well-being of trainees. It falls on the specialty as a whole to help create an ethos that supports the nurturing role of an individual educator.

The obligation to nurture also cannot be fulfilled in the absence of institutional mechanisms that enable it to thrive. For instance, some academic medical centers have implemented mechanisms for constructively addressing conflict between physicians and trainees. This type of intervention is a signal to trainees that they are not without both individual instructors' and institutional support in situations that have bearing on their future in their chosen profession.[36] Other centers have developed attractive physical space for trainees to exercise, relax, and converse; hired psychologists or others for counseling; provided day care in close proximity to the site with opportunities for parent-trainees to have more contact with their children; and implemented home-visit programs for trainees to become personally acquainted with families of physicians in their field.

Conflicts of Interest in the Surgeon's Role as Practitioner and Educator

Before leaving this discussion of trainees, we briefly address the potential conflict of interest a surgeon may face in attempting to meet his or her obligation both to patients' needs and trainees' needs. Fundamentally this issue raises questions about surgeons' choices regarding the allocation of their time and energy. Balancing one's activities to meet the high standards embedded in obligations to patients *and* students requires skill and self-consciousness about management of one's personal resources as well as a deep commitment to both patient care and training of future professionals. Not everyone is cut out for this dual role.

For those who do choose to be educators, the commitment to providing a trainee with optimum opportunities for development under the conditions we have been supporting will at times inevitably introduce an added increment of risk to the patient. Every trainee has a "first time ever" moment for every procedure. Educators understandably are committed to having the trainee gain adequate experience. The potential for compromising the standard of due care to patients is ever present in this type of situation, and is heightened in instances where availability of opportunity for students to gain experience is low. Constant awareness of this situation as an ethical dilemma *that must always be resolved by giving priority to the patient's well-being* provides a focus of loyalty for difficult decision making in this conflict of interest situation.[39] Put in the language of obligations to trainees, one could say that the surgeon-educator has an obligation to protect trainees from taking serious risks that will go against the high standards of his or her chosen profession in order to gain educational experiences.

Fortunately, the conflict of interest does not always present itself as an all-or-nothing situation. Usually the added increment of risk can be managed by ascertaining an acceptable standard of adequate supervision for a given situation. In setting such a standard, the variables of what should count as supervision, and especially who should be doing it (e.g., what should a surgeon, rather than a resident, supervise in the medical student trainee), must be decided and rigorously followed. The importance of such standards is being brought into public awareness through the new Medicare billing rules regarding documentation of attending physician work and other aspects of everyday practice where student or resident trainees are involved in direct patient care. Academic health centers would benefit by developing policy guidelines consistent with Medicare and other directives, thereby sharing the accountability with individual educators.

In the team setting, where almost all of the surgical trainee's experience is gained, the team members must have agreed-upon rules about when and under what circumstances a surgeon-trainee will conduct a procedure, what the level of supervision will be, and who will be acting as "captain."

Clinical Conclusions: A New Approach to Health Care Teams

We turn now from the specific obligations of surgeons to a brief synopsis of an evolving understanding of teamwork and how the surgeon's role obligations could continue to evolve with it. At the outset of this chapter we reviewed literature showing how the surgical as well as other health care teams have their origins in ideas of teams derived from sports and military models. The inherent tension between individual and collective responsibility for actions built into the idea of such teams has evoked thinking about alternative models that might better suit the actual situation of health care teams today.

One approach is the *individual responsibility approach* in which full responsibility and authority for decisions are vested in one person, the captain, but the person in the captain's role may vary with the situation facing the team. At no time does the team as a unit assume full responsibility for successes or failures.

The signal strengths of this approach are the many points of accountability over time, acknowledgment that expertise other than medical expertise is needed for some aspects of teamwork, and recognition of the several roles teams may be asked to play in patient care and management. Its shortcoming is that the high degree of individual accountability compromises team spirit. When push comes to shove, there is little to hold this team together.[1]

Another approach, at the opposite pole, is the *collective responsibility or participatory approach*. There may be a captain, but the captain's role is perfunctory because in all cases the group is held accountable for team outcomes by virtue of participation on the team. No one person, captain or other team member, can ever be held accountable personally to the exclusion of others. An example of this approach is a criminal conspiracy. Because each member voluntarily has joined the group and, additionally, each member of the group participates in the development of the principles and rules governing the team members' activities, accountability rests on the team as a whole. The team is radically "in it together."[40]

The strength of this approach is that the collective accountability could engage each member in working to keep the team functioning at an optimal level. Each will watch for signs of impairment, fatigue, or carelessness among teammates. There will be an investment in the rules guiding team behavior and the measurement tools used to evaluate team success or failure. Together they will try to assess the adequacy of institutional arrangements that support or compromise their possibility for more wins than losses.

But this model also has its shortcomings. We have just suggested how team spirit may be enhanced by the collective nature of this model. However, the opposite might be true when each member faces the reality that his or her well-being is welded to the other members of the team. Rather than have the positive effect of a team working together diligently to carry along the weaker members, any weak team member may be targeted unmercifully. Alternatively, the radical group identity may promote a tendency for cover-ups. One can hope that the drive to be a "winning" team will be sufficient to tip the scales in the direction of quality and accountability.

An urgent ethical question arises regarding how to allocate responsibility in cases of serious malfunction when it seems evident that one member is, in fact, responsible. In our highly individualized society we are hard-pressed to separate some level of personal responsibility from how a group as a whole functions.[41] An identifiable loose link in a chain must be corrected; the bad apple spoils the barrel.

Today a well-working surgical team probably moves from approach to approach. However, the surgeon still is captain of the team in almost all instances. A good team captain will either instill a sense of obligation on the whole team and not just the captain, or she will sense the loyalty of the other members to the team and focus on herself as a responsible leader of that team. This is particularly true when the surgeon introduces a new procedure and takes time to train everyone and get them excited and involved. The team members view the captain as legitimately having ultimate authority and accountability, but they are also aware of the need to work together and the failure of any one is viewed as a shared failure, just as success is shared. To the extent that the captain abuses this balance and takes the glory but assigns blame, the team breaks down and becomes a frightened, sometimes hateful, servant to one they view as a tyrant.

Our assessment is that as new models of teams emerge with managed care and other new arrangements, health care providers will observe that a group working together is the strongest when it can move among models. The surgeon, as traditional captain of the surgical team, has both a responsibility and opportunity to experiment with approaches that keep the patient's well-being the focus of everyone's attention.

References

1. Ruth Purtilo, "Teams, Health Care," in *Encyclopedia of Bioethics*, 2nd ed., Warren T. Reich, ed. New York, Macmillan, 1995, pp. 2469–2472.
2. Ruth Purtilo, "Ethical Issues and Teamwork," *Archives of Physical Medicine and Rehabilitation* 69 (1988): 318–326.
3. Ruth Purtilo, "Interdisciplinary Health Care Teams and Health Care Reform," *Journal of Law Medicine and Ethics* 22 (1994): 121–126.
4. John Duffy, *Healers: A History of American Medicine* Urbana, IL: University of Illinois Press, 1979.
5. Theodore M. Brown, "An Historical View on Health Care Teams," in *Responsibility in Health Care*, George J. Agich, ed. Dordrecht, Holland: D. Reidel Publishing Company, 1982, pp. 3–22.
6. Saad Nagi, "Teamwork in Health Care in the United States: A Sociological Perspective," *Milbank Memorial Fund Quarterly* 53(1975): 75–81.
7. June Rothberg, "Rehabilitation Team Practice," in *Interdisciplinary Team Practice: Issues and Trends*, Pedro Lecca and John S. McNeil, eds. New York: Praeger, 1985.
8. Edmund Erde, "Logical Confusions and Moral Dilemmas in Health Care Teams and Team Talk," in *Responsibility in Health Care* George Agich, ed. Dordrecht, Holland: D. Reidel Publishing Co., 1982, pp. 193–214.
9. John Ladd, "Legalism and Medical Ethics," *Journal of Medicine and Philosophy* 4(1979): 70–71.
10. Edmund Pellegrino and David Thomasma, *For the Patient's Good: the Restoration of Beneficence in the United States*. New York: Oxford University Press, 1988.
11. Joel Feinberg, "Supererogation and Rules," *Ethics* 71(1961) 39–46.

12. Tom L. Beauchamp and James F. Childress, *Principles of Biomedical Ethics*, 4th ed. New York: Oxford University Press, 1994.
13. American Medical Association. *AMA Principles of Medical Ethics* (1983) Chicago, IL: American Medical Association, 1983.
14. *Black's Law Dictionary*, 4th ed. Saint Paul, Minnesota, MN: West Publishing Company, 1968.
15. Charles Dougherty and Ruth Purtilo, "Physicians' Duty of Compassion," *Cambridge Quarterly of Healthcare Ethics* 4 (1995): 426–443.
16. Nelson S. Mitchell, Marilyn Kaplow and Charles McDougall, "The Surgeon's Ego: Moulding the Demon to the Needs of the 90's," *Canadian Journal of Surgery* 37 (1994): 8–9.
17. B. Booles and L. Swan, *Power Failure*. New York: St. Martin's Press, 1989.
18. Howard Brody, *The Healer's Power*. New Haven, CT: Yale University Press, 1992.
19. William F. May, *The Physician's Covenant: Images of the Healer in Medical Ethics*. Philadelphia, PA: Westminster, 1983.
20. American Medical Association, Council on Ethical and Judicial Affairs, "Reporting Impaired Incompetent or Unethical Colleagues," in *Codes of Medical Ethics: Reports of the Council on Ethical and Judicial Affairs*. Chicago, IL: American Medical Association, 1992, pp. 28–37.
21. Kenneth M. Leighton, "Tone in the Operating Room," *Canadian Medical Association Journal* 135 (1986): 443–444.
22. Betty L. Harragan, *Games Mother Never Taught You*. New York: Warner Books, 1977.
23. Amy M. Haddad, "The Nurse/Physician Relationship and Ethical Decision Making," *AORN Journal* 53 (1991): 151–156.
24. American Medical Association, Council on Ethical and Judicial Affairs, "Gender Discrimination in the Medical Profession Women's Health Issues," in *Codes of Medical Ethics: Reports of the Council on Ethical and Judicial Affairs*. Chicago, IL: American Medical Association, 1994, p. 1311.
25. U.S. President's Commission for the Study of Ethical Problems in Medicine and Bioethical and Behavioral Research, *Making Health Care Decisions: A Report on Ethical and Legal Implications of Informed Consent in the Patient-Practitioner Relationship*. Washington, D.C., U.S. Government Printing Office, 1982.
26. Diane Brahams, "Bad Professional Relations and Risks to Patients," *The Lancet* 2 (1988) 519–520.
27. Claire M. Fagin. "Collaboration Between Nurses and Physicians: No Longer a Choice," *Academic Medicine* 67 (1992): 285–303.
28. Neil Kessel, "Reassurance," *Lancet* 1 (1979): 1128–1133.
29. William D. Mattern, Donn Weinholtz, and Charles P. Friedman, "The Attending Physician as Teacher," *New England Journal of Medicine* 308 (1983): 1129–1132.
30. Arthur T. Martella and Gil Hauer Santos, "Priorities in General Surgical Training," *The American Journal of Surgery* 169 (1995): 271–272.
31. Kimberly D. Anderson and Brian E. Mans, "The Relationship Between Career Satisfaction and Fellowship Training in Academic Surgeons," *American Journal of Surgery* 169 (1995): 329–334.
32. Nancy L. York, Debra A. DaRosa, Stephen J. Markwell, et al., "Patients' Attitudes Toward the Involvement of Medical Students in Their Care," *The American Journal of Surgery* 169 (1995): 421.
33. DeWitt C. Baldwin, Jr., Steven R. Daugherty, and Edward J. Eckenfels, "Student

Perceptions of Mistreatment and Harassment During Medical School: a Survey of Ten United States Schools," *Western Journal of Medicine* 155 (1991): 140–145.

34. K. Harnett Sheehan, David V. Sheehan, Kim White, et al., "A Pilot Study of Medical Student 'Abuse': Student Perceptions of Mistreatment and Misconduct in Medical School," *Journal of the American Medical Association* 263 (1990): 533–537.

35. T. M. Wolf, H. M. Randall, K. von Almen, et al., "Perceived Mistreatment and Attitude Change by Graduating Medical Students: a Retrospective Study," *Medical Education.* 25 (1991): 182–190.

36. American Medical Association, Council on Ethical and Judicial Affairs, "Disputes Between Medical Supervisors and Trainees," *Journal of the American Medical Association* 272 (1994): 1861–1865.

37. American Medical Association, Council on Ethical and Judicial Affairs, "Sexual Harassment and Exploitation Between Medical Supervisors and Trainees," in *Codes of Medical Ethics: Reports of the Council on Ethical and Judicial Affairs.* Chicago, IL:, 1992, pp. 62–65.

38. Kathleen A. Curtis, "Attributional Analysis of Interprofessional Role Conflict," *Social Science and Medicine* 39 (1994): 255–263.

39. Ruth Purtilo, "Professional-Patient Relationship: Ethical Aspects," in *Encyclopedia of Bioethics*, 2nd ed., Warren T. Reid, ed. New York: Macmillan 1995, pp. 2094–2103.

40. Lisa Newton, "A Framework for Responsible Medicine," *Journal of Medicine and Philosophy* 4 (1979): 57–69.

41. H. Tristram Engelhardt, Jr., *The Foundations of Bioethics*, 2nd ed. New York, Oxford University Press, 1996.

17

Financial Relationships with Patients

KENNETH V. ISERSON
BRUCE E. JARRELL

Medical finances and bioethics seem to be both worlds apart and intricately intertwined. Purists claim that many issues relating money to medical practice are questions of professional etiquette rather than ethical issues. Yet within the medical profession, questions of reimbursement, payment mechanisms, and conflicts of interest have stimulated useful ethical discussions and guidelines since ancient times. As health care delivery systems and medical care itself evolves, surgeons' relationships with their patients will require even more ethical direction than this chapter describes.

Ethical Analysis of Remuneration for Surgical Services

Historical Considerations in Codes and Statements

Reimbursement as an Ethical Issue. It is appropriate for medical ethics to concern itself with the business aspects of medicine, and particularly with the surgeon's reimbursement for rendered services. Many patients believe that their doctors are more concerned about making money than with patient well-being.[1] Physicians must be concerned with generating income because, as Sohl and Bassford point out, "Except for the lucky few, the practice of medicine must be conducted by individuals who make their living by it. The mechanisms used for earning those livings will inevitably influence the practice of medicine,"[2] especially by accenting self-interest in payment and job security.

The Hippocratic Oath requires that "Whatever houses I may visit, I will come for the benefit of the sick . . ."[3] Highlighting the way physicians now work within a more legalistic and regimented health treatment system, one modern revision of the oath takes the form of a carefully defined contract between the patient and the physician. For example, it states that "The Provider (physician) undertakes to care for the health of the Purchaser (patient), to use his or her best endeavors to correct any defects therein and to prevent the development of further harm."[4] As with the original oath, it does not mention payment from the purchaser-patient to the provider-physician. Another modern version of the oath describes a view of the patient-physician covenant. It states that "physicians, are not and must never be, commercial entrepreneurs, gateclosers, or agents of fiscal policy that runs counter to our trust."[5] This statement, adopted by many medical associations, implicitly castigates the "gatekeeper" policies of managed care organizations, but never discusses the individual physician's reluctance to work without reimbursement.

Payment and the Surgeon-Patient Relationship. The surgeon-patient relationship is, as Leon Kass describes, "an asymmetric human relationship explicitly defined relative to one person's illness and health and the other's professed devotion to healing and comforting . . ."[6] This asymmetry in knowledge, power, and circumstances complicates the financial relationship. Simplistically we might ask, how much do you charge a drowning person to throw him or her a rope? How fair is the financial negotiation while he or she repeatedly sinks beneath the surface? And once rescued, do you throw the person back in if he or she cannot pay? In ancient times, when people's lives were saved, they owed their lives to their saviors. Even if the surgeon could claim to have saved a life with his or her interventions (and most surgery is not lifesaving), slavery is not in keeping with modern traditions.

Hippocrates discussed this dilemma in a typically paternalistic fashion, saying that physicians should not speak of fees to patients in dire need. "So one must not be anxious about fixing a fee. For I consider such a worry to be harmful to a troubled patient, particularly if the disease be acute. . . . Therefore, it is better to reproach a patient you have saved than to extort money from those who are at death's door."[7] The Canadian Medical Association's Code of Ethics, however, states that "An ethical physician will consider, in determining professional fees, both the nature of the service provided and the ability of the patient to pay, and will be prepared to discuss the fee with the patient."[8]

Kass goes on to say that as "doctoring, as such, benefits only the sick—justice requires wages, honor, or some other form of benefit to the practitioner, by way of reciprocation. And although it goes without saying that money-making, or more properly, the love of gain, can distort the practice or corrupt the practitioner of any activity practiced for a livelihood, the activity itself has its own independent meaning and being."[6] Consistent with this, the American Medical Association's Principles of Medical Ethics states that "A physician shall, in the provision of appropriate patient care, except in emergencies, be free to choose whom to serve."[9]

Legitimate Self-Interest in Remuneration

This brief historical reflection on and analysis of the physician-patient relationship indicates that reimbursement is surely among the surgeon's legitimate self-interests. Surgeons, no less than any other professional group, do not expect to provide their services without compensation in all cases. Over time, this general assumption has been buttressed by particular justifications.

The standards surgeons generally use to determine their fees are (1) the difficulty or uniqueness of the services performed; (2) the time, skill, and experience required; (3) the fee customarily charged locally for similar services; (4) the amount of the charges involved; (5) the quality of performance; and (6) the experience, reputation, and ability of the surgeon in performing the kind of services involved.[9]

Inadequately Reimbursed Care. Inadequately reimbursed care raises ethical challenges to this justification. Indigent care exemplifies these challenges. Poverty seems inevitable in our society. The medically indigent, often the working poor, will probably always be with us. As long as poverty exists, there will be inequities, especially in the access to health care services.[10]

Unlike virtually all other developed nations, the United States has rejected universal access to health care. Nonetheless, the medical profession has a duty to treat those in need. As the AMA says:

> Each physician has an obligation to share in providing care to indigent patients. The measure of what constitutes an appropriate contribution may vary with circumstances such as community characteristics, geographic location, the nature of the physician's practice and specialty, and other conditions. All physicians should work to ensure that the needs of the poor in their communities are met. Caring for the poor should be a regular part of the physician's practice schedule. In the poorest communities, it may not be possible to meet the needs of the indigent for physicians' services by relying solely on local physicians. The local physicians should be able to turn for assistance to their colleagues in prosperous communities, particularly those in close proximity.[9]

This statement, much more an expression of an ideal rather than a statement of fact, puts the burden of treating medically indigent patients not only on surgeons in their own communities but also on those in surrounding communities who have more resources. The practice of sending nonpaying patients to tertiary referral centers (usually teaching hospitals) because of the patients' financial rather than their medical status (known as the "wallet biopsy") exacerbates the problem.

Contract and Fiduciary Relationship in Patient-Physician Relationships. Surgeons often find themselves in an untenable situation in their treatment of patients when there will be inadequate reimbursement. The surgeon faces a conflict of interest between the patient's needs and his or her own financial interests, those of other patients, and of society[11] (see Chapter 18). Current cost-containment efforts place all physicians in the unenviable position of making patient-care decisions based on economic as well as clinical objectives. This poses five questions for surgeons: (1) To what extent may a surgeon refuse to treat a patient because of the patient's inability to pay? (2) To what extent must a surgeon seek to compel other providers, such as other physicians and hospitals, to expend resources on patients who are unable to pay for care that the surgeon believes is medically necessary? (3) To what extent can a surgeon benefit one patient at the expense of another? (4) To what extent can a surgeon withhold care from a patient to conserve scarce societal resources?[11] and (5) Are there limits on a health care institution's obligations to treat patients?

"If the patient-physician relationship were governed by a purely contractual approach, the answers to the questions raised above would be rather simple. . . . A purely contractual approach to the patient-physician relationship is suggested by two divergent theories: (1) the recent movement to increase patient autonomy and decrease physician paternalism, and (2) classic economic theory."[11] The law furnishes patients with protections comparable to other contracts, provided that the patient can find a surgeon willing to enter into a physician-patient relationship.

The economic theory describing a surgeon-patient contract assumes that rational, self-interested individuals will bargain with each other to maximize their individual welfare until they attain an efficient state. Unfortunately, this theory breaks down when the patient-surgeon relationship is examined. Unlike the theory's assumptions, in this relationship the bargainers are unequal and not at "arm's length." The surgeon has more knowledge and power, the relationship is more intimate than business-like, and the patient has little way of assessing the quality or worth of the surgeon's services.[11]

Economic theory also falls short when describing hospitals and their obligations to treat patients. Legal obligations require hospitals to at least "evaluate" and "stabilize" any patient presenting to their emergency departments. Many physicians, especially in institutions that normally serve medically indigent patients, feel that providing at least this much medical care is also their moral responsibility. This often means extensive interventions, including prolonged hospitalizations and repeated surgeries. Yet while hospitals have this obligation, it is often, even increasingly, an unfunded mandate. In some cases, such as with some trauma centers, fulfilling these obligations to their patients has moved some inner city hospitals, whose services were irreplaceable to the area, to the brink of financial collapse. Are there limits that not-for-profit institutions should place on the amount of nonreimbursed care they provide? (For-profit institutions rarely face this question.) If their services, as is usually the case, are necessary and irreplaceable for the local population, to keep operating they must restrict nonreimbursed care, in the least-harmful ways to their patients. (Those funded by governmental bodies, of course, often cannot accurately know what their budgets will be, so advance planning is almost a moot point.)

Institutions, whether hospitals, multispecialty practices, or private clinics, must develop policies that allow them to remain financially solvent. Failure to do so means that their services will no longer be available to their community. Patients in need of emergency surgical evaluation or treatment must get this care. How to balance these competing factors forms the basis of one of the knottiest ethical dilemmas facing modern U.S. medicine. Surgeons must decide for themselves and as a group how much additional financial risk they will willingly assume. The policies of the institutions in which they work may also influence these decisions (or help decide in which institutions a surgeon wishes to work). Note that if a surgeon's voluntary actions consistently accrue bad debt for an institution (e.g., hospital, managed care organization), it may consider limiting his or her privileges (financial credentialing, which may be illegal, but still occurs).[12]

Ethically Unjustified Forms of Payment. Charity care, writing off bad debts, and coercive collection methods should all be used judiciously. The surgeon is entitled to payment for services rendered, including services both as the primary surgeon and as an assistant.[12] In the office setting, he or she may also charge for missed appointments.[9] There are some fees and types of billing, however, that are ethically out of bounds.

Contingency fees are one example. The AMA states that "a physician's fee should not be made contingent on the successful outcome of medical treatment. Such arrangements are unethical because they imply that successful outcomes from treatment are guaranteed, thus creating unrealistic expectations of medicine and false promises to consumers."[9] Medicine remains an imperfect science, and it is the duty of the surgeon to remind patients of the risks involved in surgical procedures. The other problem is how patients define "success." For some patients, the success they seek is unachievable. No matter how well the neurosurgeon stabilizes the spine, if a patient has dense paraplegia before the surgery, it is likely he or she will still be afflicted postoperatively. Surgical intervention has many goals. Although surgeons should, when it is not obvious, try to ascertain these goals, patients' goals are often too nebulous or too unrealistic to be the basis of reimbursement. Similarly, reimbursement should not be contingent upon the outcome of legal or insurance claims but be based on the value of the medical service.[9] It is not the lawyer's skill that the patient (or the patient's insurance company) is paying for, but rather for the surgeon's expertise, effort, time, resources, and income otherwise forgone. Whether or not the patient gets a large monetary settlement, the surgeon should be paid fairly for the time and effort he or she has expended. (If the surgeon also spends time helping the patient in a legal dispute, this should be fairly compensated—but again not made contingent on the case's outcome.)

Likewise, excessive treatments or hospitalizations, supposedly common under fee-for-service systems, is ethically inappropriate both because it increases a patient's risk and because it is intrinsically dishonest.[9] "Cases have been reported in which clinics have conducted excessive and unnecessary medical testing while certifying to insurers that the testing is medically necessary. Such fraudulent activity exacerbates the high cost of health care . . . and is unethical."[9] Physicians may never place their own financial interests above the welfare of their patients. "The primary objective of the medical profession is to render service to humanity; reward or financial gain is a subordinate consideration. For a physician unnecessarily to hospitalize a patient, prescribe a drug, or conduct diagnostic tests for the physician's financial benefit is unethical."[9]

In the end, however, the patients (or their insurers) are responsible for paying the surgeon's bill. Even the most ardent patient advocates admit that "like almost everything else that happens to a patient, the patient is responsible for paying the bills."[13]

Clinical Topics

Setting Fees

Surgical fees are often "bundled" into a single fee for a particular procedure, such as an appendectomy. These fees normally include preoperative diagnosis, the surgery, and postoperative care. In some cases where clinical experience or technological advances have changed (usually lessened) the time, morbidity, and stress of the procedures, such as with laparoscopic cholecystectomies or coronary artery bypass grafts, the inflation-adjusted fees often continue to reflect the payments from prior years when the procedures warranted increased reimbursement.

After the first disastrous experiments in Massachusetts with resetting surgical fees based on the resource cost-based relative-value scales (RBRVS), Egdahl and Manuel devised a method to determine an appropriate relative-value for surgical procedures. This method used experienced practitioners from multiple settings who independently gave surgical procedures RVS scores from 1 to 100 (starting with pancreatoduodenectomy rated as 100). They then adjusted these scores based on face-to-face meetings over several iterations. They found that surgeons with the most experience with each procedure held sway, although compromises occurred in the process. They felt that subsequent information about the complexity-severity (C-S) scores billed by surgeons could help in the hiring process, with referral centers seeking those surgeons who normally billed the higher C-S scores.[14]

In medicine's non-market economy, most surgeons' fees are set based either on prevailing rates in a geographic area or on the fees negotiated with managed care organizations. Even if surgeons establish very high fees, they will be paid these fees only if they convince patients both that surgeons are worth the extra cost and that patients should pay the balance of the bill that their insurance does not cover.

This approach to adequate remuneration has an uncertain future. For the future there are also some, at present, unanswered questions. Should surgeons ever price their services so low as to lose money on each patient? (To calculate this, one must consider not only the surgeon's time, but also fixed expenses, such as office overhead, licensing fees, and the costs of malpractice insurance, professional meetings, publications, and associations.) Should they be a "loss-leader" for a group or institution, with these groups making up the balance? Are any ethical dilemmas involved or is this purely a "marketing strategy"? Does this type of cost-shifting undermine what health care systems exist, and what responsibility does the surgeon have to monitor this?

Medicare Payments and Surgical Services

The prospective payment system had a significant effect in reducing the growth of Medicare expenditures to surgeons. There is a question, however, about whether some of the services once provided to an inpatient (under a global fee) are appropriately done in the outpatient setting.[15] By extension, one must also question the discharge of patients who may still be quite ill ("sicker and quicker") to cut costs so that they equal or are less than the payments the surgeon receives.

The only way to maintain the same profit margin (e.g., income to the surgeon) for the same number and complexity of procedures is either to decrease costs or to increase prices. Because the "price" being paid for services is steadily decreasing, the danger is to go beyond deleting costs for "unnecessary" visits and procedures and to begin deleting those patient services necessary for adequate, if not optimal, patient care.

Yet, while OBRA 1987 lowered fees for procedures and tests, especially in ophthalmology, orthopedic surgery, thoracic surgery, urology, and gastroenterology, there was no significant change (0.09% decrease for every 1% decrease in fees) in physician services with lowered reimbursements. This contradicts HCFA's assertion that clinicians would increase their service volume and complexity to make up one half of the lost income from the lowered fees.[16] It appears that the number of clinicians, rather than the fees paid, may be the dominant factor in the number of procedures performed. The best way to decrease the number of procedures may be to decrease the number of specialists trained to do those procedures. Market forces appear to have initiated this process already.

Surgeon Availability versus Use of Services

There is a positive association between the supply of surgeons and specific operative rates,[17,18] the total surgery rate,[19] and aggregate measures of use.[20] For example, back surgery rates are at least 40% higher in the United States than in any of 11 other developed countries, and is five times higher than in England and Scotland. The rate goes up linearly with the number of orthopedic surgeons and neurosurgeons. Managed care patients in the United States have about half the number of spine operations as do fee-for-service patients. The question remains whether fee-for-service patients in the United States receive too many back surgeries or citizens in other countries and in managed care organizations receive too few.[21]

Other studies found that the frequency of CABG was nearly twice as high for fee-for-service patients as for HMO patients or Medicaid recipients. Whether this represents more appropriate use of CABG for the HMO/Medicaid group or simply cost cutting at the expense of patient welfare is uncertain. If the excess operations in fee-for-service patients represent a misuse of cardiac surgery, the HMO/Medicaid patients may actually have been better off than their cohorts.[22]

One study, looking at ophthalmology, general surgery, orthopedic surgery, and urology, found that more patients "receive care in areas with a high supply of surgeons, but those who receive care are not treated any more intensely." The authors suggested that this was due to the greater ease of seeing a surgeon coupled with stronger preferences for referrals to surgeons in these areas.[23] Also, the statistical relationship of physician density to physician-initiated visits may not show inappropriate services but rather reflect the clustering of sick patients around medical centers.[24]

Patients suffer when surgeons are motivated by financial considerations and alter their advice or recommend services to their patients above and beyond what is in patients' interests. But where too few surgeons exist, patients also suffer. Therefore, analysts suggest "that the net impact on welfare of a high and growing surgeon supply is not so clear."[23]

Part of the problem of "overuse" of surgical services also stems from the nature of medical practice. The greatest variations in surgical rates and hospital use occur in conditions for which there is less consensus on criteria for a firm diagnosis and for optimal treatments.[25] Cost reduction in these clinical contexts may be difficult to achieve without injuring many patients. Surgeons should serve as advocates to protect patients from such injury.

Billing for "Ghost Surgery"

The public, and sometimes lawyers, loosely use the term "ghost surgery" to indicate anytime that another surgeon, usually a resident, performs an operation. Both legal and ethical opinion agree, however, that this term and its implications apply only when the surgeon is not "scrubbed in" to an operation and the other surgeon operates unsupervised. As with all medical training, residents need to perform procedures to learn and become proficient in them. The surgeons who directly supervise them are there both to teach the resident and to protect the patient. This supervising role often takes a great deal more skill, emotional toll, and effort than would be expended by simply performing the procedure oneself. Contrary to the current practice, serious consideration should be given to reimbursing supervising physicians at a higher level.

True "ghost surgery," where the surgeon of record—who, the patient believes, will perform the operation—is not present at the operating table, should normally not be billed by the "supervising" surgeon. As the AMA says:

> The surgeon's obligation to the patient requires the surgeon to perform the surgical operation: (1) within the scope of authority granted by the consent to the operation; (2) in accordance with the terms of the contractual relationship; (3) with complete disclosure of facts relevant to the need and the performance of the operation; and (4) utilizing best skill.[9]

In many cases, residents will "open" and "close" without the supervising surgeon present. If this routine procedure is well within the resident's capabilities, this should not raise the specter of "ghost surgery." Similarly, when a patient's condition warrants an emergency procedure and the attending surgeon arrives as soon as possible (but after the procedure has commenced), the attending surgeon need not be reluctant to bill for the procedure.

Managed Care and the Surgeon

Angell says that now "Many of us . . . believe that doctors have other obligations that compete with their obligation to the patient. Doctors are increasingly being asked, in one way or another, to save money for a third party—and sometimes for themselves—by scrimping on the medical care they deliver."[26] In his 1991 address to the Southern Thoracic Surgical Association, Robert Sade stated that a surgeon cannot be both an unlimited patient advocate and a cost-cutter. To deny any procedure or device to any patient based upon cost is to subvert patient welfare and make the physician a "double agent."[27] By contrast, Bahn urges others to become more active as gatekeepers.[28]

Managed care organizations (MCOs) achieve some of their cost savings by avoiding "discretionary" surgery and hospitalization, although MCO patients generally have the same rates of nondiscretionary surgery as non-MCO patients.[29] As institutions evolve, managed care and other large physician groups are measuring physician productivity in relative-value units, patients per hour, or similar measures, rather than simply billings and collections. This puts more financial risk at the institutional level, and would, ideally, allow physicians to practice without conflicts relating to patient finances. Few, if any, groups have yet evolved to that point.

In some cases, high fees and availability of certain practitioners are causing some specialties to be subsumed by others. This is especially true of surgery because surgeons are more expensive than most other specialists. Payers know this and, whenever possible, have other physicians do some of the work that the surgeons once did. This may severely limit or eliminate some surgical specialties, such as general thoracic surgery. From 1991 to 1996, for example, there was a predicted 27% decrease in payments to thoracic surgeons, primarily because many cases they once saw were being treated by pulmonologists.[30] The practice patterns of related surgical and nonsurgical specialists (such as ophthalmologists and optometrists or neurologists and neurosurgeons) depend on the availability of these practitioners. Where there are insufficient numbers of particular specialists, others take over where they can.[31]

Changes in technology, biology, societal culture, and surgical practice may also positively alter the course of many specialties and their incomes. For example, in the future neurosurgeons may have markedly increased workloads due to the possibility of spinal grafting to treat paralysis and neural implants to treat Parkinson's and Alzheimer's diseases. Successful surgical management of these diseases may alter population demographics enough so that orthopedic and vascular surgeons increase their workloads. Some have also posited that MCOs will better use general surgeons, revitalizing the specialty by expanding their practices and "keeping patients 'down on the farm.'"[32]

In the future, providers wishing to be competitive under a managed care system will need to be cost-effective. To do this, they will need accurate and timely financial information to relate their true costs to reimbursement and to calculate the value of their services. Financial data are necessary to implement financial continuous quality improvement to contain costs while maintaining quality. Not all managed care contracts are profitable, and providers should evaluate each contract separately. Some plans have begun to measure the cost differences among physicians providing care to similar patients (physician profiling). "Those physicians whose costs are high with no corresponding difference in the quality of the outcomes in their patients may be identified as a drain on the managed care system. When hospital privileges are tied to such data, this process is termed economic credentialing."[33]

As specialist services, including surgical services, are capitated (a set fee to supply services for an entire population) under managed care, the quality of care may suffer. Surgeons may not be willing to perform the appendectomy at 2 AM or come in to set the fracture on a holiday. Fee-for-service, despite its many shortcomings, does provide a motivation to "go the extra mile."

Self-Referral and Conflicts of Interest

The potential for conflicts of interest abounds in medical practice (see Chapter 18). Since the late nineteenth century, national medical leaders have condemned one form of conflict of interest, fee splitting, in all of its various forms. From its formation in 1913, the American College of Surgeons actively tried to eradicate this practice, as well as all other "dishonest money-seeking." In the past, American medical professionals received money for referring patients to other practitioners, pharmacies, medical equipment suppliers, hospitals, sanitaria, and undertakers. In turn they paid commissions to both medical professionals and laymen who steered patients their way.[34]

While such obvious "kickbacks" have disappeared from the medical scene, referring patients to facilities in which the surgeon has partial or complete ownership seems to have generated new questions about conflicts of interest. While no one wants to restrict physicians' ability to make legitimate investments, there are restrictions on referring patients to facilities that will generate additional income for the practitioner. The AMA says that:

> . . . when physicians refer patients to health care facilities in which they have an ownership interest, a potential conflict of interest exists. In general, physicians should not refer patients to a health care facility which is outside their office practice and at which they do not directly provide care or services when they have an investment interest in that facility. The requirement that the physician directly provide care or services should be interpreted as commonly understood. The physician needs to have personal involvement with the provision of care on site.[9]

This injunction applies both to medical facilities and medical services, such as home health care agencies.[9]

One exception exists when a community needs a unique medical service and the only way to provide it is through physician investment. Many physician investors have used this justification for their own behavior (and referral patterns), but few can fulfill the AMA's rigid ethical guidelines for such investments. These standards include complete disclosure to patients and third-party payers, opening the project to wider investment than just referring physicians, no require-ment for investors to refer patients, returns based on equity rather than refer-rals or facility use, no non-compete clauses concerning similar investments, and safeguards for patients through utilization review of referrals.[9]

One self-referral conflict that has become politically incorrect to discuss is that of referring only within one's own physician group. This is, in fact, a basis for many managed care organizations, group practices, and university physician groups. Although patients may assume that these referrals represent the best possible choice (medically and financially) for additional care, that may not neces-sarily be true. A closer look at such arrangements is certainly justified, although it will be unpopular with managed care organizations, physician groups, academic medicine, and most third-party payers. This stance alone should make closer scrutiny worthwhile (see Chapter 18).

Medicaid Patients

Medicaid and other public medical assistance programs at the local level vary tremendously among states in their eligibility requirements, mechanisms of payment, and willingness of providers to take patients. It was often assumed that the low reimbursement rates under most Medicaid programs kept many practi-tioners from seeing these patients, however, a study in Maryland showed that increasing Medicaid physician fees (for obstetric care) to the level of private third-party payers did not guarantee patients equal access to private physicians.[35]

Because one goal of many Medicaid administrators is to decrease usage (and supposedly, costs), one technique they have employed is case management or a managed care approach. First used in Arizona and copied in other states, such as Tennessee, this system begins reducing costs by making enrollment very dif-ficult. The system's restrictions, poor physician reimbursement, and bureaucracy all serve to reduce the number of patients in the system and payment for ser-vices rendered. (At least in Arizona, many physicians and administrators also became wealthy from the money not paid for patient services and by control-ling contracts for large numbers of patients.)

In less sophisticated systems, case management has decreased at least some inappropriate usage of Medicaid services. One system had a marked drop in pediatric emergency department use by Medicaid patients after a preauthori-zation requirement was initiated. However, there was no decrease in the num-ber of patients admitted to hospital through the emergency department.[36] Simi-larly, another study found that, while indigent women present at a later stage of breast cancer, their outcome from that point on is independent of their insur-ance status.[37]

Surgeons working in trauma centers, especially in larger cities, have a high proportion of Medicaid (and other medically indigent) patients. A study of patients admitted to New York trauma centers showed that 71% of patients with penetrating trauma are Medicaid or self-pay, compared to 21% of blunt-trauma patients. Level 1 trauma centers received approximately equal numbers of blunt and penetrating trauma, while community hospitals had four times more blunt than penetrating trauma. However, it is not just the mix of patients and payers, but the higher costs associated with trauma care and the relatively low levels of reimbursement that have increased operating losses for trauma centers.[38]

Trauma centers in many large cities, including Chicago and Los Angeles, have closed because of the trauma patients' financial drain on their system. How much longer hospitals can finance unfunded fiduciary obligations has become an urgent ethical and public policy issue.

Collecting Fees

Surgeons collect patient-related fees from four groups: governments, insurance companies, managed care organizations, and patients or families. As with any worker in a capitalist society, surgeons should get paid for their work. How aggressively should they seek payment from the various groups? Governments pay their bills slowly, as do some MCOs. The time-value of money (the interest earned when you keep it, rather than sending it to creditors) motivates them to hold payments for as long as possible. This is the nature of all non-cash businesses. When government entities don't pay or pay less than agreed on, there is often little the surgeon can do. The only recourses are the court system (slow and expensive) or working with organized professional groups to proactively change the system.

Insurance companies normally pay their bills on the schedule mandated by their system. Some MCOs, however, adjust or retrospectively deny claims for physicians who bill them fee-for-service (even under a specified contract). In our view, this behavior, seen with some MCOs, represents dishonest business practices. Because the managed care industry is so poorly regulated, however, the practices persist. Aggressive pursuit of the surgeon's legitimate business interests is the best solution to these problems, in our judgment.

Acquiring bad debts is one of the tribulations of being in business. Businesses normally try to avoid bad debts by screening customers, requiring prepayment for goods or services, or refusing to serve customers in arrears on their payments. The nature of surgical practice, including on-call responsibilities to hospitals, does not allow this. Surgical emergencies require immediate treatment. If a surgeon is responsible for providing that treatment, the prospect of not getting paid does not relieve the surgeon of the ethical, professional, or legal (COBRA federal law) responsibility to provide this treatment. This also holds true for the immediate postoperative period. In non-emergency situations, surgeons may choose not to initiate or to terminate relationships with patients for, among other reasons, probable or proven nonpayment.

Economic Abandonment and Cost-Shifting

Indigent and other patients at risk for not paying their bills are often told to seek care (or a "consultation") at the university, county, or other regional health care facility known to generally accept such patients, regardless of their ability to pay. In some cases, these patients, who have been surgeons' long-term patients, have suddenly lost their insurance. How unacceptably far behind in payment a patient is before the surgeon refuses further care varies. Some will continue to care for long-term patients. Others have little tolerance for this situation and "refer" such patients to publicly operated facilities. This allows such surgeons (or the groups who employ them) to skim paying patients from the general population, deny that they have a duty to help provide indigent care (in conflict with the AMA guidelines discussed above), and force society to subsidize their incomes and lifestyles by making others pay for the care of the patients they turn away.

Should the financial interests of one or more patients be sacrificed for those of another? In circumstances of absolute scarcity, such as in triage situations, this is necessary. But the traditional way of paying for much indigent medical care over at least the past several decades—increasing costs to patients who could afford them to pay for those who could not—is being thwarted by third-party payers who are no longer willing to do this. The "cherry-picking" behavior of many managed care organizations, where they select only patients who statistically have the least risk of costing them money (the young, healthy teenager and adult) is the extreme expression of this behavior.

The "heroic" cost-shifting behavior by physicians contradicts legal principles not to expend one person's assets to benefit another without explicit permission.[11] One must, however, have something at risk to be heroic. Physicians themselves do not exhibit any heroism when they shift costs between those who can pay and those who cannot pay. Only third-party payers seem to lose when surgeons cost-shift between their paying patients and the medically indigent. Physicians and hospitals lose only if these costs cannot be shifted, and as described above, hospitals generally suffer the greatest economic losses, as a consequence of their mandate to treat medically indigent patients, a mandate based in the assumption of fiduciary responsibility for patients regardless of their ability to pay.

The conflict between the economic interests of the physician trying to preferentially attract paying (or high-reimbursement) patients diminishes the profession's trustworthiness. It also violates the profession's virtues of truthfulness, loyalty, and respect for persons.[39]

Copayments, Balance Billing, and Collection Practice

Medicare's previous payment scheme (customary, prevailing, and reasonable charges) to reimburse physicians, basing the next year's payments on the current year's charges, encouraged physicians to constantly raise their fees. In addition, Medicare overpaid for many technical procedures, such as surgery, while underpaying for office visits and similar cognitive services.[40]

Although recent laws have increased patients' Medicare copayments, this seems to be offset by balance billing limits. It is estimated that rural and African-American patients have suffered the most from these changes, while those with large medical expenses have benefited.[41]

The AMA states that ". . . in some cases, financial hardship may deter patients from seeking necessary care if they would be responsible for a copayment for the care. . . . When a copayment is a barrier to needed care because of financial hardship, physicians should forgive or waive the copayment. . . . Physicians should ensure that their policies on copayments are consistent with applicable law and with the requirements of their agreements with insurers."[9]

"Although harsh or commercial collection practices are discouraged in the practice of medicine, a physician who has experienced problems with delinquent accounts may properly choose to request that payment be made at the time of treatment or add interest or other reasonable charges to delinquent accounts."[9] Surgeons should use discretion in hardship cases. Patients should be notified of these policies in advance and of any bills sent to collection agencies.[9] Although it is a drastic step rarely used, even the AMA's Ethical and Judicial Council agrees that in states with lien laws, a physician may file a lien to assure payment of his or her fees.[9]

Charity Care and Bad Debts

There is a difference, both ethically and economically, between those patients who cannot pay without extraordinary personal sacrifices (charity care) and those who can but are unwilling to pay (uncompensated care or bad debt). This amount may be the entire bill or the amount not covered by a third-party payer. Not-for-profit status (most academic medical centers, for example) requires delivering charity care, although the exact amount is usually not specified in law or regulation. They must also have a sliding payment scale so that patients pay for their health care services according to their financial state.

A large study showed that general surgeons have more patients with bad debts than would be expected, whereas orthopedic surgeons generated considerably more charity care. (The distribution of charity versus bad debt may, however, be a function of the physicians surveyed.) Unemployed patients (9.9% of the total) had disproportionate amounts of bad debt (31.8%) and charity care (25.8%). Retired individuals (37% of total patients) also had a high rate of charity care (57.1%). Other markers for patients with disproportionately high bad debt or charity care were "self-pay" patients and those on Medicare or Medicaid.[42]

The number of patients or the amount of charity and unreimbursed care surgeons generate may stem from their attitudes toward the financial aspects of health treatments and the direct effect that payment (or nonpayment) for patient services has on their income. The attitude of many surgeons working at not-for-profit hospitals is notable for their lack of interest in the financial status of the patient and finances in general. In part, that is due to these institutions' attracting practitioners who have little interest in their patients' finances, only in their health. This attitude is enhanced in large multispecialty groups where physicians lose perspective of the relationship of their income to any particular patient's payment for their services. This relationship is much more evident in smaller groups or individual practice.

Accounting rules, however, require that care rendered as charity be identified in advance, not retrospectively. They also require that charity care not be included as revenue (decreasing total income but lowering tax liability), whereas bad debts are reported as expenses against income.[43] Some hospitals, however, believe that these rules are in error and include all revenue they never attempt to collect under "charity" care. Some hospitals also question whether they should also include those expenses for Medicaid patients that do not equal the revenues for these patients. Even with this altered accounting method, these hospitals still accrue bad debts, because they are unwilling to simply write off bills for those who can pay, but won't—including insurers. The amount of time the bad debt is on their books at any time is a function of how quickly accounts are "aged," that is, written off as uncollectable. The clinician and institution have multiple opportunities, especially for hospitalized patients, to identify which patients should be considered "charity" cases before billing them.[44]

A strange group to be receiving charity care are other physicians and their families. Professional courtesy, reduced or no fees, was originally discussed in the Hippocratic oath, and both Percival's *Medical Ethics* (1803) and the AMA's first code of ethics in 1847 specifically required it (see Chapter 10). While professional courtesy to physician colleagues and their families "is a long-standing tradition, it is not an ethical requirement."[9] A large national survey showed that 98% of physicians (80% for psychiatrists) support this practice. General surgeons (98%) and surgical subspecialists (99%) fully support professional courtesy.[45] However, this time-honored practice has the potential for interfering with the doctor-patient relationship and increases physician insensitivity to the costs of medical care.

Managing Financial Aspects of the Surgeon-Patient Relationship

Many surgeons now practice under managed care systems; most will do so in the future. Financial arrangements with their patients, therefore, operate on a level somewhat removed from the individual practitioner. The surgeon is salaried and ideally operates or sees patients only on the basis of medical need. When the surgeon participates in any form of remuneration from the managed care system where decisions are based on cost savings, his or her fiduciary relationship with patients is jeopardized. Whether or not treatment decisions change because of this reimbursement pattern, the perception that they could do so colors any decisions that the surgeon makes—especially those not to perform requested services.

Fee-for-service (indemnity) arrangements, of course, have always had that drawback—but in the opposite direction. The financial incentive was to do more operations, rather than fewer. Procedures are well reimbursed, office visits are not. Most patients now have some form of payment system, whether it be an insurance carrier, Medicare, Medicaid, or a combination. These payers most commonly base reimbursements on fee-for-service charges, although some are now moving aggressively to managed care systems, including capitation for some populations. True fee-for-service payments are becoming rarer, except for the "notch group," those people who fail to qualify for any insurance or Medicaid.

In the past, many surgeons accepted "self-pay" or non-paying patients (often the same group) with the understanding that high fees generated by paying patients would cover the costs of treating these patients. Such cost-shifting has become less tenable under new payment systems. It still occurs, however, especially where surgeons have leeway in what they charge patients. Without a national health care system, each surgeon or group must look to their own consciences when deciding how many such patients they can take.

Clinical Conclusions

Medicine is a beneficent endeavor. Surgeons, though, need to profit from medical practice to fulfill their own legitimate interests. What is fair to charge patients and society for these services becomes a central question that we have addressed in this chapter. Fair compensation to surgeons is based on their expertise, effort, time, and the years they spent learning their craft. Surgeons, the institutions in which they practice, and society perform an intricate dance around many of the ethical issues regarding reimbursement for medical care. Cost-shifting, care for the medically indigent, and prepaid health care programs all complicate the issues. Yet guidelines exist and are well disseminated for setting and collecting surgical fees. These preclude reimbursement for work not done (including "ghost surgery") and compromising their patient-surgeon relationships with self-referrals or performing unwarranted procedures. Many other issues, including the conflicts raised by referrals within closed panels of physicians, are less clear.

References

1. Gina Kolata, "Wariness is Replacing Trust between Healer and Patient," *New York Times* (February 20, 1990): A1. (National Edition)
2. P. Sohl and H. A. Bassford, "Codes of Medical Ethics: Traditional Foundations and Contemporary Practice," *Social Science and Medicine* 22 (1986): 1175–1179.
3. Kenneth V. Iserson, Sanders AB, Mathieu D, *Ethics in Emergency Medicine*, 2nd ed. Tucson, AZ: Galen Press, 1995.
4. J. Rosalki, "The Hippocratic Contract: A Revision of the Hippocratic Oath with a Contract-Based Orientation," *Journal of Medical Ethics* 19 (1993): 154–156.
5. Ralph D. Crawshaw, David E. Rogers, Edmund D. Pellegrino, et al., "Patient-Physician Covenant," *Journal of the American Medical Association* 273 (1995): 1553.
6. Leon R. Kass, "Professing Ethically: On the Place of Ethics in Defining Medicine," *Journal of the American Medical Association* 249 (1983): 1305–1310.
7. Hippocrates, "The Oath," in *The Loeb Classical Library*, Vol. 1., W. H. S. Jones, trans. Cambridge, MA: Harvard University Press, 1962.
8. Canadian Medical Association, *Canadian Medical Association Code of Ethics*. Toronto, Ontario, Canada: Canadian Medical Association, 1990.
9. American Medical Association, *Code of Medical Ethics, Current Opinions of the Council on Ethical and Judicial Affairs*. Chicago, IL: American Medical Association, 1996.
10. Charlotte Muller, "Review of Twenty Years of Research on Medical Care Utilization, " *Health Services Research* 21 (1986): 129–144.
11. Maxwell J. Mehlman and Susan R. Massey, "The Patient-Physician Relationship and the Allocation of Scarce Resources: A Law and Economics Approach," *Kennedy Institute of Ethics Journal* 4 (1994): 291–308.
12. Charles W. Bailey, Jr., "How to Avoid Being Dropped from Managed Care Plans," *Postgraduate Medicine* 95 (1994): 59–62.
13. George J. Annas, *The Rights of Patients: The Basic ACLU Guide to Patient Rights*, 2nd ed. Carbondale, IL: Southern Illinois University, 1989.
14. Richard H. Egdahl and Barry Manuel, "A Consensus Process to Determine the Relative Complexity-Severity of Frequently Performed Surgical Services," *Surgery, Gynecology, and Obstetrics* 160 (1985): 403–406.
15. Gerald F. Kominski and Andrea K. Biddle, "Changes in Follow-Up for Medicare Surgical Patients under the Prospective Payment System," *Medical Care* 31 (1993): 230–246.
16. José J. Escarce,' "Effects of Lower Surgical Fees on the Use of Physician Services under Medicare," *Journal of the American Medical Association* 269 (1993): 2513.
17. Charles E. Lewis, "Variations in the Incidence of Surgery," *New England Journal of Medicine* 281 (1969): 880–884.
18. Beverly Pasley, Philip Vernon, Geoffrey Gibson, et al., "Geographic Variations in

Elderly Hospital and Surgical Discharge Rates, New York State," *American Journal of Public Health* 77 (1987): 679–684.

19. J. Cromwell and J. B. Mitchell, "Physician-Induced Demand for Surgery," *Journal of Health Economics* 5 (1986): 293–313.

20. M. Stano, "An Analysis of the Evidence on Competition in the Physician Services Markets," *Journal of Health Economics* 4 (1985): 197–211.

21. Daniel C. Cherkin, Richard A. Deyo, John D. Loeser, et al., "An International Comparison of Back Surgery Rates," *Spine* 19 (1994): 1201–1206.

22. Kenneth M. Langa and Elliott J. Sussman, "The Effect of Cost-Containment Policies on Rates of Coronary Revascularization in California," *New England Journal of Medicine* 329 (1993): 1784–1789.

23. José J. Escarce, "Explaining the Association between Surgeon Supply and Utilization," *Inquiry* 29 (1992): 403–415.

24. J. Hay and M. Leahy, "Physician-Induced Demand: An Empirical Analysis of the Consumer Information Gap," *Journal of Health Economics* 1 (1982): 231–244.

25. John E. Wennberg, Kim McPherson, and Philip P. Caper, "Will Payment Based on Diagnosis-Related Groups Control Hospital Costs?" *New England Journal of Medicine* 311 (1984): 295–300.

26. Marcia Angell, "The Doctor as Double Agent," *Kennedy Institute of Ethics Journal* 3 (1994): 279–286.

27. Robert M. Sade, "The Different Drummer, the Double Agent, and Future Dilemmas in Bioethics," *Annals of Thoracic Surgery* 53 (1992): 183–190.

28. Cordell H. Bahn, "The Surgeon as Gatekeeper," *American Journal of Surgery* 165 (1993): 550–553.

29. Allbert L. Siu, Arleen Leibowitz, Robert H. Brook, et al., "Use of the Hospital in a Randomized Trial of Prepaid Care," *Journal of the American Medical Association* 259 (1988): 1343–1346.

30. L. Penfield Faber, "General Thoracic Surgery in the Year 2010," *Annals of Thoracic Surgery* 55 (1993): 1326–1331.

31. Matthew Menken, "The Workload of Neurosurgeons: Implications of the 1987 Practice Survey in the USA," *Journal of Neurology, Neurosurgery & Psychiatry* 54 (1991): 921–924.

32. Andrew L. Warshaw, "Pancreatic Surgery. A Paradigm for Progress in the Age of the Bottom Line," *Archives of Surgery* 130 (1995): 240–246.

33. Timothy A. Denton, Aurelio Chaux, and Jack M. Matloff, "A Cardiothoracic Surgery Information System for the Next Century: Implications for Managed Care," *Annals of Thoracic Surgery* 59 (1995): 486–493

34. Marc A. Rodwin, "The Organized American Medical Profession's Response to Financial Conflicts of Interest: 1890–1992," *The Milbank Quarterly* 70 (1992): 703–741.

35. Michael H. Fox and Kai L. Phua, "Using Medicaid Claims Data to Evaluate a Large Physician Fee Increase," *Health Services Research* 29 (1994): 315–340.

36. J. Thomas Badgett, "Can Medicaid Format Alter Emergency Department Utilization Patterns?" *Pediatric Emergency Care* 2 (1986): 67–70.

37. R. T. Osteen, D. P. Winchester, D. H. Hussey, et al., "Insurance Coverage of Patients with Breast Cancer in the 1991 Commission on Cancer Patient Care Evaluation Study," *Annals of Surgical Oncology* 1 (1994): 462–467.

38. Sharm A. Joy, Leo Lichtig, Robert A. Knauf, et al., "Identification and Categorization of and Cost for Care of Trauma Patients: A Study of 12 Trauma Centers and 43,219 Statewide Patients," *Journal of Trauma* 37 (1994): 303–308.

39. Susan S. Braithwaite, "The Courtship of the Paying Patient," *Journal of Clinical Ethics* 4 (1993): 124–133.
40. Physician Payment Review Commission, *Annual Report to Congress*. Washington, DC: U.S. Government Printing Office, 1988.
41. Janet B. Mitchell and Terri Menke, "How the Physician Fee Schedule Affects Medicare Patients' Out-of-Pocket Spending,"*Inquiry* 27 (1990): 108–113.
42. Kerry E. Kilpatrick, Michael K. Miller, Jeffrey W. Dwyer, et al., "Uncompensated Care Provided by Private Practice Physicians in Florida," *Health Services Research* 26 (1991): 277–302.
43. American Institute of Certified Public Accountants. Health Care Audit Guide. New York: AICPA, 1990.
44. Patrice Ferko, "Managing Bad Debt and Charity Care Accounts," *Topics in Health Care Financing* 20 (1993): 66–70.
45. Mark A. Levy, Robert M. Arnold, Michael J. Fine, et al., "Professional Courtesy— Current Practices and Attitudes," *New England Journal of Medicine* 329 (1993): 1627–1631.

18

Understanding, Assessing,
and Managing Conflicts of Interest

GEORGE KHUSHF
ROBERT GIFFORD

Certain types of financial arrangements have long been frowned upon by the medical profession.[1,2] Many of these were grouped under the heading of "fee splitting" and directly prohibited. Thus, for example, a generalist could not obtain a kickback for referring a patient to a surgeon; a surgeon could not use an agent to "drum up" business, and so forth. The reason generally given for prohibiting such practices was that financial arrangements were inappropriately introduced into a decision-making process that should be exclusively directed by medical factors. However, the various discouraged financial arrangements were addressed independently of one another, and they were discussed under the name of the particular practice in question (e.g., advertising, fee splitting). They were not grouped together under a principle that accounted for why the practice was ethically problematic. Recently this has changed. The previously prohibited financial arrangements have been grouped together with a host of other types of practices, and they are now addressed under the rubric of conflicts of interest.[2-6]

We draw on the extensive literature assessing conflicts of interest and provide: (1) a brief history of attempts at dealing with the problem, leading up to recent accounts that provide a more integrated and sustained analysis of the issues involved; (2) a conceptual analysis of the nature of a conflict of interest and why this is ethically problematic in medicine; (3) an overview of the types of conflicts one can have, illustrated by examples drawn from surgery; and (4) an account of how to manage conflicts and thus mitigate the harms associated with them.

Ethical Analysis of Conflicts of Interest

The Context: Changing Market Realities

In a previous era, surgery was separated from the rest of medicine, disparaged as a trade to be practiced by barbers and butchers.[7] In taking the Hippocratic Oath, medical doctors were to forswear the knife. At that time, the financial arrangements for the payment and provision of services were also quite simple, and surgeons were not very well reimbursed for their services. Obviously, this state of affairs was to change dramatically. Following the important role that surgery played in the rise of the clinicopathological school that grounded modern medicine,[8] this previously frowned upon "trade" gradually emerged as one of the more prominent specialties of medicine.

In the late nineteenth century surgery came to symbolize the pinnacle of medical knowledge and power, a status well exemplified in Thomas Eakins' famous painting, *The Gross Clinic*.[9] There the noted American surgeon Samuel Gross holds a bloody scalpel, and looks out with cool power and brilliance, as attendants assist him. The mother of the patient sits cringing, unable to fathom or stomach the marvel taking place in the operating room. With this prestige and mystique also came a commensurate remuneration. As medicine entered the twentieth century, surgery came to be one of the highest paid of all specialties.

The increased wealth that came to surgery brought with it new problems. The surgeon depended on referrals from general practitioners, who often felt underpaid and underappreciated and who sometimes resented the surgeon's prestige. The generalist's ability to refer thus gave some power to negotiate. Often, as a result, as much as 50% of the surgeon's fee would go to the referring physician. The financial practice was called *fee splitting*.

Fee splitting was used broadly to refer to a number of practices that were considered to be inappropriate by many physicians.[2] Included were the practice by some physicians of receiving a commission from apothecaries for prescriptions; the "drumming" of business, which involved agents who would receive payment for generating patients; and "steering," which involved arrangements with individuals who would guide clients to a particular physician.

In addition to fee splitting, there were other strategies available for generalists to obtain a part of the surgeon's fee. One of the more prominent methods was referred to as "ghost surgery."[10] Today, this phrase describes the practice whereby an attending surgeon gets credit for an operation performed by a resident (see Chapter 17). However, at the beginning of the twentieth century, it meant that a generalist would claim to do the surgery, but would instead have an anonymous itinerant surgeon perform the critical part of the operation. The generalist would thus maintain control over the process, obtaining a considerable part of the remuneration.

At the end of the nineteenth and beginning of the twentieth century, these practices were common. However, about the same time as the Flexner Report (1910), as physicians sought to eliminate any influence that would compromise medical judgment, the American Medical Association (AMA) and the newly formed American College of Surgeons (ACS, formed 1913) came together to condemn them.[2] It was argued that physicians should be remunerated only for services that they actually performed. Fee splitting provided an inappropriate incentive to refer even when this was not needed. Similarly, itinerant surgery compromised a surgeon's ability to optimally direct the surgery, because the generalist would maintain considerable control over the operation. Such strategies led physicians to act on the basis of self-interest, rather than the interest of the patient. Although critics of fee splitting and itinerant surgery did not use the language of conflict of interest, this, in part, was the problem.

This was not the only problem, however. In fact, similar types of incentives to overtreat were found in fee-for-service medicine generally, a fact that led George Bernard Shaw to quip:

> That any sane nation, having observed that you could provide for the supply of bread by giving bakers a pecuniary interest in baking for you, should go on to give a surgeon a pecuniary interest in cutting off your leg, is enough to make one despair of political humanity.[11]

If the prohibitions against fee splitting were motivated simply by a concern about the role of economic incentives in medical decision making, then consistency seemed to call for a more radical critique, extending to fee-for-service medicine itself. While many physicians condemned fee splitting because of the convoluted incentives it introduced, others condemned it because of the way it weakened the authority of the profession, and thus undermined the long-term interests of physicians. It was this coalescence of the ideals and self-interest of physicians that enabled the prohibition.[1]

As long as some surgeons broke ranks and were willing to engage in fee splitting or serve as ghost surgeons, generalists, with their capacity of referral, would have greater bargaining power. In order to protect the independence of surgery and maintain a solidarity among surgeons, the ACS required its members to abstain from those types of practices. This prohibition is still a part of the ACS Statement on Principles (1994).[12] The Fellowship Pledge involves the commitment, "I will take no part in any arrangement, such as fee splitting or itinerant surgery, which induces referral or treatment for reason other than the patient's best welfare." It is interesting to note, however, that even the current ACS Statement does not directly mention conflicts of interest, restricting its scope to the century-old condemnation of fee splitting and itinerant surgery.

When these practices were proscribed, generalists still had one outlet available for obtaining a part of the surgeon's fee, a method that satisfied even the requirement that physicians not bill for any services they did not directly provide (a common criticism of fee splitting). The generalist could be the first assistant during an operation, and thus be reimbursed for that service. This practice could not be outright condemned, especially in rural contexts where a surgeon assistant might not be available. The ACS response is also still apparent in its most recent Statement on Principles:

> Obviously, proper care of a patient on occasion may demand that a surgeon engage in practice outside usual specialty limits when no appropriately trained physician is available. This should not be a frequent or continuing occurrence.[12]

However, in this case, in contrast to that of ghost surgery, the surgeon maintains control over the operation.

While the ACS may have been a bit more zealous than the AMA in its condemnation of market mechanisms in medicine, the two organizations were in general agreement until the 1950s. At that time the AMA began to soften its stance, especially with respect to self-referral.[2] This was in response to requests by physicians to own pharmacies and requests by ophthalmologists to hire opticians. In response, the ACS, led by Paul Hawley, launched a vigorous, public campaign against fee splitting and against the softening AMA position. There was also a call by the ACS to introduce legal prohibitions against fee splitting. The AMA resisted this, arguing that these concerns should be addressed by the professional societies, not by the legislature.

These were just the first rumblings in a major earthquake that was to shake medicine. Increasingly, medicine moved from being a relatively low cost, low technology profession to a high cost endeavor, which required the coordination of large amounts of capital and an increasingly complex network of services.[3,13,14] Hospitals came to be organized along market interests and that market ethos worked its way into all areas of medicine.

One of the most significant developments involved the rise of third party reimbursement.[1] Its influence was further heightened when the government become a major insurer, with the introduction of Medicare and Medicaid. As a result of insurance, the immediate interest a patient had in cost effectiveness was increasingly lost, because the patient and physician were buffered from costs. Third-party payers would reimburse whatever costs were incurred, without any role in determining what services were appropriate; that would be done by the physician, who had the clinical skills to evaluate what was medically indicated. Since patients had little or no out-of-pocket expense, it was now in their interest to do any and everything that the physician recommended.[15]

Because of the incentives introduced through fee-for-service (FFS), indemnity-based medicine, costs rose astronomically in the health care sector. The types of incentives Shaw quipped at, where it was in the interest of a physician to provide increased services, now were exacerbated. Although fee splitting was officially condemned, there was a sense in which all of medicine involved the incentives to overtreat that one found in such financial mechanisms. As capital flowed into the health care sector, medicine had to increasingly work with business interests. The result was a new "medical industrial complex."[16]

The rate of increase in costs could not be indefinitely sustained. In order to counter the trends, several strategies were used by public and private payers. First, it was recognized by governmental payers that medicine was now a large market, but it did not have within it the types of market mechanisms and competition that led to efficiency in other sectors of the economy; there was "market failure." This resulted, in part, from an ad hoc combination of professional codes and norms that discouraged entrepreneurialism in medicine (e.g., prohibitions against advertising, etc.) and an increasingly entrepreneurial context. In order to overcome this, the courts, in the name of antitrust concerns, broke down some of the remaining barriers against the introduction of market mechanisms.[17–19]

In this new context, practices such as the following became common. (1) Physicians would invest in diagnostic facilities, to which they would refer their patients; such "self-referral" would then lead to further overutilization of services.[20–24] (2) Hospitals would pay physicians for referrals, purchase practices in order to have a regular base, and provide extensive benefits to physicians, in order to attract them to their facility; this would introduce incentives similar to fee splitting, only now it was the hospital that pays the commission, rather than a surgeon.[2] (3) Pharmaceutical companies would provide gifts, including generous vacation packages, in order to increase their sales. In all these cases, the question of physician bias in medical decision making was raised.[3]

In addition to such incentives to increase utilization and costs, pressures were introduced to decrease costs, and these often involved altered incentive structures that led physicians' interests into tension with the interests of patients. Attempting to lower costs, the government introduced as a part of its payment structure the Prospective Payment System.[25,26] Through diagnostic related groups (DRGs), a set payment would be provided to hospitals for each particular diagnosis. Because the hospital would receive the same amount no matter how much it spent on a patient, it now became in the financial interest of the institution to provide less care rather than more. Because the physician was to some extent independent from the hospital, and the physician still controlled decisions, it was assumed that such a mechanism would not adversely affect the patient. However, hospitals found ways to pass on their altered incentives to physicians, who now felt some pressure to decrease utilization of services.[2]

In some ways, DRGs can be viewed as "mini managed care."[26] In health maintenance organizations (HMOs) and other managed care organizations (MCOs), the incentives found in DRGs are generalized; physicians are now discouraged from using rather than encouraged to use services. This often involves payment by capitation, requirements that physicians pay for certain lab tests themselves, and withholding and bonus structures that penalize or reward physicians, depending on their utilization patterns.[27]

It is in this context, where there are complex incentives to over- and undertreat, that the questions about the relation between physician interests and obligations are raised with new force.[3] However, now the scenarios found in the market-oriented medical industry are too diverse and complex to formulate norms for each problematic practice. In the past, one could identify the particular practices and formulate norms to direct them. Thus, physicians addressed fee splitting, itinerant surgery, and so on. However, now one would need to also talk about DRGs, MCOs (with their many and complex incentive structures), hospital-physician relations, and so on. Although this is still the approach usually taken, it is very unwieldy and often does not sufficiently convey the basis for any proposed guidelines. Instead, it is better to formulate the core principle behind the traditional condemnation of fee splitting, and attempt to generalize the ethical concerns so that they can be applied in diverse situations. In order to do this, we turn to a detailed consideration of conflicts of interest.

Defining Conflicts of Interest

What is a conflict of interest? Simply defined, a conflict of interest involves a situation in which the self-interest of an individual is in tension with an obligation. In medicine, the classic conflict takes place when a physician's financial self-interest motivates behavior that is contrary to the needs and interests of a patient; in other words, a physician must choose between the good of the patient and the physician's own good. There is thus a discord between self-interest and the interests of others.

In its most general use, a conflict of interest involves both conflicts between two or more roles or obligations (where there is a hierarchy of obligations) and conflicts between self-interest and obligation.[28-30] Most accounts of conflicts of interest in medicine will separate these two and focus strictly on the conflicts between self-interest and obligation.[2,13,14,31] However, this fails to appreciate the way in which institutions use self-interest to provide incentives for the fulfillment of obligation. Behind a conflict between self-interest and obligation one thus often finds a conflict of obligations, with an attendant dispute about the ranking of those obligations.[32,33] A conflict of interest does not take place when there are two equal obligations or interests; in such cases one has "conflicting interests"[29] or "conflicts of commitment."[34]

Generally, a surgeon has an obligation to provide whatever is in a patient's interest. However, if a surgeon is an employee in an HMO, that surgeon also has an obligation to that institution to control costs. In some cases, for example, when a lab test or treatment may conceivably provide some marginal benefit, but at a very high cost, there is a tension between the obligation to the patient and the obligation to the institution.[35] This conflict of obligations is transformed into a more traditional conflict of interest when the HMO provides a surgeon with a financial incentive for fulfilling her or his obligation to the institution. Behind that conflict of interest and its appropriateness thus lies a broader question about whether it is appropriate for a surgeon to have an obligation to an institution that may come into tension with the surgeon's obligation to the patient.[32,33,36]

Similarly, a surgeon in an academic center may have multiple obligations, including obligations to the students and residents being taught, obligations to the professional and scientific community to engage in productive research, and the traditional obligation to the patient.[37,38] In subtle and not so subtle ways, personal rewards (in the form of respect, financial remuneration, tenure) that an academic surgeon receives for fulfilling research and teaching responsibilities transform the conflict of obligations into a conflict of interest.[39] For this reason, when evaluating conflicts of interest, it is important not to focus exclusively on the relation between the particular self-interest and the obligation with which it is in tension; one should also consider the obligations that are reinforced by the incentives that create that conflict, and ask in a more general way about the appropriateness of (1) the conflict of obligations and (2) the mechanisms by which the fulfillment of obligation is reinforced by incentives that lead to the more traditional conflicts of interest.

In this chapter, we will use the phrase "conflicts of interest" in the narrower sense, to speak of a conflict between self-interest and an obligation.[35] Thus, for example, we will not directly consider the types of conflicts that arise when obligations to different patients are in tension (see Chapter 19). However, even in this narrower sense, it is helpful, following a recent AMA statement, to make a further distinction between potential and actual conflicts of interest.[40] In a potential conflict of interest, there is a financial or other self-interest that *may* come into tension with an obligation. The potential conflict raises a flag, but there is not yet a divergence between self-interest and obligation. In an actual conflict of interest, the divergence takes place; one cannot simultaneously maximize the self-interest and obligation at the same time.

While potential conflicts do not raise an immediate problem, they are important to consider for two reasons. First, they point to areas that could be a problem in the future and thus which should be monitored. Second, they can provide the *appearance* of an actual conflict of interest. In some contexts, even such an appearance can cause problems for an individual or the profession, and thus should be avoided.[2,40,41]

Even when there is an actual conflict of interest, that does not yet mean that a wrong has taken place. Conflicts of interest may lead to inappropriate actions, but they do not necessarily imply wrong action. They are better regarded as temptations that should, if possible, be avoided. In actual conflicts of interest, the world is structured such that it is in a person's self-interest to do that which goes contrary to obligation, and thus the interests of others. Individual interest and common good are not in accord.

In other sectors of the economy there are often situations in which the interests of two parties of a transaction are not necessarily in accord. For example, the interest of the car salesperson overlaps, but is not fully synchronous, with that of the car buyer. In these contexts there is a somewhat antagonistic relation, expressed in the saying "buyer beware," which leads to a process of negotiation. Through that process of interaction, the interests of buyer and seller come into accord, and a transaction takes place that is in the interests of all concerned; a Pareto optimal exchange. It is the possibility of such negotiation, and the mutual awareness of the possible incompatibility of interests, that allows such a transaction to work out in favor of all parties.

In the practice of surgery, however, one cannot assume that such negotiation will take place. The patient is vulnerable as a result of the illness experience and the asymmetry of the surgeon-patient relation.[35] As a result, the patient places trust in the surgeon, who is supposed to act as an agent of the patient. Through the process of diagnosis, the surgeon determines the patient's demand for services; but the surgeon is also the supplier and works together with other suppliers. As a result of the asymmetry of the relation, the patient does not (because he or she is not situated where he or she is able to) radically question the recommendation of the surgeon, as a consumer of services normally would in other market transactions.[42]

Because of the patient's trust, arising from the unique vulnerability, and the role of the surgeon as the patient's agent in determining the demand for services, the surgeon has traditionally been understood as accruing an *obligation* to act in the patient's interest, when determining the use of services, and so forth. However, as the Shaw quip shows, when the surgeon profits from supply, it is also in the financial interest of the surgeon to supply more, rather than fewer services. This is an incentive that is operative not just in fee splitting, but in all of fee-for-service medicine. There is thus a potential conflict of interest inherent in all fee-for-service medicine; namely, a possible divergence between the financial self-interest of the surgeon and the good of the patient (especially if the good involved fewer rather than more services).

At least since the time of the Hippocratic Oath, there has been a recognition within the medical community that the patient's illness makes him or her especially vulnerable, and thus ripe for exploitation. Because, additionally, the surgeon has access to confidential and sensitive information about the patient, the surgeon is in a unique position to take advantage of that patient. Thus, there has been a strong obligation to give priority to the patient's interest and not manipulate the situation for undue profit. While there may be a potential conflict of interest at the heart of fee-for-service medicine (which was the major approach to financing), and while there are often even actual conflicts of interest, there was also a strong professional ethos against any violation of a surgeon's obligation, and a confidence in the virtue and character of the surgeon.[2] Some of the most problematic conflicts such as those found in fee splitting were generally proscribed.

In addition to strong ethical statements, which sought to positively motivate appropriate surgeon behavior, there were also professional sanctions for the more egregious violations. Thus, for example, the ACS Statement on Principles states:

> Whether due to repeated ineptness, lack of knowledge, or willful failure to apply acceptable indications for operations or other procedures, the performance of unnecessary surgery is an extremely serious violation of ethical principles for which disciplinary action is indicated. Committees in hospitals are organized to guard against such violations or repeated mistakes.[12]

In the final section of this chapter, we will consider how such sanctions and professional statements can work to mitigate conflicts. However, before doing that it will be important to briefly overview some of the types of conflicts found in the current context of health care payment and provision.

The Geography of Conflicting Allegiances

Conflicts arise through the intersection of different domains of interest, allegiance, and obligation. Any grouping of them is somewhat arbitrary because the grouping can be by a practice in question (e.g., self-referral, capitation) or by the types of interests and obligations (e.g., teaching conflicts, research conflicts). Here, we will group conflicts into three categories, financial, faculty (teaching and research), and institutional. However, most attention will be given to financial conflicts because these are currently of greatest concern.

Financial Conflicts of Interest. In most essays on conflicts of interest, the primary focus is on financial conflicts in which a surgeon's obligation is in tension with the surgeon's own financial self-interest.

Consider self-referral—for example, an orthopedic surgeon who owns a large building that houses diagnostic x-rays, a CT scanner, and a physical therapy facility. This surgeon may see a patient who has a knee injury and send her down the hallway for plain x-rays. After reviewing these, the patient may be sent for a CT scan of the knee. The surgeon may then decide that the patient needs physical therapy, sending her to a physical therapist who is also housed in the same facility. In this case the orthopedic surgeon makes a profit at every step and there are strong financial incentives to use all these resources in clinical decision making.

The incentives operating are similar to those found in all of fee-for-service, indemnity-based medicine.[43] The surgeon has an interest in providing more. However, in this case the surgeon also profits from the activities of others involved in the patient's care, and thus, to some extent, benefits from services that were not fully provided by the surgeon. This was a central issue in early discussions of fee splitting,[2] and it is explicitly condemned in some ethical codes.[44]

This scenario can be slightly altered by moving the x-ray, CT scanner, and physical therapy outside of the office of the surgeon. If the orthopedic surgeon has ownership in the facilities where the services are being provided, then incentives to provide services are similar to the initial scenario.

Several studies have shown that self-referring physicians utilize x-rays and other diagnostic imaging services as much as 4.5 times more often than non-self-referring physicians, and they also use physical therapy services in which they have a financial interest as much as 45% more often.[20–24,45,46] The large discrepancy in utilization and costs between self- referring and non-self-referring physicians shows that financial incentives do play a significant role in influencing physician behavior.

In response to rising costs and the strong empirical evidence that financial incentives do play a significant role in influencing surgeons' behavior,[46] MCOs have introduced alternative incentive structures to reduce utilization. For example, a primary care physician may be given a financial incentive not to refer patients to specialists. A specialty financial pool may be established, with whatever is remaining at the end of the year split among primary care physicians as a bonus.[27,47] The primary care physician then has a clear financial incentive not to refer patients for specialist evaluation. At times, this may work against a patient's interest in obtaining care from the most competent surgeon.

Specialists also may find themselves under financial incentives that similarly lead to a reduction of services. When surgical care is capitated, for example, the surgeon gets paid whether or not she operates. In this case, when a patient is in a gray zone, where the indications for surgery are not clear, surgeons will be less inclined to intervene (see Chapter 17).

In addition to payment by capitation and the use of primary physician gatekeepers,[48] MCOs use mechanisms such as requiring physicians to pay for certain lab tests themselves, withholdings and bonus payments, and regular practice reviews that consider the costs of physician practice patterns. All of these mechanisms reduce costs by providing the physician with financial incentives to reduce utilization. This introduces a potential conflict between the patient's interests and those of the physician.[27,36,49]

Hospitals depend on physicians for their economic well-being and this has led to physician-hospital agreements. It is the physician who determines where a patient will go for treatment and what treatment should be provided. Additionally, physicians can establish ambulatory surgical facilities or diagnostic centers that can compete with hospitals. In order to protect their financial interests, hospitals seek ways to solidify a physician's commitment to their institution. A common and longstanding mechanism used is to provide physicians with free office space and use of facilities, a practice taken for granted by many physicians, but quite unusual in the business world. By making a physician at home in the institution, hospitals establish patterns of behavior that are more likely to lead to increased referrals, and thus more money.

Ideally, surgeons will choose the hospital or other facility that is best equipped and, all things being equal, the least expensive for the patient. And it seems that offering free office space does not gravely compromise a surgeon's ability to do that, especially because all hospitals offer similar benefits. However, other mechanisms are used by hospitals that may not be as innocent and that may place a physician in a conflict of interest. Problematic practices often used include kickbacks, joint ventures, and hospital purchase of physician practices.[2]

Kickbacks usually are not given directly, because this is prohibited in many states and in all cases where government money is used (Medicaid and Medicare). However, physicians may be paid for consulting or for interpreting diagnostic tests, even in cases where this is not needed or even provided.[2] Such additional remuneration gives physicians an added financial incentive to stay with a given institution.

Another common practice involves the formation of joint ventures with surgeons. For example, a hospital may offer physicians an investment opportunity in surgical facilities, and provide a rate of return on that investment that is very high. They may restrict the investment opportunity to surgeons using those facilities. Surgeons then have a double financial interest: they would lose the investment opportunity if they practice in another institution, and, if they stay in their joint venture, they benefit from the increased use of the facilities.[2] This introduces the same types of incentives found in self-referral, and it assures to a hospital regular referrals.

Instead of forming joint ventures with surgeons, a hospital may choose simply to purchase surgeon practices. This is a strategy financial consultants are advocating.[2] Although the practices tend to lose money when they are purchased, the increased referrals to the hospital more than makes up for the loss. It also gives hospitals increased control over surgeon behavior. Such administrative and financial control is important in the current, changing market of health care.

In the context of fee-for-service, indemnity-based medicine, the incentives were roughly the same for surgeons and hospitals. Both benefitted when a large number and volume of services were provided. However, with the introduction of the Prospective Payment System in 1983, and now with increased managed care penetration, hospitals often benefit from doing less.[34] With DRGs, hospital interest diverged from surgeon interest because the latter still benefited from providing more, whereas the former had incentives to do less. When surgeons were still relatively independent, DRGs did not pose a significant threat to patient care. However, with joint ventures and especially with the purchasing of practices, hospitals obtained the leverage to pass on their new incentives to surgeons. The direct employment of surgeons and the use of mechanisms such as capitation and evaluation of practice profiles, further increases this leverage.[50] In the future, it is likely that hospitals, which always actively sought surgeons, may now turn away surgeons who have expensive styles of practice or who have too high a caseload of Medicaid, Medicare, and indigent patients (see Chapter 17).

In the current, increasingly market-oriented context, previously frowned-upon practices such as advertising and the acceptance of gifts from pharmaceutical and biotechnology companies is becoming increasingly accepted. In part, these changes have been brought about by legal rulings that interpreted previous prohibitions as a violation of antitrust policies.[17-19] There are also a host of entrepreneurial practices such as the purchasing of stocks and investing in new technologies that can, in some contexts, lead to actual conflicts of interest.

There is a large literature on gift giving and conflicts of interest.[2,51,52] We cannot consider this in any detail here. Nor can we provide even a cursory overview of the diverse entrepreneurial ventures that may lead to conflicts of interest. Such an overview requires not only an account of the ventures, but of the situations where they become problematic. For example, a physician may own stock in a surgical equipment company. This, by itself, says nothing about whether there is a conflict of interest. However, if that physician is part of a professional society committee evaluating new equipment, or if he or she plays a role in purchasing equipment for a hospital, then the stock interest raises important concerns.

Similarly, when considering advertising,[53] it is important to consider not only the general practice, but also the context. Done responsibly, advertising may serve an appropriate social function. However, in a context where a physician charges for different components of an operation, and there are alternative ways of performing the operation that are equally successful, and one of the ways uses new, expensive technology, then it is problematic to advertise the use of the new technology. Patients are tempted by the high-cost gadgetry, and physicians could then exploit this for profit.[54] Even though the patient would not be harmed medically (we assume the morbidity and mortality is equal for the different strategies), he or she would be harmed financially. However, a slight change in the context may change the appraisal of the advertising. For example, if one moves into a managed care context where physicians are paid a set fee for the operation or by capitation, then advertisement may serve to inform the public that new technology is available, but used only under certain conditions where it is needed. There is still a potential conflict of interest even in this altered context, but the change in financial arrangements may bring patient interest and physician self-interest into greater accord, so that an actual conflict is avoided (see Chapter 19). One need not be aware of all the possible scenarios for entrepreneurial ventures because we will instead develop general strategies for evaluating any conflicts of interest, and these strategies can be applied to each new case as it arises.

Research and Teaching Conflicts. There is now a considerable body of literature on faculty conflicts of interest, much of this addressing research conflicts.[34,40,52,55–57] In considering these conflicts, it is important to consider not just financial interests but other interests such as fame, security, and power. These additional interests may also compromise obligations, and an attempt to mitigate a financial conflict may actually introduce a more egregious nonfinancial conflict of interest.

For faculty, there are conflicts of obligation, which may be translated into more traditional conflicts of interest by considering the mechanisms of evaluation used in assessing and rewarding the fulfillment of obligations.[34] It is often difficult to balance teaching, research, and clinical obligations. If a nonfinancial interest in security such as attaining tenure is based too heavily on research to the exclusion of teaching and clinical work, then a physician may have too strong an incentive to compromise obligations in those areas. Similarly, there are conflicting obligations between teaching and clinic, which are often very difficult to balance. For example, Newton notes that in cataract extraction "[s]everal of the most delicate and critical manoeuvres . . . are under the complete control of one operator and, once begun, can be neither interrupted nor transferred to more skilled hands." How does one weigh the risk to the patient (and thus the patient's interest) against the interest of society in passing on the skills of surgery, and the interest of the resident in performing the surgery? The delicate balance of such conflicting obligations of the surgical faculty can be easily disturbed by the introduction of a relatively modest self-interest, which may be used by a given medical school as a way of rewarding its clinical faculty. Institutions must thus be careful regarding the ways in which they assess and reward their faculty, lest they introduce conflicts of interest that compromise obligations.

In the case of research, there are also many nonfinancial interests, which may compromise scientific protocols.[58] These may play as significant, or more significant a role, when compared to financial conflicts. For example, a physician who has a vested career or prestige interest in a given technology or procedure may have just as strong an interest in a positive outcome as others who would only have a financial interest (e.g., stock options) in such an outcome.

Among the myriad financial interests that may lead to conflicts of interest in research, one finds the following:

1. A physician or surgeon who holds a patent, or who has investments in a company that seeks to manufacture or market the product of research, has an individual interest that may play a role in the research.[34,41,59,60]
2. When research is funded by a company that has a direct stake in the outcome, researchers may be influenced in subtle ways.[61]
3. When a physician or surgeon is provided with remuneration for enrolling a patient in a clinical trial, then the incentive may lead to recommendations that are not in the patient's best interest and that may compromise the research.[62]
4. A researcher who knows that honoraria for speaking engagements will be provided, should research lead to positive results, has an individual interest that may compromise protocols.[57]
5. A physician or surgeon who is concerned about the patient's well-being, and who has a style of practice that involves much experimentation with different treatments, may compromise a clinical trial by not carefully following protocols. This happened in the case of breast cancer trials.[63] Such concerns may also lead physicians and surgeons to not enter patients in trials.[64]

For a more detailed assessment of the types of conflicts of obligation and interest faculty may encounter, the reader is referred to the Association of American Medical Colleges' "Guideline for Dealing with Faculty Conflicts of Commitment and Conflicts of Interest in Research."[34]

Institutional Conflicts of Interest. Just as individuals have interests that may come into tension with their obligations, so also institutions may have institutional interests that come into tension with their broader mission and obligations.[41,65] Such institutional self-interest may include owning a patent in a product being evaluated by researchers at that institution; having an ownership interest in biotechnology or pharmaceuticals[59]; or simply a financial interest (profits) that is given priority over obligations traditionally associated with health care institutions. Physicians who have administrative responsibilities should be aware of such conflicts and the role that institutional interests may have in compromising obligations. The same principles used to evaluate individual conflicts can also be used for institutional ones.

Clinical Topics: Managing Conflicts of Interest

Surgeons play a role in crafting the contexts in which they practice. To the degree they have control, they should structure their environment so that they avoid a divergence of self-interest and professional obligation. To the degree that surgeons do not have control, they should be aware of the way self-interest may motivate inappropriate action, and they should cultivate the character that assures virtuous conduct.

In the past, conflicts of interest were addressed largely through professional codes and sanctions, with heavy reliance on the virtue of individual physicians and surgeons. Today, however, there are reasons to believe that this by itself is not enough.[13] There is a growing body of empirical evidence that the profession has not been sufficiently effective in self-policing.[20–24] This evidence, together with a concern about the ways in which the market is transforming medicine, has led organizations such as the ACS to favor legislation that eliminates some of the more egregious conflicts.[2] Nevertheless, other medical professional organizations, such as the AMA, oppose addressing these problems by state legislation. They feel that legislation will inappropriately intrude upon the discretion of physicians, and the approach will further erode professional virtue, because ethical ideals cannot be legislated. The law will only assure conformity to external standards and do nothing about motivation and character.[66] The question is thus: what should be done about conflicts of interest that arise in an increasingly commercial context of medicine?

One thing is clear: not all conflicts of interest can be eliminated.[13] Whether potential or actual, they are all-pervasive in medicine.[58] It is thus unrealistic to think that a simple change, such as paying surgeons by salary, will solve the problem. When one pays by salary, one simply changes the types of conflicts that arise, and the new conflicts may be worse than those eliminated.[67–69]

Similarly, one should not focus just on financial conflicts.[58] Many such conflicts arise in the context of conflicting obligations; therefore, eliminating the financial incentive that is used to reward the fulfillment of a certain obligation will not eliminate the deeper conflict. One may actually introduce a worse nonfinancial conflict of interest when replacing a financial conflict.[13] One must thus realistically assess the possibilities of mitigating conflicts and avoid overly zealous attempts at expunging all financial self-interest from medicine. An unrealistic campaign to eliminate financial self-interest may actually hinder good medical practice; minimally, it will inappropriately harm a surgeon's livelihood, and this too is an important and legitimate concern that should be weighed together with other factors. When we appreciate the additional factors related to self-interest—factors such as job security, reputation, and tenure—and when we consider the ways in which conflicting obligations can be translated into conflicts of interest, then the futility of any attempt at doing away with all conflicts becomes clear.

Obviously, not all conflicts of interest have the same intensity. Most are benign, failing to present serious temptations. The questions thus become: what conflicts of interest are sufficiently problematic that they should be eliminated, and how can these be separated from those more benign conflicts that pervade all of medicine? In answering these there will be two main considerations.

First, one must ask how easily a conflict can be eliminated without requiring major structural changes in the way health care is financed, and without creating new, alternative conflicts or undermining some valuable goal. There are some conflicts that are just too difficult to avoid; for example, the incentive to overtreat that is at the heart of fee-for-service medicine. The easier it is to eliminate an actual conflict without some loss, the more incumbent it is upon one to do so. All things being equal, the approach that avoids a conflict of interest would be preferable. Second, one must consider the intensity of a conflict. This will be a measure of (1) the likelihood that the conflict will lead to a breach of obligation and (2) the harm that results should a breach take place.[4] One may not be able to eliminate certain types of conflicts, but one can mitigate their intensity.

Several guidelines have been formulated to address conflicts of interest.[34,40,43,52,70] These are rarely developed in general terms that apply to all conflicts. Instead, they address particular areas such as self-referral, pharmaceutical gift-giving, research, and managed care incentives. Unfortunately, we cannot provide a detailed discussion or even an outline of the results of these guidelines. (The reader is referred to the above citations for additional information and for samples of the way management of conflicts can be operationalized.) Here we shall restrict ourselves to a brief overview of two sample guidelines provided by the AMA. These have been chosen because they address the two factors mentioned in the previous paragraph, namely, difficulty of elimination and intensity. Then we shall consider some general principles for assessing and managing all conflicts.

One of the most significant areas of concern is that of physician self-referral. This has been the focus of several recent legislative and regulatory efforts, most conspicuously those advanced by Representative Pete Stark, leading to restrictions on self-referral for Medicare patients.[2] However, as the AMA noted in a 1986 report, the types of conflicts found in self- referral are "not significantly different in principle from other conflicts presented by fee-for-service medicine."[43] Yet in 1992, as a response to growing empirical data indicating that self-referral led to much higher utilization rates, the AMA went on to declare that self-referral is "presumptively inconsistent with the physician's fiduciary duty when adequate alternative facilities exist."[43] At the same time, a distinction was made between in-house self-referral and external self-referral. This is an interesting distinction, because the data on overutilization for in-house versus external self-referral is the same.[20-24] Why was a distinction made? The answers are instructive.

The AMA was not moved primarily by the empirical studies on overutilization, arguing that all of them were flawed. Instead, the Council referred to the "symbolic significance . . . with regard to which of two alternative conceptualizations of the physician's role—that of professional or that of entrepreneur—the medical profession will move toward in the era of health care reform."[43] In the report on self-referral, it also becomes clear that the Council was more concerned about the deleterious impact an *appearance* of conflict has on the profession, than it was about actual conflicts. This was the primary factor motivating the stronger guidelines. However, at the same time, it was too difficult to eliminate in-house self-referral; physicians regularly benefit from ownership in facilities where they practice. Thus, as long as there is "personal involvement with the provision of care on site" one does not have the type of self-referral that is the focus of the AMA report. Again, this is despite the empirical data that showed similar types of overutilization in both cases. Obviously, the ease of eliminating a given conflict, and the degree to which it is intimately intertwined with the way medicine is regularly practiced played a role in the formulation of the guidelines.

With self-referral, the problem is overutilization. Physicians have a financial interest in providing treatment that the patient does not necessarily need. With managed care, the problem is the opposite one of underutilization. Whereas the AMA dealt with the former problem grudgingly, concerned more about the appearance of a conflict and its symbolic significance, the AMA was earnest about the latter one.[70] The 1995 guidelines on managed care thus began by asserting the need to maintain patient advocacy, long considered central among physician obligations. Managed care was also perceived as a threat to another core ethical motif, that of informed consent (an obvious reference to so-called "gag rules" that prohibit physicians from informing patients of "experimental" treatments that are not covered by the health plan). But most important for our purposes here, the guidelines attempted to address the intensity of a conflict by pointing to the strength of a physician's financial interest. Thus "[l]imits should be placed on the magnitude of fee withholds, bonuses, and other financial incentives to limit care."[70] Recognizing that the alternative incentive structures could not be eliminated outright (and an attempt to do this may have been regarded as a violation of anti-trust), the Council on Ethical and Judicial Affairs of the AMA sought to mitigate conflicts by reducing the likelihood of a transgression of obligation.

In the case of the AMA guidelines, there was no general reflection on how one can measure the intensity of a conflict, or on how one could tell when the magnitude of a financial incentive was too great. This was left up to intuition. However, it is important to be able to assess this directly, at least in a relative way that enables a weighing of alternative scenarios. To assess which conflicts should be eliminated, one should consider the intensity of a conflict and measure it against the intensity of any conflicts that would arise in alternative contexts. Further, one should also consider the negative impact of any attempt at legislating these concerns and the uncertainty of predicting the harms, so that one avoids an overly restrictive and intrusive approach. With this in mind, the following approach to measuring intensity can be helpful in the formulation of guidelines.

The intensity of a conflict is a measure of how likely a conflict, as a temptation, will lead to a violation of the obligation, and the intensity of the harm, should such a violation take place. The probability of transgression multiplied by the intensity of harm will yield the intensity (or severity) of the conflict of interest.[4]

In measuring the probability of transgression, the following factors will be relevant.

1. Strength and immediacy of self-interest. The greater the personal benefit, and the more immediately that benefit is conferred, the more likely it will motivate.[4]

2. Vector measuring degree of overlap between self-interest and obligation. If a financial self-interest is in accord with an obligation, so that it motivates action that is in accord with duty, then one may have a potential conflict, but one does not have an actual conflict of interest. In that case, the self-interest does not lead to a transgression of obligation. However, as self-interest diverges from obligation, the probability of transgression increases. There is no neat line between potential and actual conflicts. It is thus better to view them on a continuum, ranging from perfect accord between self-interest and obligation to a complete discord. As discord increases, the probability of a transgression of obligation increases.

3. Surgeon character. The greater a surgeon's virtue, the less likely will that physician be motivated by self-interest to violate an obligation. One can thus look to the character of an individual physician or institution for an indication of the probability of transgression.

4. Uncertainty of normative boundaries. The greater the uncertainty and ambiguity of a norm, and the more latitude a surgeon has for variable judgment, the greater the likelihood that self-interest will play a significant role in motivating the physician.[4,13] For example, if there is considerable uncertainty in determining whether a surgeon should order an x-ray, then, if a physician benefits financially from the x-ray, it will be more likely that the x-ray will be performed when it is not needed.

5. Probability, strength and immediacy of sanction, should a violation of obligation occur. A surgeon may be positively motivated by professional ideals. However, surgeons are also motivated by self-interest, seeking to obtain individual benefits and avoid harms. The problem in conflicts of interest is that an individual benefit may play a greater role in motivation than the professional ideal. In order to alter the likelihood of such a transgression, one may introduce sanctions that alter the egoistic utility calculus. The

greater the probability that a violation of obligation is detected and sanction applied, and the greater and more immediate that sanction, the lower the probability of a transgression initially taking place.

In order to calculate the intensity of a conflict, one should multiply the probability of transgression by the harm that results from the violation of obligation. When considering legislation, it is also important to ask whether one has the type of harm that should be legislatively prohibited, and whether the costs associated with legislation, monitor, and sanction are proportional to the harms that would be eliminated. In some cases the costs of legislating conflicts of interest may be much greater than the benefits.

From this all too quick overview of measuring intensity of conflicts of interest, we can readily see some of the ways in which conflicts can be mitigated.

1. Reduce the strength and immediacy of self-interest.[47] This is the focus of the AMA guidelines on managed care incentives and HCFA Medicare regulations.[70] For example, physicians negotiating a contract with a managed care organization can reduce the strength of self-interest that leads to under-utilization of services by reducing the percent of the physician's income at risk (withholdings) from 30% to 20%. One could also reduce the immediacy of self-interest by spreading risk among other physicians and surgeons in a group, or by having bonuses provided annually rather than quarterly. Similarly, one can address self-referral by setting limits on the percent of ownership in a diagnostic facility and regulating the way in which the surgeon receives profits. For example, orthopedic surgeons who share ownership in an out-of-house facility may actually have a smaller incentive to refer than those who have a 100% ownership interest in in-house diagnostic equipment, because the benefit to that surgeon of each of his or her referrals will be smaller—the total profit from the referral is spread among the other owners. However, if the surgeon were provided a profit proportional to referrals, then one would lose the mitigation of the conflict that could result from the joint ownership. One could also reduce the role that the benefits of self-referral play in motivation by having the dividends paid annually, rather than over shorter periods or after each referral.

2. Bring self-interest into greater accord with obligation.[47] As outcomes information on physicians is developed, this information can be introduced into reimbursement considerations in order to reduce the probability of violating obligations to patients. In the case of managed care, instead of reducing the strength of withholdings, one could maintain or increase their intensity, but directly tie reimbursements to quality of care.

3. Promote virtue among surgeons and institutions.[3,50] By developing forums for reflection on ethical issues (a function that may be performed by eth-

ics committees), and by advancing professional ideals, the probability of transgression decreases.[40,51] There is a clear benefit in reminding physicians of their ethical obligations, and regularly showing how the ethical ideals of the profession can be operationalized in clinical contexts. It would thus be valuable to have regular conferences for physicians, discussing the ways in which new financial incentive structures may compromise obligations by subtly influencing the behavior of physicians.

4. Reduce uncertainty of obligations and norms. The lack of clear professional norms about when a diagnostic test is needed leads to considerable variability in the use of such tests. Further, many tests have little or no morbidity associated with them, and, however small the likelihood, they may yield some useful information. When there is such uncertainty and variability associated with professional norms, financial incentives can play a very large role in determining utilization rates. Physicians can reduce this uncertainty by developing practice standards and guidelines. Further, institutional committees and peer review of practice patterns can provide feedback on the appropriateness of certain patterns. By providing peer information on utilization, some information on standards of practice can be developed. The clearer the information on norms, the less likely that they will be transgressed.

5. Monitor practice and provide strong and immediate sanction should a violation of obligation occur. The ACS Statement on Principles states that "the performance of unnecessary surgery is an extremely serious violation of ethical principles for which disciplinary action is indicated. Committees in hospitals are organized to guard against such violations or repeated mistakes."[12] However, such monitoring and sanctions have not been actively pursued in most contexts. The more carefully a situation is monitored, and the greater the rapidity and strength of a transgression's punishment, the more will a conflict's intensity be reduced.

These different strategies can be used individually or in tandem to manage conflicts of interest, and thus reduce their intensity.

The factors that play a role in determining the intensity of a conflict vary considerably in different contexts. It is thus important to manage conflicts as closely as possible to their local context, called the principle of subsidiarity. This principle should be operative in the formulation of policies: one should respond to conflicts at the most immediate level possible. As a result, one should generally avoid formulating policies at the federal or state legislative levels. It is preferable to address conflicts at the institutional level, although one may look for ways to hold institutions accountable for failing to sufficiently mitigate conflicts. Ethics committees or committees explicitly focusing on conflicts have been recommended by some medical society guidelines.

Finally, it should be noted that disclosure is often advocated as a central means for managing conflicts. There are many who are advocating that disclosure of financial incentives and surgeon interests should be made a part of the informed consent process.[39,71] However, there are some problems with this proposal, and it is unlikely that it could be regarded as the complete solution.[4,58] The disclosure of conflicts of interest (e.g., those in self-referral) may further erode patient trust and the fiduciary relation, and it is not clear that a patient is in a position to make full use of that information.[13] As we noted earlier, there are important differences between the surgeon-patient relationship and a normal market interaction between consumer and supplier. Further, the disclosure of potential (as opposed to actual) conflicts would be counterproductive because there would not be a reason for suspecting transgression of physician obligations. Also, how would one address in the disclosure and consent process the complex issues associated with measuring a conflict's intensity? Of course, all this does not mean that disclosure is not important. And in contexts such as sponsorship of research and conferences, disclosure of conflicts can alert participants or reviewers to potential biases. However, even there, disclosure should be viewed only as a small part of managing conflicts, and one should avoid demanding it under any and all circumstances. In some of the literature, one gets the impression that because disclosure is relatively easy, it should always be done. Such an approach fails to appreciate that harms may result from disclosure, especially if the information disclosed could be easily misunderstood.

Clinical Conclusions

Changes taking place in the health care sector, especially the introduction of new financial incentives associated with entrepreneurial medical practices and managed care, have led to a heightened concern with conflicts of interest. The self-interest of surgeons may lead to a compromise of professional obligation. This possibility threatens the fiduciary character of the surgeon-patient relation by undermining the patient's trust.

In order to avoid these harms, we have recommended that physicians attempt personally to avoid conflicts whenever possible. Generally, if one can eliminate a personal conflict, one should attempt to do so. One should also personally avoid entering situations where conflicts are introduced. However, this does not mean that institutions or the law should prohibit all conflicts. They are all-pervasive in surgical practice, research, and education. Institutions should thus focus on the most severe conflicts, attempting to mitigate them when possible, but weighing the costs of such intervention against potential benefits.

The intensity of a conflict of interest is a measure of the probability that it will lead to a transgression of fiduciary obligations to the patient. This is a function of several factors, including the strength and immediacy of a surgeon's self-interest, the degree of overlap between self-interest and obligation, the moral character of the surgeon, the uncertainty of the norms, and the strength and immediacy of the sanction, should a violation of obligation occur. A conflict of interest can be managed by altering one or more of these factors.

References

1. Paul Starr, *The Social Transformation of American Medicine*. New York: Basic Books, 1982.
2. Marc A. Rodwin, *Medicine, Money, & Morals*. Oxford: Oxford University Press, 1993.
3. Arnold S. Relman, "Dealing With Conflicts of Interest," *New England Journal of Medicine* 313 (1985): 749–751.
4. Dennis F. Thompson, "Understanding Financial Conflicts of Interest," *New England Journal of Medicine* 329 (1993): 573–576.
5. Janicemarie K. Vinicky, Sue Shevlin Edwards, and James P. Orlowski, "Conflicts of Interest, Conflicting Interests, and Interesting Conflicts," *The Journal of Clinical Ethics* 6 (1995): 358–366.
6. Janicemarie K. Vinicky, Sue Shevlin Edwards, and James P. Orlowski, "Conflicts of Interest, Conflicting Interests, and Interesting Conflicts, Part 2," *The Journal of Clinical Ethics* 7 (1996):69–76.
7. Erwin Ackerknecht, *A Short History of Medicine*. Baltimore and London: The Johns Hopkins University Press, 1982.
8. Owsei Temkin, "The Role of Surgery in the Rise of Modern Medical Thought," in *The Double Face of Janus*, Owsei Temkin. Baltimore: The Johns Hopkins University Press, 1977, pp. 487–496.
9. William Innes Homer, *Thomas Eakins, His Life and Art*. New York: Abbeville Press, 1992.
10. Margaret Keller Holmes, "Ghost Surgery," *Bulletin of the New York Academy of Medicine* 56 (1980): 412–419.
11. George Bernard Shaw, *The Doctor's Dilemma: A Tragedy*. Baltimore, MD: Penguin Books.
12. American College of Surgeons, *Statement on Principles*. Chicago: American College of Surgeons, 1994.
13. E. Haavi Morreim, "Conflicts of Interest, Profits and Problems in Physician Referrals," *Journal of the American Medical Association* 262 (1989): 390–394.
14. E. Haavi Morreim, *Balancing Act, The New Medical Ethics of Medicine's New Economics*. Washington, D.C.: Georgetown University Press, 1995.
15. John Goodman and Gerald Musgrave, *Patient Power: Solving America's Health Care Crisis*. Washington, D.C.: Cato Institute, 1992.
16. Arnold Relman, "The New Medical-Industrial Complex," *New England Journal of Medicine* 303 (1980):963–970.
17. Bernard Hirsh, "Antitrust and Professional Activities," *Journal of the American Medical Association* 250 (1983): 491–492.
18. Bernard Hirsh, "Antitrust and Medical Ethics," *Journal of the American Medical Association* 250 (1983): 2759–2760.
19. Stephen Miles and Robert Koepp, "Comments on the AMA Report 'Ethical Issues in Managed Care,'" *The Journal of Clinical Ethics* (1995): 306–311.

20. Bruce J. Hillman et al., "Frequency and Costs of Diagnostic Imaging in Office Practice—A Comparison of Self-Referring and Radiologist-Referring Physicians," *New England Journal of Medicine* 323 (1990): 1604–1608.

21. Bruce J. Hillman et al., "Physicians' Utilization and Charges for Outpatient Diagnostic Imaging in a Medicare Population," *Journal of the American Medical Association* 268 (1992): 2050–2054.

22. Jean M. Mitchell and Elton Scott, " New Evidence of the Prevalence and Scope of Physician Joint Ventures," *Journal of the American Medical Association* 268 (1992): 80–84.

23. Jean M. Mitchell and Elton Scott, " Physician Ownership of Physical Therapy Services," *Journal of the American Medical Association* 268 (1992): 2055–2059.

24. Jean M. Mitchell and Jonathan H. Sunshine, " Consequences of Physicians' Ownership of Health Care Facilities—Joint Ventures in Radiation Therapy," *New England Journal of Medicine* 327 (1992); 1497–1506.

25. Charles E. Begley, "Prospective Payment and Medical Ethics," *The Journal of Medicine and Philosophy* 12 (1987): 107–122.

26. Leonard Fleck, "DRGs: Justice and the Invisible Rationing of Health Care Resources," *The Journal of Medicine and Philosophy* 19 (1994): 367–368.

27. Alan L. Hillman, "Financial Incentives for Physicians in HMOs," *New England Journal of Medicine* 317 (1987):1743–1748.

28. Kenneth Kipnis, *Legal Ethics*. Englewood Cliffs, NJ.: Prentice-Hall, 1986.

29. Joseph Margolis, "Conflict of Interest and Conflicting Interests," in *Ethical Theory and Business*, Tom L. Beauchamp and Norman E. Bowie, eds. Englewood Cliffs, NJ: Prentice-Hall, Inc., 1979, 361–372.

30. Joseph M. McGuire, " Conflict of Interest: Whose Interest? And What Conflict?" in *Ethics, Free Enterprise, & Public Policy*, Richard T. De George and Joseph A. Pichler, eds. New York: Oxford University Press, 1978, pp. 214–231.

31. Michael Davis, "Conflict of Interest," *Business and Professional Ethics Journal* 4 (1982):17–27.

32. American College of Physicians, "American College of Physicians Ethics Manual," *Annals of Internal Medicine* 117 (1992): 947–960.

33. Marcia Angell, "Medicine: The Endangered Patient-Centered Ethic," *Hastings Center Report* 17 (1987):12–13.

34. Association of American Medical Colleges, "Guidelines for Dealing With Faculty Conflicts of Commitment and Conflicts of Interest in Research," *Academic Medicine* 65 (1990): 487–496.

35. E. Haavi Morreim, "Conflicts of Interest" in *Encyclopedia of Bioethics*, 2nd ed., Warren T. Reich, ed. New York: Macmillan, 1995, pp. 459–465.

36. Robert M. Sade, "The Different Drummer, the Double Agent, and the Future Dilemmas in Bioethics," *Annals of Thoracic Surgery* 53 (1992): 183–190.

37. Francis D. Moore, "The Surgical Internship and Residency," *Bulletin of the New York Academy of Medicine* 54 (1978): 648–656.

38. Michael J. Newton, "Moral Dilemmas in Surgical Training: Intent and the Case for Ethical Ambiguity," *Journal of Medical Ethics* 12 (1986): 207–209.

39. Clifton B. Perry, "Conflicts of Interest and the Physician's Duty to Inform," *American Journal of Medicine* 96 (1994): 375–380.

40. American Medical Association, Council on Scientific Affairs and Council on Ethical and Judicial Affairs, "Conflicts of Interest in Medical Center/Industry Research Relationships," *Journal of the American Medical Association* 263 (1990): 2790–2793.

41. E. M., "The Florida Case: Appearances Matter," *Science* 248 (1990):153–154.

42. George Khushf, " Proportional Coinsurance: A Market-Based, Ethically Sound Alternative to Medical Savings Accounts," *American Philosophical Association Newsletter* 93 (1994): 84–87.

43. American Medical Association, Council on Ethical and Judicial Affairs, "Conflicts of Interest, Physician Ownership of Medical Facilities," *Journal of the American Medical Association* 267 (1992):2366–2369.

44. Association of American Physicians and Surgeons, *Principles of the Association of American Physicians and Surgeons*. Tucson, AZ: Association of American Physicians and Surgeons, 1991.

45. Alfred W. Childs and E. Diane Hunter, " Non-Medical Factors Influencing Use of Diagnostic X-ray by Physicians," *Medical Care* 10 (1972): 323–335.

46. David Hemenway et al., "Physicians' Responses to Financial Incentives," *New England Journal of Medicine* 322 (1990): 1059–1063.

47. Alan L. Hillman et al., "HMO Managers' Views on Financial Incentives and Quality," *Health Affairs* 10 (1991): 207–219.

48. Michael D. Reagan, "Physicians as Gatekeepers: A Complex Challenge," *New England Journal of Medicine* 317 (1987): 1731–1734.

49. Robert A. Berenson, " Capitation and Conflict of Interest," *Health Affairs* 5 (1986): 141–146.

50. Alexander M. Capron, " Containing Health Care Costs: Ethical and Legal Implications of Changes in the Methods of Paying Physicians," *Case Western Law Review* 36 (1985–86): 708–759.

51. James P. Orlowski, " The HEC and Conflicts of Interest in the Health Care Environment," *HEC Forum* 6 (1994): 3–11.

52. Royal College of Physicians of London, "The Relationship Between Physicians and the Pharmaceutical Industry," *Journal of the Royal College of Physicians of London* 20 (1986): 235–242.

53. Cutis E. Margo, "Selling Surgery," *New England Journal of Medicine* 314 (1986): 1575–1576.

54. David A. Grimes, "Technology Follies, The Uncritical Acceptance of Medical Innovation," *Journal of the American Medical Association* 269 (1993): 3030–3033.

55. Baruch A. Brody, *Ethical Issues in Drug Testing, Approval, and Pricing*. Oxford: Oxford University Press, 1995.

56. Colin Norman, "Clinical Trial Stirs Legal Matters," *Science* 227 (1985): 1316–1318.

57. Eric J. Topol, et al., "Confronting the Issues of Patient Safety and Investigator Conflict of Interest in an International Clinical Trial of Myocardial Reperfusion," *Journal of the American College of Cardiology* 19 (1992): 1123–1128.

58. Kenneth J. Rothman, "Conflict of Interest, The New McCarthyism in Science," *The Journal of the American Medical Association* 269 (1993): 2782–2784.

59. William Booth, "Conflict of Interest Eyed at Harvard," *Science* 242 (1988): 1497–1499.

60. Leonard G. Wilson, "The Crime of Saving Lives," *Archives of Surgery* 130 (1995): 1035–1039.

61. Deborah E. Barnes and Lisa A. Bero, "Industry Funded Research and Conflict of Interest: An Analysis of Research Sponsored by the Tobacco Industry through the Center for Indoor Air Research," *Journal of Health Politics, Policy and Law* 21 (1996): 515–542.

62. David S. Shimm and Roy G. Spece, "Industry Reimbursement for Entering Patients

into Clinical Trials: Legal and Ethical Issues," *Annals of Internal Medicine* 115 (1991): 148–151.

63. C. Barbara Mueller, "Breast Cancer Trials on Trial," *Cancer* 75 (1995): 2403–2411.

64. Kathryn M. Taylor, Richard G. Margolese, and Colin L. Soskolne, "Physicians' Reasons for Not Entering Eligible Patients in a Randomized Clinical Trial of Surgery for Breast Cancer," *New England Journal of Medicine* 310 (1984): 1363–1367.

65. Ezekiel J. Emanuel and Daniel Steiner, "Institutional Conflict of Interest," *New England Journal of Medicine* 332 (1995): 262–267.

66. James S. Todd, "Must the Law Assure Ethical Behavior?," *The Journal of the American Medical Association* 268 (1992): 98.

67. Randall S. Bock, "The Pressure to Keep Prices High at a Walk-In Clinic," *New England Journal of Medicine* 319 (1988): 785–787.

68. Arnold S. Relman, "Salaried Physicians and Economic Incentives," *New England Journal of Medicine* 319 (1988): 784.

69. Henry Scovern, " A Physician's Experiences in a For-Profit Staff-Model HMO," *New England Journal of Medicine* 319 (1988): 787–790.

70. American Medical Association, Council on Ethical and Judicial Affairs, "Ethical Issues in Managed Care," *Journal of the American Medical Association* 273 (1995): 330–335.

71. Douglas Levinson, "Toward Full Disclosure of Referral Restrictions and Financial Incentives by Prepaid Health Plans," *New England Journal of Medicine* 317 (1987): 1729–1731.

19

Relationships with Payers and Institutions that Manage and Deliver Patient Services

KEVIN WM. WILDES
ROBERT B. WALLACE

The rapidly changing nature of health care finance has opened a host of ethical questions for physicians, patients, hospitals, and payers. Surgeons are no exception to these questions. Each day physicians and surgeons find themselves caught in a maze of changing financial structures that influence surgical practice (see Chapter 17). The changes from fee-for-service structures to those of managed care raise a number of ethical issues about the patient-physician relationship and how patients ought to be treated. These structural changes also raise potential conflicts of interests and conflicts of obligations, or the perception of such conflicts, in the surgeon's relationships to patients, hospitals, and payers (see Chapter 18). There are other ethical questions for hospitals and health care institutions and the surgical services they offer. As hospitals attempt to compete for market share, conflicts may arise between an institutional interest in offering economically efficient services and the fiduciary obligation of providing quality care to patients. Hospitals are no longer simply points of delivery for surgical care. They are, increasingly, financiers of medical and surgical services as well as providers of such services so they cannot escape such conflicts of interest.

It should be noted at the outset of this chapter that the ethical issues surrounding health care finance and delivery are not unique to managed care. One can easily identify similar ethical issues in a fee-for-service system. However, the transition from fee-for-service to managed care provides a contrast that high-lights these ethical problems.

This chapter analyzes the legitimate moral interests of patients, surgeons, hospitals, and payers. It focuses on the surgeon's relationship to these different parties. We must recognize that in a world of limited resources there will be conflicts among these interests because not all needs and interests can be met. Recognizing that there will be conflicts among legitimate moral interests and the surgeon's obligations to patients, we support an overall strategy of preventive ethics and institutional analysis that seeks to anticipate these conflicts. The obligation to inform all parties on how resources will or will not be used is crucial to prevent ethical conflicts. Success or failure in managing them will depend on open, frank, honest communication as well as the development and communication of policy guidelines by institutions and payers.[1] These ethical concerns are not only the concerns of surgeons but ought to be part of the whole culture of medicine. All parties need to understand the limits, rights, and options in using health care resources. At the same time many of the issues in this chapter make it clear that a number of important ethical questions in contemporary surgical practices are not simply questions for individual agents because the practice of surgery is situated in institutional contexts. The institutional context calls both for structural solutions to ethical dilemmas at the level of policy, as well as individual choices by surgeons about how it is appropriate to act in particular cases.

Ethical Analysis

Like all contemporary physician-patient encounters, the relationship between surgeon and patient is encompassed within wider contexts that have direct and indirect effects on it. The practice of surgery is embedded in relationships to provider institutions, such as hospitals and surgical centers, to payer institutions, such as insurance companies, managed care organizations (MCOs), government programs, and, increasingly, to providers of services. These institutional settings provide the necessary financial resources and institutional support for modern surgery. They provide the place, the support personnel, and the financial support for surgical practice, as well as the care of the patient before and after the surgery. Payers, in whatever form they take, provide the resources necessary for the surgery and the care of surgical patients. The relationships of surgeons, patients, hospitals, and other patients affected by allocation decisions form a complex web of relationships with ethical dimensions. In recognition of the institutional context of medicine and surgery, Emanuel has argued that physicians and bioethicists "must stop being case oriented and become institutionally oriented."[1]

These wider and more complex social and institutional structures provide support not only for the care of surgical patients but also for a variety of other health care services. These institutions have legitimate interests, both moral and economic, that influence, and go beyond, the practice of surgery. Institutions and payers act to support the relationship of surgeons, physicians, and patients. These payer institutions also have ethical obligations to support the work of many physicians and surgeons as well as to provide care to a broad range of patients. It is often forgotten that payers have ethical obligations to all their subscribers and investors. These long-term interests and obligations have ethical significance because they influence an institution's ability to keep present commitments and obligations as well as future ones. Institutions such as hospitals have long-term interests in their own survival and their own ability to serve future generations. In a changing economic climate hospitals increasingly are financiers of services as well as points of delivery. As hospitals bid for contracts with little or no margin in order to maintain market share and still hope to survive, they have to finance the difference from other revenue sources. In such situations hospitals are likely to have conflicts between obligations to provide standard of care services and their own legitimate interest in fiscal responsibility and stability. Surgeons may find themselves caught between hospitals and patients as they are often involved in the types of services hospitals like to market.

Surgeons and physicians are likely to find themselves in two types of ethical conflicts with payers, patients, and institutions. It is helpful to classify these conflicts as falling under one of two categories: conflicts of obligation and conflicts of interest (see Chapter 18). If one looks at surgery as part of a complex web of structures and embedded within institutional arrangements, then it will be obvious that surgeons play different roles within the different set of structures.

Conflicts of Obligation

Surgeons find themselves with a number of ethical obligations that may conflict. They have a primary obligation to the patient that is created by the fiduciary nature of the relationship. It is possible to view the surgeon-patient relationship in economic terms in which the patient, understood as a consumer, is purchasing the services of the surgeon. However, such a view overlooks the reality of the patient's vulnerability brought on by the illness or disease. Because of the patient's vulnerability, the relationship of patient and surgeon is more completely captured in the language of a fiduciary relationship. The fiduciary nature of the relationship has been guided traditionally by a principle of beneficence—that is, acting in a way that protects and promotes the health-related interests of the patient, with the consent of the patient.[2,3]

The ethical obligations of physicians and surgeons toward patients often obscure other ethical obligations. Surgeons need institutional support for their work and their relationships with institutions create still further ethical obligations. Institutions and payers do not have unlimited resources, and they must steward their resources in such a manner as to fulfill their obligations to other patients, present and future. For-profit institutions may also have obligations to their investors. To recognize the obligations of stewardship, for institutions and payers, is to recognize that surgery, like all of medicine and health care, is not the act of a single person or simply the relationship of the surgeon and the patient. It is, rather, the result of the collaboration of many people and institutions working together with limited resources. The surgeon will have conflicting obligations to the patient and to the institution and to other patients regarding the prudent management of resources.

Decisions about how resources are allocated are not simply choices about efficiency and the maximization of outcomes. Decisions about the efficient use of resources are made within the context of prior choices about appropriate and inappropriate goals to be pursued. Institutions, such as hospitals and payers, have certain fiduciary obligations in the management and use of resources. While their primary ethical obligations are to their patients, surgeons also have ethical obligations to the institution in which they work. For surgeons, institutional responsibility involves participation in developing guidelines for treatment that most effectively utilizes resources without compromising patient care. There is much to be gained by developing such treatment guidelines, but too often a cooperative effort between hospital, administration, physicians and payers has not been achieved.

The ethical issues discussed in this chapter are the result of the successes and sophistication of contemporary surgery. The developments in surgery in this century have created new surgical and therapeutic opportunities that have, in turn, created great demands on resources. The success of contemporary surgery has moved it from a "cottage industry" to the complex institutional setting in which it is now situated.[4] Those who administer such institutions and payment systems have fiduciary obligations toward those who have entrusted resources to them. Just as surgeons have ethical and fiduciary obligations to patients, so too institutions and payers have ethical obligations to many patients, surgeons, physicians, and investors. These obligations must be met in the context of limited resources.

In recent years the rapid development of MCOs has dramatically transformed the way medicine and surgery are delivered.[5] These developments reflect the wider context of health care delivery and surgery. The institutional context is not new to surgery. However, managed care, driven by the goal of containing costs, has brought the concerns of this wider context to bear on the practices of medicine and surgery in a way that a fee-for-service structure did not. Managed care has institutional goals different from those of fee-for-service. MCOs respond in an economically rational way to the cost-control goals of payers, especially those of private employers, and, increasingly, of public payers (e.g., Medicare and Medicaid, the Department of Veterans Affairs, and military medicine).

The restructuring of health care finances has led to radical changes for all health care institutions and for surgeons. In a fee-for-service structure, surgeons were able to isolate their relationship with the patient from the other structures of health care. In this practice setting surgeons could understand their ethical obligations in terms of beneficence toward the patient, contextualized by the patient's consent and autonomy.[6,7] In a managed-care environment surgeons no longer control the system of resources; control rests in the hands of payers and institutional managers. Surgeons will have many different obligations to patients, provider organizations, and payers. At times these obligations will conflict.

Conflicts of Interest

Here it is helpful to develop more carefully the second type of conflict that a surgeon may experience, a conflict of interest, which is discussed in considerable detail in Chapter 18. As Rodwin points out, "conflict of interest" is a term that is more often an analytical tool than the subject of analysis.[8] To have an interest in something is to have a stake or a claim in it. For example, in the practice of medicine there is the assumption that physicians and surgeons have a professional obligation to act on behalf of the patient's interests. At the same time, surgeons also have interests in being good professionals, in protecting their professional reputation, and in being reimbursed for their services (see Chapter 17). It is possible to identify a number of conflicts of interest in medicine as well as in other areas of life. The difficult issue is to distinguish those conflicts of interest that are acceptable from those that are not.

Different reimbursement systems raise the question of whether or not the systems may not engender conflicts of these interests, or the appearance of such conflicts, in particular the conflict between the obligation to act on behalf of the patient's interest and the surgeon's interest in reimbursement. It is often charged that reimbursement schemes in managed care create conflicts of interest for surgeons insofar as there is an incentive to undertreat, which conflicts with fiduciary obligations. However, the potential conflicts over reimbursement and the patient's interests are not the exclusive property of managed care. The possible conflict between a patient's interest and physician interest in reimbursement is not new. In fee-for-service structures there are incentives for physicians and surgeons to render services that may not be in the best interest of the patient (e.g., unnecessary surgery) but which may be in the financial self-interest of the surgeon. Surgical procedures, such as hysterectomies and tonsillectomies, were often performed when they were not in the patient's medical interest but in the financial interest of the surgeon.

Challenging conflicts of interest arise from the way the surgeon is reimbursed by the payer, when surgeons have their economic well-being tied to the interests of the payers through risk-sharing arrangements with MCOs. MCOs are classified as health maintenance organizations (HMOs), preferred-provider organizations (PPOs), or various mixes of the two.[9] There are two major forms of HMOs, the group or staff model and the network or independent-practice-association (IPA). In the IPA model a group of physicians agrees to provide services to a plan's patients for a discounted fee. IPA HMOs use community physicians in private practice. The staff or group model HMO fully integrates physicians into the structure. Physicians are reimbursed in a variety of ways. The group or staff HMO tends to pay on a salary or capitation basis, whereas the IPA HMO uses some kind of risk sharing as incentive.

There is real diversity among MCOs. Some MCOs are well capitalized and well managed with real commitments to quality over the long term. Others, however, are poorly capitalized and poorly managed with a weak commitment to quality of care. These often aim at cost reduction as the major goal without a long-term commitment to the quality of care. The status of an MCO as "for profit" or "not for profit" is not as crucial to the ethical questions as many seem to think; rather, the capitalization, mission, and management are central to ethical issues. Those MCOs that are well managed and well capitalized will be more likely to provide appropriate information and disclosure to patients and surgeons. They are often more likely to promote the quality of care as well as the cost of care.

Another source of conflict of interest is the relationship of the surgeon to health care institutions. This relationship will have an impact on the supportive care and resources for the patient-surgeon relationship. Hospitals and surgical centers have legitimate ethical interests in reimbursement and the use of resources. They also have ethical obligations to other patients, present and future, and in conducting research. Academic medical centers have additional obligations, at the heart of their identity, in the training of physicians and surgeons, present and future. Institutional interests in preserving the stability and health of the institution may, at times, conflict with the surgeon's care of a patient. Institutions such as hospitals will also have relationships with payers that will have an impact on the surgeon-patient relationship.

Hospitals and surgical centers will have interests in developing surgical packages to offer to different payers. Surgeons have a responsibility to work with provider institutions and payers to develop protocols and guidelines that result in the most efficient use of resources without compromising quality. The perception of many is that MCOs have been concerned primarily with reducing costs with only a secondary concern for the quality of care. Surgeons must continue as advocates for their patients in these situations. Indeed, not to do so exposes the surgeon to malpractice action.[10] Surgeons cannot accept the ruling of a payer when it may affect adversely the welfare of their patients. Surgeons will therefore have legitimate ethical and professional concerns in how a package of surgical services is assembled (e.g., specifications, materials to be used).

Consideration of how to manage conflicting obligations and conflicts of interest is essential to our ethical analysis. This management concerns the surgeon-patient relationship, potential conflicts in the use of resources, the relationships of surgeons to payers, and the relationships between surgeons and institutions. We turn now to a brief analysis of each and how to manage them prospectively, with a view toward preventing the ethical conflicts they can engender. The institutional setting provides a structural way to address different ethical concerns can be addressed. For each of the following topics it is possible to conceive of institutional ethics committees taking a role in which economic arrangements and their effect on institutional services can be reviewed and discussed, a topic that we take up in greater detail later in this chapter.

Surgeon-Patient Relationship

Conflicting obligations and conflicts of interest should be addressed from the ethical perspective of the surgeon-patient relationship, which is based on respect for patient autonomy, beneficence, and trust. The relationship rests on the assumption that the surgeon is dedicated to protecting and promoting the health-related interests of the patient, an ethical commitment captured by the principles of beneficence and autonomy. With appropriate respect for the autonomy of each patient, the surgeon acts on the patient's behalf to promote the good of the patient as articulated by the patient. While the surgeon-patient relationship is crafted around the surgeon's obligation to protect and promote the interest of the patient, it is not always clear which clinical strategies can be expected to achieve this goal. Medical and surgical choices are made within the web of values and interests that shape the life of a patient. Out of respect for each patient, physicians and surgeons seek the consent and authorization of the patient.[6] It is the balance of beneficence and respect for the patient's autonomy that shapes the ethical contours of the surgeon-patient relationship. Respect for the patient's autonomy and a commitment to beneficence are central to fostering an attitude of trust. Patients trust that surgeons will use their competence and skills in the best interest of the patient. This trust depends on a fiduciary obligation on the part of the surgeon toward the patient. Medical authority and social position are tied to the assumption of trust.

Potential Conflicts Regarding the Use of Resources

In contemporary health care structures the surgeon-patient relationship can no longer be viewed in isolation from other relations and ethical interests. Just as there were ethical issues in fee-for-service medicine, so too the emerging structures of managed care create a number of ethical conflicts for the surgeon-patient relationship.

First, like other physicians, the surgeon will increasingly have to balance the interests of one patient with the interests of other patients. Realizing that systems constrain the use of procedures, a surgeon will be forced to think about whether or not to use a resource for one patient or save the resource for another (i.e., to ration resources). Limits on resources may lead a surgeon to think how to perform hip replacement surgery more efficiently—for example, using shorter-life materials in patients in their eighties, or whether to do screening mammograms on low-risk patients.

Second, many of the emerging institutional structures and payment systems potentially put the interests of the patients in conflict with the interests of their physicians and surgeons. Many new structures provide incentives to surgeons to minimize the use of resources. The recommendations in favor of performing procedures may have an impact on the financial well-being of the surgeon.

Third, many of the new payment structures constrain the freedom of patients and surgeons. Restrictions on the length of stay, for example, direct the way surgeons can care for their patients. Such constraints are evident when a patient wants a particular surgeon who may be part of the managed care plan. Within networks of physicians, surgeons, and institutions, surgeons may be constrained in the recommendations they can make to patients for both the procedures they should have and who should perform the surgery (if the best person is someone outside the referral network). These kinds of dilemmas make it clear that the issue of limits is best dealt with honestly and preventively when possible. That is, patients should be informed honestly about limitations in their coverage.

Woolhandler and Himmelstein have taken issue with restrictions placed on physicians as a condition of hire by insurers. They quote their own contract: "Physician shall agree not to take any action or make any communication which undermines or could undermine the confidence of enrollees, potential enrollees, their employers, their unions, or the public" in the company for which they worked.[11] In the aftermath of the public controversy surrounding the publishing of this essay, US Health Care has dropped this requirement. Since then there has also been state and federal legislation proposed to promote full disclosure, as well as federal regulation of Medicare and Medicaid MCOs. The controversy illustrates the ethical concern over "gag rules" and the practice of informed consent.[12] One ethical way to approach such limits is openly and honestly. That is, one way to avoid apparent conflicts of interest and obligation is to be sure that patients are informed about their choices and the limits on those choices. When done in advance, such open and honest disclosure can prevent ethical conflicts and help surgeons fulfill their obligations to patients and payers.

One can argue that these problems, and many others, stem from the question, for whom does the surgeon work?[13] In the older fee-for-service model, the surgeon was reimbursed for the procedures he or she thought best for the patient. This often led to overtreatment and the mismanagement of resources. Today, however, in the emerging models of payment, the surgeon finds himself or herself part of an institutional network that limits what can and cannot be done. Patients may rightly worry if surgeons are making recommendations and acting on the patient's interests or on the interests of the payer, the institution, or the surgeon—threatening the ability of patients to trust surgeons.

Surgeons and Payers

It is difficult to capture the rapidly changing payment structures in health care under a single heading (see Chapter 17). However, the dominant current model seems to fall under the heading of "managed care." The goal of managed care systems is to constrain the costs of health care by controlling the use of resources by physicians. Physician referral for services is a crucial resource for any insurance plan. Insurer institutions need surgeons as a resource to offer enrollees. Surgeons and physicians will be crucial to the control of the use of resources. Surgical interventions potentially involve significant expenditures of resources. In the managed care environment, physician services are not reimbursed simply for services rendered as in the fee-for-service model. Primary care physicians assess patients and make treatment recommendations for patients in consultation with payer guidelines. *Under this model, physicians and surgeons are now more like employees than independent businessmen and businesswomen.* Surgeons have incentives to control the use of resources. Their ability to act on behalf of patients depends on the payer's approval. These changes raise obvious questions about the assumptions one can make about the surgeon-patient relationship.

Another set of issues can be understood in terms of incentives to surgeons to limit care. Even when this is not an actual ethical problem, the public perception of these incentives may erode the basic trust in the surgeon-patient relationship. One approach to the problem of inappropriate conflicts is to be sure that the financial structures reward quality, not quantity, of services. One can argue that both fee-for-service and managed care structures focus too much on quantity of services rather than quality of service. Rewarding quality can be achieved through the use of clinimetrics to assess a patient's condition, outcome data, and practice guidelines. One can also include judgment of patient satisfaction and peer review. It would seem that the surgeon's immediate responsibility is to be accountable within such criteria for his or her own practice.

Forms of payment must be examined as to their impact on the surgeon-patient relationship. *If not doing something for a patient, in order to save money, results in a greater balance of harms over goods, the fiduciary obligation of beneficence is violated.* Such structures threaten the surgeon's primary role as a fiduciary of the patient. As a fiduciary the surgeon should not practice below a standard of care or an ethical standard of beneficence and of autonomy.[2,3] For example, because of limits on resources, it may be easy not to recommend surgical procedures such as joint replacements or transplants that would benefit the patient.

Managed care ought not be seen simply as a mechanism for containing costs. There are also ethical dimensions of how the managed care system can best manage resources to provide quality care for all its members. Physicians, as part of the network, share in these obligations.

Surgeons and Health Care Institutions

The shift in payment structures affects health care institutions (hospitals, surgical centers) as well as surgeons. Payers have sought to limit the use of hospital beds by restricting the length of reimbursable stays for patients in hospitals as well as the procedures that can be done. This has meant that institutions such as same-day surgical centers, both as free-standing units and as part of traditional hospital structures, are quickly becoming an essential part in the practice of contemporary surgery.

Such changes mean that surgeons have found their relationship with institutions radically changed. They now must work as part of an institution and not beyond its pale. The choices available to surgeons in treating patients will depend on institutional policies and payer policies. Furthermore, this changed relationship to the institution, as well as the limitations on what the institution can offer, means that surgeons must adjust the type of care and instructions they give to patients for the after-surgery period. Patients will need to realize what their condition will be like after the surgery, the type of care they will need, and the limitations they will face.

Surgeons become part of the services offered by institutions to health care payers. Many hospitals and other health care institutions have responded to changes in the economic order by marketing differing packages of services to different health care plans. Many of the services offered are surgical, in which a total package is offered at a fixed price. Such arrangements may raise questions about the surgeon's loyalty to patients. It becomes important for surgeons and physicians to be involved in the development of the packages in which they will participate. Issues such as length of stay, or the use of intensive care medical resources, testing, or the type of antibiotics that are used, are important elements of any package. The participation of surgeons in developing medically good packages is crucial to the honesty and integrity of the surgical package.

Summary

The changing social and economic structures of health care have created important ethical challenges for surgeons and their patients as well as for institutions. Surgeons have obligations not only to their patients but to the institutions and payers for whom and with whom they work. Health care institutions and payers have their own ethical obligations for the stewardship of resources as well as to patients. Surgeons find themselves with obligations to their patients. But these obligations cannot be fulfilled in isolation; rather, they are set within the institutional context of payers and health care institutions.

It is entirely possible that there may be direct conflicts of moral obligations. There may also be the *perception* of conflict on the part of patients. Surgeons can act to alleviate such conflict and the perception of conflict. First, surgeons should, in our view, avoid acting as the "gatekeeper" as some evolving MCO structures seek to decentralize the role of gatekeeping.[7] The AMA Council on Ethical and Judicial Affairs has written "[W]hile this responsibility to guard society's resources is an important one, physicians must remain primarily dedicated to the health care needs of their individual patients."[7,14] Allocation decisions are within the ambit of those charged with the stewardship of resources. However, surgeons can play an important role in the shaping of guidelines and policies about the use of resources. Furthermore they can act as advocates for their patients within the system. Failure to undertake these three tasks is tantamount to abandoning the surgeon's fiduciary obligations. Surgeons can also act to inform and educate patients concerning all available treatment alternatives including those not available within their plan. Once these fiduciary obligations are satisfied, the surgeon should avoid ethical conflicts, or the perception of conflicts, by following a policy of "economic informed consent."[8,15,16]

Clinical Topics

Physician-Hospital Networks

The development of managed care networks has complicated obligations for surgeons. These relationships can be structured in a number of ways. Surgeons can have a number of different relationships to hospitals and networks. Physicians and surgeons may be, essentially, employees of hospitals. Or, they can have contractual, capitation-based arrangements that carry incentives to lower costs in the care of patients. They can also be involved in a variety of profit-sharing arrangements. Or surgeons might be involved as part owners of the institutions.

Hospitals may be owned by managed care corporations, be publicly held, government owned and operated, or operated as nonprofit corporations. Ownership of the institution will have an impact on the way the institution understands itself, its mission, and how it will use its resources. In turn, this self-understanding has an impact on the practice of surgery within the institution. It is essential that surgeons understand their own relationships to institutions, their impact on surgical practice, and the way the relationship might be perceived, and then to protect the fiduciary nature of surgical practice.

Patients need to understand the relationship of their surgeon to the institution and to the payer insofar as such relationships will affect the care of patients. They need to understand how this relationship will influence the care they will receive and the limits to care. Such information will allow them to seek treatment alternatives should they desire them. One strategy for avoiding ethical conflicts of obligation or conflicts of interest is to explicate all assumptions, expectations, and arrangements. For example, hospitals should make clear their mission and their way of proceeding. Insurers should explain health plans to enrollees. Information should be made available in clear and honest ways. Surgeons should understand the limits and boundaries placed on their practice and be sure that their patients also understand the context of this relationship.

Advertising

Advertising raises a number of ethical issues for the surgeon and the health care institution. One issue is stewardship. That is, if, as we assume, the stewardship of resources is an important ethical goal for health care institutions, then one will have to examine the use of resources for advertising. This is not to say, a priori, that advertising ought not to be done. It is to say, however, that such practices need to be examined for their need and effectiveness for the institution. There must be an honest assessment of the effectiveness of advertising for the institution. Does it actually attract patients? Does it actually make the community more aware of the institution? Such advertisement should be assessed in terms of its effectiveness and the investment it represents. This is the type of question that must be asked in the obligation to use resources well.

A second question raised by advertising deals with the question of what is being communicated in the advertising. That is, are claims that are made true and warranted? Are false fears being generated? Are false hopes being raised? For example, in advertising for surgical services, claims are often made that institutions offer surgery done by the "leaders in the field" as if no one else in the community adequately preformed the procedure (e.g., laser surgery). Or advertising may use raw, uninterpreted statistical information that may be misleading in such a form. Advertising needs to communicate honestly and fully because any type of misleading information runs the risk of fraud and thus endangers both fiduciary obligations and ethical obligations of adequate disclosure required by informed consent.

There has been an important discussion about enrollment disclosure and managed care. A general concern has been that subscribers not be misled by advertising that emphasizes positive features without mentioning the built-in constraints that lead to a denial of beneficial care.[7,17,18]

Alternative Remuneration

Systems and institutions can remunerate surgeons in a number of ways outside the traditional fee-for-service model. They might be remunerated on some type of capitation system or a system of utilization review. The potential ethical conflicts here have to do with the patient's well-being and the interests of the surgeon. Under capitation or utilization review, there is a financial interest to be economically disciplined. Such arrangements could mean that the surgeon is only authorized to do less than the standard of care. In instances when there may be financial interests to provide excessive services or to provide less than the standard of care, the surgeon, as fiduciary, should not accept such a relationship even if the patient consents, because a fiduciary surgeon is ethically prohibited from allowing conflicts of interest to result in substandard care. Such structures can put the interests of the surgeon in conflict with the interests of the patient. An alternative model is a salary model, in which the surgeon is paid an annual salary by the institution. Such a model reduces the intensity of conflicts of interest and therefore make them more manageable ethically (see Chapter 18).

Abuses of the Coding System

Surgeons and hospitals are in many instances ranked on the basis of short-term results of treatment, such as mortality and morbidity in the surgical treatment of coronary artery disease. These results may be adjusted based on risk stratification, or severity of illness, thus producing incentive to inflate the severity of illness. Because many of the factors used to determine severity of illness are subjective, this potential exists. Similarly, hospital reimbursement is frequently affected by severity of illness, which provides incentives for hospitals to inflate the severity of illness. The physician has the ultimate responsibility for this determination, and thus an ethical responsibility to be as objective as possible, even if doing so diminishes revenues.

Referral Outside the Managed Care Network

Just as many of the choices in treating a patient are conditioned by the resources available within the managed care network, so too are such choices conditioned by the resources that exist outside the network. It may well be that a physician or surgeon may think that a patient would benefit from a particular procedure or treatment that is best done by someone outside the network. In the best situation, those who perform such procedures within the system are sufficiently competent. In the worst situation, those who perform such procedures within the system are marginally competent. In either case the person who best performs the procedure is outside the system. The question becomes whether or not the surgeon can make the referral or even tell the patient about other possibilities, so that the patient may seek treatment beyond the limits of that provided by the network if so desired.

The referral issue involves not only referral to surgeons or other medical personnel but the lack of availability of a particular procedure within the managed care plan. Some people might respond that withholding information is appropriate because the procedure would not be reimbursed. However, patients may choose to pay for the procedure out of pocket, raise the money, find a benefactor, or appeal the MCO's decision not to provide reimbursement.

In either type of case, the question for the surgeon or physician is directed by the surgeon's fiduciary obligations to the patient. Does acting on this obligation to protect and promote the patient's interests involve the additional ethical obligation to inform him or her of alternative treatments or surgeons? Do the ethical obligations of informed consent lead to obligations to inform the patient about a surgeon or procedures that are not available under his or her plan? What are the surgeon's obligations to the managed care plan? Our response to these questions is based on the ethics of informed consent (see Chapter 2). The best strategy is to be sure that the patient has access to the best medical opinion about his or her medical situation, along with information about the options, as well as the limits, for treatment. Such knowledge is essential for consent and essential for fulfilling one's fiduciary obligations to the patient. Surgeons can prevent such ethical dilemmas by being sure, ahead of time, that they are free to communicate freely and completely with patients. In this way they can fulfill their obligations to give the best medical assessment and advice to their patents.

Surgeon-Lawyer/Risk Manager Relationship

In dealing with patients the surgeon manages several roles and relationships simultaneously. He or she is surgeon for the patient. But he or she is also an agent of the health care institution or the MCO. Surgeons will have to keep these different relationships distinct in dealing with different agents of hospitals, health care institutions, and payers. Attorneys and risk managers, now fixtures in different institutional structures, tend to be concerned primarily with welfare and interests of the institutions. Surgeons should, therefore, clarify for themselves the extent and limits of obligations to each of the different parties. In particular surgeons have obligations to patients that institutional lawyers and risk managers may not always sufficiently appreciate. The fiduciary obligation to the patient should not be compromised by lawyer-directed medicine.

An effective way to do this is to inform institutional counsel and other risk managers, in advance, of plans for surgical management of types that might involve increased risk of malpractice (e.g., on patients who are high surgical risks (see Chapter 9) and tell these managers to prepare to manage that risk well. The alternative is to ask risk managers what to do, opening the door to unnecessary compromise of the surgeon's fiduciary obligations.

The Role of Ethics Committees and Ethics Consultants

Until recently it was plausible to hold the position that the best way to avoid ethical dilemmas with patients was to establish a good, honest relationship with them. This is, no doubt, still a wise position. However, with the changing economic structures of health care, there may be a new role for ethics committees to review the web of relationships in patient care.

One structural way to deal with such conflicts is through the use of institutional ethics committees or some type of ethics consultation. A health care institution may have an ethics committee established. These committees can play a variety of roles in the life of an institution. They can educate, help create policy, and become directly involved in a consultation process in a clinical setting. In these roles ethics committees and ethics consultants can be of service to surgeons and patients when the proactive use of institutional resources conflicts with the management of particular cases. The committee should concern itself with the development of policies to manage conflicting obligations and conflicts of interest in ways that preserve the fiduciary obligations of both surgeons and the institution. In this way, an ethics committee would strengthen both physician's and institution's commitment to being fiduciaries of the patients served by the institution.

Obligations of Department Chairs and Section Chiefs

Surgical leaders, whether departmental chairs, chiefs of service, or division chiefs, have a responsibility to oversee the quality of care provided, as well as the efficiency with which it is provided. They have a responsibility to participate in the development of methods of evaluating quality of care and the effects of various alterations in practice. How does one measure the effect of hospital length of stay, or the restricted use of resources, on the quality of care? Thus far, we believe, measurement has been primarily financial without proven means of measuring quality.

Teaching institutions have the responsibility of instructing trainees and students in the changing patterns of practice, the methods of evaluating these changes, and the limitations of these methods. Excessive utilization in teaching programs has been the norm; in the future, students and residents must learn the importance of effective and efficient resource utilization.

Surgical leaders must provide the example of ethically justified practice in the relationship with the institutions, the payers, and the patient. The interposition of the payer between the patient and surgeon can be confusing to the patient and raise questions about the surgeon's loyalty to the patient. This requires that surgeons make a greater effort to gain the confidence and trust of their patients and to reaffirm that their loyalty is to the patient.

Education and Training

The future of medical education and training in a managed care environment is, at least, uncertain. In the past, financial support has come from the government and private payers. Many private payers currently question their responsibility for support of medical education. Although it is possible that physicians can be educated and trained without direct government or private support, it is not certain that the quality of surgeons produced in the future will be the same. This is a decision that will have to be made as our health care system continues to evolve.

Clinical Conclusions

Contemporary surgery is practiced in the context of many different relationships. The central relationship is that of surgeon and patient. This fundamental relationship, however, requires the support of payers and hospitals who have legitimate moral interests. These institutions have obligations to use resources for other patients and to support the work of other physicians and surgeons. There are also obligations to maintain the fiscal stability of the institutions. The obligations of stewardship and management will have an undoubted impact on how physicians and surgeons are able to treat particular, individual patients. At times surgeons may think that they are being hindered in giving care to patients. Or, patients may feel compromised by the relationships of surgeons and physicians to payers.

In a world of limited resources, such as ours, choices will have to be made about how resources are allocated. One method of minimizing ethical conflict, and the perception of conflict, is to make sure that everyone involved is committed to fulfilling fiduciary obligations and understands the different relationships and the way resources are allocated. Patients should be given full disclosure by employers and institutional providers about the particular type of health coverage they have. This calls for an expanded understanding of informed consent to include "economic informed consent." They should also understand the reimbursement relationship of payers to physicians and to institutions. Surgeons ought, we have argued, to talk openly and honestly with patients and actively resist the imposition of limits on information surgeons can share with patients. Patients need to understand the context of the information and recommendations they are given and not given.

References

1. Ezekiel J. Emanuel, "Medical Ethics in the Era of Managed Care: The Need for Institutional Structures Instead of Principles for Individual Cases," *Journal of Clinical Ethics* 6 (1995): 335–338.
2. Frank A. Chervenak and Laurence B. McCullough, "The Threat of the New Managed Practice of Medicine to Patients' Autonomy," *The Journal of Clinical Ethics* 6 (1995): 320–323.
3. Edmund Pellegrino and David Thomasma, *For the Patient's Good: The Restoration of Beneficence in Health Care*. New York: Oxford University Press, 1988.
4. Frederick L. Grover, "The Bright Future of Cardiothoracic Surgery in the Era of Changing Health Care Delivery," *Annals of Thoracic Surgery* 61 (1996):499–510.
5. John K. Ingelhardt, "The American Health Care System: Managed Care," *New England Journal of Medicine*, 327 (1992):742–747.
6. Joseph Margolis, "Conflicts of Interest and Conflicting Interests," in *Ethical Theory and Business*, Tom L. Beauchamp and Norman Bowie, eds., Englewood Cliffs, NJ, Prentice- Hall, 1979, pp. 361–372.
7. Edmund Pellegrino, "Rationing Health Care: The Ethics of Medical Gatekeeping," *Journal of Contemporary Health Law Policy* 2 (1986):23–45.
8. Marc Rodwin, *Medicine, Money, and Morals*. New York: Oxford University Press, 1993.
9. Jonathan P. Weiner and Gregory de Lissovoy, "Razing a Tower of Babel: A Taxonomy for Managed Care and Health Insurance Plans," *Journal of Health Politics, Policy, and Law* 18 (1993): 75–103.
10. *Wickline v. The State of California*, 192 California Appellate, 3rd 1630, 1986.
11. Stephen Woolhandler and David Himmelstein, "Extreme Risk: The New Corporate Proposition for Physicians," *New England Journal of Medicine* 335 (1995): 1706–1708.
12. American Medical Association, "AMA calls on managed care providers to cancel gag clauses and submit contracts for ethical review," *News Release, American Medical Association*, 23 January 1996.
13. Marcia Angell, "The Doctor as Double Agent," *Kennedy Institute of Ethics Journal*, 3 (1993): 279–86.
14. American Medical Association, Council on Ethical and Judicial Affairs, "Ethical Issues in Managed Care," *Journal of the American Medical Association*, 273 (1995): 330–335.
15. Mark Hall, "Informed Consent to Rationing Decisions," *The Millbank Quarterly* 71 (1993): 645–676.
16. David Mechanic, Therese Ettel, and Diane Davis, "Choosing Among Health Insurance Options: A Study of New Employees," *Inquiry* 27 (1990): 14–22.
17. Alan S.Brett, "The Case Against Persuasive Advertising by Health Maintenance Organizations", *New England Journal of Medicine* 326 (1992): 1353–1355.
18. F. S. Figa and H. M. Figa, "Redefining Full and Fair Disclosure of HMO Benefits and Limitations," *Seaton Hall Legislative Journal* 14 (1990): 151, 152–154.

Index